Comprehensive Approach to Psychiatry 1

Series Editors

Bernardo Carpiniello
Department of Medical Science and Public Health
University of Cagliari
Cagliari, Italy

Antonio Vita
Department of Clinical and Experimental Science
University of Brescia
Brescia, Italy

Claudio Mencacci
Department of Neuroscience
Luigi Sacco Hospital
Milano, Italy

This book series will cover a broad range of topics with each volume providing an up-to-date overview of subject matters of particular interest for psychiatrists and other professionals in the field of mental health, through a comprehensive approach, including clinical, therapeutical, forensic and psychosocial points of view.

The topics addressed will be selected in collaboration with the Italian Society of Psychiatry.

The book series is aimed at psychiatrists, psychotherapists, psychologists, social workers, nurses, psychiatric rehabilitation technicians, students and researchers.

More information about this series at http://www.springer.com/series/16231

Bernardo Carpiniello
Antonio Vita · Claudio Mencacci
Editors

Violence and Mental Disorders

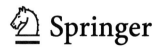 Springer

Editors
Bernardo Carpiniello
Department of Medical Science
and Public Health
University of Cagliari
Cagliari
Italy

Antonio Vita
Department of Clinical and Experimental
Science
University of Brescia
Brescia
Italy

Claudio Mencacci
Department of Neuroscience
Luigi Sacco Hospital
Milano
Italy

ISSN 2524-8405   ISSN 2524-8413   (electronic)
Comprehensive Approach to Psychiatry 1
ISBN 978-3-030-33190-0   ISBN 978-3-030-33188-7   (eBook)
https://doi.org/10.1007/978-3-030-33188-7

This Springer imprint is published by the registered company Springer Nature Switzerland AG
The registered company address is: Gewerbestrasse 11, 6330 Cham, Switzerland

Foreword

This volume on *Violence and Mental Disorders* is the first in a series entitled *Comprehensive Approach to Psychiatry* edited by the Italian Psychiatric Association (Società Italiana di Psichiatria, SIP) in collaboration with Springer. One of the main goals of our Association is to promote scientific knowledge at an international level based on the contribution provided by Italian Psychiatry. The identification of violence as an opening issue for the series is not a fortuitous choice. Indeed, although mental disorders contribute to overall societal violence to a limited extent, this involvement unfortunately continues to be associated with a disproportionate degree of social alarm. Violent behaviors are frequently associated with mental disorder, eliciting fear among both the general population and healthcare professionals. In all honesty we should acknowledge how mental disorder and violence are still today perceived as being closely connected, leading to an unbearably heavy stigma for both patients and psychiatrists. A major step forward introduced in 1978 with the Italian Psychiatric Reform related to removal of the wording "danger to oneself or to others ..." from the criteria for coercive psychiatric treatment, and the abolition of Psychiatric Hospitals, a process of deinstitutionalization which recently concluded with the dismantling of the Judicial Psychiatric Hospitals. Indeed, the highly debated Law 81/2014 saw Italy resolutely opt to go beyond the administration of large forensic institutes, replacing them with a network of small residential facilities known as "REMS" (Residences for the execution of safety measures), now managed by the National Health Service. On these grounds, the issue of the social dangerousness of patients with a mental disorder has been the focus of recent debate in Italy, investigating the appropriateness of refocusing the issue on the treatability of the disorder in those who commit a criminal act. To contribute towards reducing the stigma that accompanies mental disorder, for years our Association has been soliciting the Italian Judicial System to abolish the inclusion of "social dangerousness" from mandatory psychiatric assessments for patients who commit crimes. Indeed, the Association advocates that psychiatrists should be asked to evaluate solely the need for care of the subject, suggesting the potential outcomes of the disorder in relation to treatment prescribed, leaving the task of evaluating the social dangerousness of the perpetrator up to the legal system, based on the same criteria routinely adopted to define as socially dangerous a criminal with no history of mental disorders. We trust that this volume edited by Carpiniello, Vita, and Mencacci, through a comprehensive overview of the complicated issue of violence in mental disorders and input from a series of leading international experts in the field, may provide a significant contribution towards a better understanding of the multifaceted nature of this intricate problem.

Enrico Zanalda
President
Italian Psychiatric Association

Massimo di Giannantonio
President Elected
Italian Psychiatric Association

Contents

Part I   General Aspects

1   **Violence as a Social, Clinical, and Forensic Problem**   3
    Bernardo Carpiniello, Claudio Mencacci, and Antonio Vita

2   **Neurobiology of Violence**   25
    Mirko Manchia, Linda Booij, Federica Pinna, Janice Wong,
    Florian Zepf, and Stefano Comai

3   **Epidemiology and Risk Factors for Violence in People
    with Mental Disorders**   49
    Daniel Whiting and Seena Fazel

**Part II   Risk Factors, Phenomenology and Characteristics
            of Violence in Mental Disorders**

4   **Violence in Major Mental Disorders**   65
    Mario Amore, Andrea Aguglia, Francesca Santi,
    and Gianluca Serafini

5   **Psychopathy, Personality Disorders, and Violence**   81
    Stefano Ferracuti, Gabriele Mandarelli, and Antonio Del Casale

6   **Substance-Use Disorders and Violence**   95
    Fabrizio Schifano, Caroline Zangani, Stefania Chiappini,
    Amira Guirguis, Stefania Bonaccorso, and John M. Corkery

7   **Posttraumatic Stress Disorder, Intimate Partner
    Violence, and Trauma-Informed Intervention** 115
    Ohad Gilbar, Katherine E. Gnall, Hannah E. Cole,
    and Casey T. Taft

8   **Major Neurocognitive Disorders and Violence** 135
    Tracy Wharton and Daniel Paulson

Part III The Contexts of Violence

**9 Studying Patients with Severe Mental Disorders
Who Act Violently: Italian and European Projects** 155
Giovanni de Girolamo, Giorgio Bianconi, Maria Elena Boero,
Giuseppe Carrà, Massimo Clerici, Maria Teresa Ferla,
Gian Marco Giobbio, Giovanni Battista Tura, Antonio Vita,
and Clarissa Ferrari

**10 Prevalence and Risk Factors of Violence by Psychiatric
Acute Inpatients: Systematic Review
and Meta-Analysis—A 2019 Update** 181
Ester di Giacomo, Laura Iozzino, Clarissa Ferrari, Cosmo Strozza,
Matthew Large, Olav Nielssen, and Giovanni de Girolamo

11 Violence and Mental Disorders in Jails. 203
Ester di Giacomo and Massimo Clerici

**12 Violent Behavior in Forensic Residential Facilities: The Italian
Experience After the Closure of Forensic Psychiatric Hospitals** 211
Enrico Zanalda, David De Cori, Grazia Ala,
Alessandro Jaretti Sodano, and Marco Zuffranieri

Part IV Prevention and Management of Violence in Mental Health

13 Violence Risk Assessment in Mental Health. 231
Liliana Lorettu, Alessandra M. A. Nivoli, Paolo Milia,
and Giancarlo Nivoli

**14 Psychopharmacology of Violent Behavior Among People
with Severe Mental Disorders** 253
Leslie Citrome and Jan Volavka

**15 Non-pharmacological Approaches to Violence Among People
with Severe Mental Disorders** 269
Antonio Vita, Valentina Stanga, Anna Ceraso, Giacomo Deste,
and Stefano Barlati

Part I

General Aspects

Violence as a Social, Clinical, and Forensic Problem

Bernardo Carpiniello, Claudio Mencacci, and Antonio Vita

1.1 Violence as a Social Problem

1.1.1 Violence as a Social and Public Health Problem

In 1996, the 9th World Health Assembly adopted Resolution WHA49.25, "noting with great concern the dramatic worldwide increase in the incidence of intentional injuries affecting people of all ages and both sexes," and declared violence an outstanding and growing public health problem worldwide [1]. In the first report on violence released in 1996, the World Health Organization defined violence [2] as "the intentional use of physical force or power, threatened or actual, against oneself, another person, or against a group or community, that either results in or has a high likelihood of resulting in injury, death, psychological harm, maldevelopment or deprivation."

According to a WHO Report published in 2002 [3] violence is an integral part of human life, which assumes a series of forms, such as self-directed violence, interpersonal violence, and collective violence. Overall, violence is one of the leading causes of death worldwide for people aged 15–44 years. The rate of deaths per year due to violence is 28.8 per 100,000 persons, 31.3% represented by homicides, and 49.1% by suicides. Over the period 2000–2012, homicide rates declined by just over 16% globally (from 8.0 to 6.7 per 100,000 population), and in high-income countries by 39%

B. Carpiniello (✉)
Public Health-Unit of Psychiatry and Psychiatric Clinic, Department of Medical Sciences, University Hospital of Cagliari, Cagliari, Italy
e-mail: bcarpini@iol.it

C. Mencacci
Department of Neurosciences, Fatebenefratelli and Sacco Hospital, Milan, Italy

A. Vita
Division of Psychiatry, Department of Clinical and Experimental Sciences, Spedali Civili, University of Brescia, Brescia, Italy
e-mail: antonio.vita@unibs.it

© Springer Nature Switzerland AG 2020
B. Carpiniello et al. (eds.), *Violence and Mental Disorders*, Comprehensive Approach to Psychiatry 1, https://doi.org/10.1007/978-3-030-33188-7_1

(from 6.2 to 3.8 per 100,000 population). By contrast, homicide rates in low- and middle-income countries featured a lower decline over the same period [4]. More than a million people a year, approximately 4400 people every day, die, and a much higher number suffer from nonfatal injuries as a result of intentional violence. The health of thousands of people is affected by the consequences of having been the victim of or witness to acts of violence. Moreover, thousands of lives are destroyed and families shattered, with huge costs deriving from the treatment of victims, support for families, damage repair, prosecution of perpetrators of violence, or missed productivity and investment [5]. Deaths are of course only the most visible consequence of violence, as the human cost in terms of grief and pain is incalculable. Indeed, "invisible" violence frequently occurs out of sight in homes, workplaces, and even medical and social care setting. Interpersonal violence, including child abuse, youth violence, intimate partner violence, sexual abuse, and abuse of the elderly, occurs largely in a family context and is committed by siblings, intimate partners, and friends. A quarter of all adults have reportedly been physically abused as children, while one-fifth of women report having been sexually abused during childhood or adolescence; one-third have been subjected to physical or sexual abuse by an intimate partner in their lifetime and finally approx. 6% of older adults have reported abuse over the past month. This violence contributes to health impairment, with premature deaths from physical illnesses including heart disease, stroke, cancer, and HIV/AIDS in victims of violence being frequently related to unhealthy behaviors such as smoking, alcohol and drug misuse, and unsafe sex, which are, at least in part, an expression of attempting to cope with the stress produced by the violence. No single factor is sufficient to explain violence, the result of a complex interplay of individual, relationship, social, cultural, and environmental factors [5] including social inequalities, in particular in low- and middle-income countries [6]. Understanding how these factors are related to violence represents a fundamental approach, viewing the issue as a public health problem and identifying the means of preventing it. In this context, the psychopathological origin of violence constitutes only one aspect of this multifaceted issue.

1.1.2   Mental Disorders as a Risk Factor for Violence

The association between mental disorders and violence has long been debated [7]. Data from literature, independent of the samples studied (population studies, treated samples), indicate a major risk of violence among people affected by a mental disorder. Studies of subjects treated for their disorder, the majority of which conducted on inpatients, show prevalence rates that vary according to the setting and time frame considered, with higher rates of violent behaviors among inpatients affected by severe mental illness (17–50%), and lower rates among outpatients (2–13%); however, studies based on both outpatients and inpatients reported that 12–22% had perpetrated violence [8]. A recent national census of patients in the charge of mental health services in Norway, which included 65% of all inpatients (N 2358) and 60% of all outpatients (N 23,124), found a 32% risk of violence among inpatients and 8% among outpatients, with the latter comprising 80% of all patients followed by mental health services [9]. These data are consistent with a meta-analysis showing the lowest rates of violence in studies conducted on outpatients (8%) and the highest rates among involuntarily committed inpatients (36%) [10]. With regard to community samples, studies based on the US Epidemiological Catchment Area Study [11–13] found a prevalence of any violent behavior over the past year ranging from 6.8% to 8.3% [14–16], up to four times higher than among those with no mental disorder. In a study based on data from the National Comorbidity Study [17], the prevalence of violence ranged from 4.6% in the past year for a lifetime diagnosis of major depressive disorder to 16.0% for a past-year diagnosis of bipolar disorder, two to eight times higher than for people without a mental disorder. Although evidence from published literature supports an association between mental disorders and increased risk of violence, several aspects should be taken into consideration to gain a more in-depth knowledge of the problem. Firstly, the fact that the majority of studies were conducted on inpatients may have contributed towards inflating the magnitude of the problem [8]. Indeed, the above-cited study performed in Norway revealed how, when prevalence rates were weighted taking into account the respective rates of in- and outpatients, less than 2% of patients displayed a high risk of violent behavior; in particular, the study showed how 87% of patients had no risk of violent behavior, and 11% a low/moderate risk, with only 1.4% of patients displaying a high risk and 0.4% a very high risk. Significantly, an outpatient study in Italy demonstrated the absence of severe acts of violence among the 10% of patients who had manifested aggressive behavior over the previous year [18]. Moreover, on considering the population-attributable risk percent (PAR%) (in other terms, the percentage of violence in the population that can be ascribed to a mental disorder), an extremely important parameter in terms of public health, we observe that only a limited amount of overall societal violence, ranging from 2 to 10%, is attributable to schizophrenia, the mental disorder public opinion most frequently associates with violence [19]. Data from the NESARC Study estimated a reduction of 0.19 new cases of violence per 100 people when removing severe mental disorder from the total population, corresponding to a 19% reduction in the incidence of violence in the population (i.e., population attributable risk percent) [20]. Finally, the association of violence and mental disorder may be, at least in part, mediated by the living conditions of affected subjects [21]. Being affected by a severe mental illness does not per se appear to be associated with a major risk of violence in the absence of historical (e.g., past violence, physical abuse), clinical (e.g., substance abuse, perceived threats), dispositional (e.g., age, sex, income), and contextual variables (e.g., recent divorce, unemployment) [22], or it is only associated to a slightly increased risk, which rises considerably when severe mental disorders are linked to substance use and/or adverse living conditions [20].

1.1.3 Mental Disorder as a Risk Factor for Becoming Victims of Violence

Further to the well-known association between mental disorders and risk of committing violence, the risk of becoming victims of violence for people affected by severe mental disorders, although less emphasized, is equally worthy of consideration. Choe et al. reported [8] how 20–34% of outpatients had been violently victimized in their lifetime, a considerably higher percentage than that relating to the perpetrators of violence (2–13%); a series of studies including both outpatients and inpatients reported a 35% rate of victims of violence, but only 12–22% of violence perpetrated. Overall, the risk of violent victimization among subjects affected by mental disorders has been estimated to be between 2- and 100-fold more common than in the general population [23, 24], depending on the study methods used. People with schizophrenia are undoubtedly at increased risk of becoming victims of violence in the community, with a risk of being victimized up to 14 times higher than the risk of being arrested as a perpetrator [25]. A recent review of 30 studies (including 6 on domestic violence and 11 on sexual violence) comprising 16,140 subjects affected by severe mental disorders reported a prevalence of recent domestic violence ranging from 15 to 22% in women and 4 to 10% in men or mixed samples; median prevalence of sexual violence was 9.9% in women and 3.1% in men, with a sixfold higher odds of victimization compared with the general population [26]. Another review of 42 studies regarding different types of domestic abuse experienced by men and women receiving psychiatric treatment found a 30% median prevalence of lifetime partner violence among female inpatients and 33% among female outpatients; among males only one high-quality study reported a lifetime prevalence of 32% across mixed psychiatric settings [27]. Taking into account the results published in recent studies, both perpetration of violence and victimization are more common among those affected by severe mental illness than in the general population, although victimization should be viewed as a greater public health concern than perpetration.

1.1.4 Violence Related to Mental Disorders as Cause of Public Alarm and Increased Stigma

Although a trend towards a higher mental health literacy and a greater acceptance of professional help has been observed in recent years, negative attitudes towards people with mental disorders continue to persist [28]. The prevalent focus on the perpetration of violence by people affected by mental disorders seems to be a major factor contributing to the negative stereotypes held of people with severe mental illness. Adverse media coverage of isolated incidents [29] and a tendency of the media to attribute violent crimes to the mentally ill, together with a particular emphasis on describing violence when attributed to a mental disorder [30], affect the public perception of the risk of violent behavior among those affected by mental illnesses [31], representing an important contributing factor to the stigma attached to these people [32]. However, recent anti-stigma interventions targeting the media seem to have elicited some improvement in the style of reporting [33]. Conflicting results are however present in literature as to the effective changes in the perception of people with mental disorders in recent years [34–38], highlighting the persistence of a negative sense of the potential danger linked to a propensity to violence among the mentally ill. Thus, as has been befittingly reported "the stigmatization of people with mental disorders is alive and well, despite decades of campaigning to improve public understanding and to reduce discrimination" [39].

1.1.5 Violence and Deinstitutionalization

It has been argued that stigma has increased, at least in some Western countries such as the USA and northern European countries, due to increasing violence among people with a mental illness. This is considered as largely caused by inadequate treatment resulting from the deinstitutionalization of psychiatric hospitals and reduction in number of psychiatric beds, and ensuant difficulties for community psychiatric services to effectively care for people with a mental illness [40–43]. However, Penrose's law, maintaining how the size of the prison population is inversely related to the number of psychiatric beds, has been disputed on methodological grounds, particularly as only very limited conclusions can be drawn from the sparse and non-comprehensive data available [44]. Other authors however have revealed how although Penrose's law has been proven remarkably robust in the longitudinal perspective, the rise in crime rates may only be attributed to a very limited extent to the deinstitutionalization [45]. Moreover, no conclusive evidence currently supports either side of the debate, given that a series of counter-arguments contrast the validity of Penrose's law, such as the fact that the characteristics of detained subjects affected by severe mental illness differ from the characteristics of deinstitutionalized individuals [46]. A comparative study of a series of European countries between 2002 and 2006 revealed how the number of conventional psychiatric inpatient beds had tended to fall with inconsistent changes in involuntary admissions, while the number of forensic beds in supervised and supported housing, as well as the prison population, had increased in the majority, although not all, of the countries studied. Interestingly, data from the latter study relating to Italy, where a radical deinstitutionalization process had taken place with the Reform Act in 1978, highlighted no substantial variation in the number of people detained in jails between 1990 and 2006, together with a lack of significant change in forensic bed rate [47]. To ascertain whether or not the process of deinstitutionalization has gone too far, a comparative study was conducted using data from the areas of general psychiatry, forensic psychiatry, and penitentiaries as interlocked systems, combining epidemiological and service utilization data; the results obtained revealed how time series from EU member states suggested that civil detention rates had remained more or less stable during the 1990s, although on rather different levels, while admissions to forensic psychiatric facilities had increased over the same period; no data relating to psychiatric morbidity in European prison populations were available [48]. Also in this study, time series of forensic prevalence rates for Italy were significantly lower compared to all countries considered and had remained stable from 1990 to 2002 [48]. Overall data for Italy showed how 40 years after the Reform, concomitant to the progressive decline of psychiatric beds, the population of psychiatric patients placed in Italian forensic psychiatry hospitals had progressively declined [49]. Some authors were of the opinion that deinstitutionalization in Italy had not only failed to result in an increase in compulsory psychiatric hospitalizations, but also to cause any increase in the number of suicides among the mentally ill and in the number of crimes committed by the same [50]. The most important evidence contrasting the assumption that crime rates increase in relation with the reduction of hospital beds likely derives from data on homicides. Indeed, data from England and Wales show not only the presence of little fluctuation in numbers of people with a mental illness committing criminal homicide over the 38 years studied, but also the observation of a 3% annual decline in their contribution to the official statistics [51]. A subsequent study focusing on homicide in the same countries over a 50-year period underlined how the rate of total homicides and rate of homicides due to mental disorders had risen steadily until the mid-1970s, from then on only registering a reversal in the rate of homicides attributed to mental disorders, which declined to historically low levels, while other homicides continued to rise [52]. Further data from New Zealand reported how the percentage of all homicides committed by the mentally ill fell from 19.5% in 1970 to 5.0% in 2000 [53]. Although no national data relating to rates of homicide committed by the mentally ill are available in Italy, indirect data on violence evidence the low and decreasing rates of admission into forensic units, and no increase in self-directed violence, given that the age-adjusted suicide rate remained stable, ranging from 7·1/100,000 population in 1978 to 6·3/100,000 population in 2012 [49], and a slow reduction of overall homicide rates over time, to date among the lowest in Europe (less than 1 per 100,000 inhabitants) [54]. Taken together, these data seem to indicate the lack of any increase in violence attributed to the mentally ill, even in a largely community-based system of care such as the Italian mental health system.

1.1.6   Violence and Family Burden

Family burden, one of the most widely acknowledged issues related to mental health, is a multifactorial phenomenon linked to caregiving. Violence towards others is one of the factors producing a significant contribution to family distress, producing a deterioration in the quality of life of caregivers, and disrupting warmth and positive relationships between family members, as shown in families both of patients affected by long-term psychotic illness [11, 55] and of subjects at their first episode [12, 13, 56–58]. Even family members who no longer live with their affected siblings may experience distress [59]. In Italy, where patients are more likely to live with their families of origin, a feeling of heavy burden and dissatisfaction with the services received is frequent, particularly in the presence of a family member who is highly disabled, resulting in a high level of interpersonal friction and a higher risk of aggressive behaviors. The latter patient group, accounting for approx. 12% of all patients affected by schizophrenia in community care, was frequently admitted to hospital, with half being admitted during the year prior to evaluation (one in ten involuntarily), and resorting to an intensive use of community and residential facilities [60].

1.2 Violence as a Clinical Problem

1.2.1 The Challenging Duty of Assessing Violence Risk

Although community studies show an association between any mental disorder and an increased risk of violent behavior [16], in clinical practice schizophrenia and related disorders [61], bipolar disorder [62], and personality disorders [63] are most commonly associated with a higher risk of violence. Given that the large majority of people affected by severe mental disorders will not perpetrate any form of violence throughout their life, the usefulness of diagnosis per se seems to be of relative importance in recognizing patients who are truly at risk, an extremely difficult task even for an expert psychiatrist. Indeed, assessing the risk of violence implies a highly comprehensive evaluation of psychopathology, personal history, and contextual factors. The case of schizophrenia and psychotic disorders is emblematic in this regard. Psychotic symptoms are traditionally considered of paramount importance to explain not only why a person may become violent, but also the severity of the violence; however, taking into account the high frequency of positive symptoms in contrast with the substantially low rate of acts of violence in psychotic subjects, the need to take into account an interactional effect with other symptoms, social/interpersonal factors, past and current living circumstances, and contextual factors and events is mandatory [64]. Indeed, the interplay between a wide set of clinical and extra-clinical factors is undoubtedly fundamental in explaining violence [65, 66]. With regard to clinical aspects, the interactive role of positive and negative symptoms should be considered, as well as the occurrence of neurocognitive and/or social cognition deficits, of some specific psychopathological experiences (e.g., intense emotional distress, threat/control, override symptoms, command hallucinations, hallucinations of threatening content) together with co-occurring borderline or antisocial personality/psychopathic traits or disorders and/or substance abuse [65–70]. Clinical stage of the disorder is of specific importance, in light of the well-established higher risk of violence among first-episode patients and patients with longer duration of untreated psychosis [71–73]. Moreover, factors such as low treatment adherence [66] and inpatient setting of treatment [65, 66] are significant variables that should be considered. Among extra-clinical factors, sociodemographic data such as male sex and younger age, and historical data, in particular antecedent violent acts and childhood experiences of domestic violence, are of significant importance [65, 66, 74, 75], as well as the presence of triggers (e.g., exposure to violence, parental bereavement, self-harm, traumatic brain injury, unintentional injuries, substance intoxication) [76]. Some authors hypothesize different pathways to violence: psychotic symptoms per se do not seem to be significantly related to violence in adults with early-onset antisocial behavior; on the contrary, they could be specifically related to violence in those with no reported history of childhood antisocial behavior, thus suggesting at least two different developmental trajectories in schizophrenia-associated violence [65]. In this regard, a recent study has shown that only premorbid juvenile delinquency of moderate level predicts violent acts during the first psychotic episode, with an indirect effect mediated by positive symptoms, while a high level of previous delinquency directly predicted violence without mediating factors [77]. An even more complex picture has been proposed in a recent study in which 41 possible causal pathways between risk factors and violence are described [66]. All these aspects clearly illustrate the complexity involved in assessing the risk of violence, a task that general psychiatrists are nowadays required to perform as frequently as forensic psychiatrists. This explains the growing interest in the use of structured means of assessment in common practice, based on a combination of clinical and actuarial data [78]. These structured assessment tools are to be preferred over unstructured clinical judgement due to their higher reliability and transparency. Unfortunately, meta-analytic data reveal that the ability of these tools to predict violence is not sufficiently evidence based in the majority of cases, and that at best they may be used to classify single subjects at a group level, not allowing a real prognosis in individual cases; thus, considering their higher negative predictive value, they could conveniently be used to screen out low-risk individuals [79, 80]. Moreover, on a practical ground, it should be borne in mind how the assessment tools available are extremely time consuming and unsuitable for use in common clinical practice [81]. It has indeed been argued that although use of predictive assessment tools is significantly better than leaving things to chance, in practical terms this means very little for staff members working in a community mental health center. For example, it was calculated [82] that in an inner city area in which a 6% rate of violence among people with mental disorders could be expected over a 6-month period, the rate of wrong prediction using structured tools would correspond to 90%; this rate increases to 97% when predicting severe violence, which occurs in approx. 1% of the mentally ill per year. The prediction goes on to become totally meaningless with regard to homicides committed by persons with a mental disorder at a rate of approx. 1/10,000 per year, thus underlining the inherent difficulty or impossibility of predicting rare events [82]. Even a relatively user-friendly scalable risk prediction score, recently developed following the example of cardiology, proved to be valid only in identifying subjects at low risk of violence, implying how in clinical practice the tool would only be of use as an adjunct to the decision-making process, necessitating further clinical evaluation to identify subjects at higher risk [83].

1.2.2   Critical Issues in Management of Violence

1.2.2.1 Violence and Involuntary Admissions

Violence is frequently used to justify psychiatric hospitalization. Physically violent behaviors are highly prevalent immediately prior to hospitalization, being reported in about one-third of cases [84, 85] and representing one of the main reasons for involuntary admission [86, 87]. In psychiatry the issue of compulsory admissions remains controversial, although being deemed necessary in order to facilitate treatment and prevent harm. In Europe, the mental health laws enforced in many countries explicitly envisage compulsory admission to prevent harm in the case of "dangerousness to self or others"; while in many others this is only to ensure due care to severely mentally ill people who refuse treatments [88], as occurs in Italy, where involuntary inpatient treatment is justified only when the person is in a situation of mental alteration such as to require urgent therapeutic interventions, these interventions are rejected and it is deemed impossible to take timely extra-hospital measures. However, even in countries such as Italy where the criterion of dangerousness in justifying involuntary admissions has been abolished after the Reform Law in 1978, the issue still remains one of the main aspects driving the decision-making process in clinical practice [89]. Another puzzling issue is that the criteria developed in several countries to regulate practices are criticized as leaving scope for discretion, with values and beliefs of staff a crucial factor for decisions [90]. Interestingly, although compulsory admission is an almost universally adopted practice with a very high inter-country variability, proof of its effectiveness and presence of standard regulations are still lacking [91]. Indeed, a systematic literature review found that involuntary admissions were associated to no better or even worse outcomes with respect to voluntary admissions (e.g., suicide risk was higher, social functioning was lower, and dissatisfaction with treatment was higher due to the feeling that hospitalization was not justified) [92]. Aggressions occur frequently even during hospitalization, with compulsory admissions representing one of the most significant risk factors [93]; indeed, up to 40% of subjects admitted involuntarily due to recent aggressive behavior become physically aggressive during compulsory hospitalization [85]. Unfortunately, healthcare workers are the most frequent victims of violence in inpatient units, a serious occupational issue that involves both staff and patients, with negative consequences on the psychological well-being of workers, service costs, and standards of care [94]. To this regard, a recent survey of Italian psychiatrists found that 91% had been subjected to verbal aggression, 72% had been threatened with dangerous objects, and 65% had been victims of physical assaults; the main consequences were a significant increase of feelings such as fear, vulnerability, and inadequacy, and a 50% higher probability of a negative modification of the therapeutic relationship with patients [95].

1.2.2.2 Violence and Coercive Measures

Undoubtedly, the use of coercive measures is one of most challenging aspects of psychiatric practice, and probably the main reason underlying criticism of the entire discipline. The EUNOMIA study reported how coercive measures were applied in a substantial group of involuntarily admitted patients across Europe, ranging between 21% and 59%, with an average rate of 38%; aggression towards others is the most frequent reason for adopting coercive measures, with forced medication being the most frequent measure used in eight of the countries studied; mechanical restraint was used in two, while seclusion was adopted in only six countries; the use of these measures was largely dependent on diagnosis and severity of illness, while large variations across countries seem to reflect very different societal attitudes and clinical traditions [96]. A comparison of involuntarily admitted patients who underwent coercive measures with patients who were not subjected to this form of treatment, taking into account not only clinical factors, such as high levels of psychotic symptoms, but also high levels of perceived coercion at admission, was found to be associated, on controlling for a country-related effect, with the use of coercive measures, thus suggesting that these factors should be taken into consideration by programs aimed at reducing similar practices in psychiatric wards [97]. Marked differences between countries also emerged with regard to the use of forced medication, largely due to legal and policy-making aspects rather than to clinical reasons, thus underlining the need to develop specific guidelines; however, forced medication should always be considered as a last resort, to be adopted when all other therapeutic options have failed [98]. Exploring the outcomes of coercive measures in the context of the Eunomia Study, forced medication appears to be unique in its significant impact on patient disapproval of treatment received as a coercive measure; however, all measures, in particular seclusion, were found to be associated with a longer stay in hospital, although the association was not fully explained by a higher severity of patients coerced on admission [99]. Negative experiences elicited in patients submitted to coercive measures undoubtedly represent the most relevant reason for avoiding the latter. Research studies clearly indicate that patients associate very negative emotions and feelings to forced medication, restraint, and seclusion, expressing a desire to be treated with respect rather than submitted to any form of control; however, sensitivity towards patients' views while trying to respond to their needs at each point of the coercive process and improving empathy and communication may represent moderating factors in scaling down the negative impact of coercion [100]. Care staff-related factors (e.g., de-escalation, communication, knowledge and experience, limit setting, intervention timing, and containment) and organizational/environmental factors (e.g., staff mix, staff training, patient mix, organized activity, physical environment, policy, and rules) are deemed crucial factors in the prevention of violence and subsequent coercive measures [101].

Unfortunately, despite the emphasis placed on de-escalation and use of noncoercive strategies or coping skills [99], evidence derived from the limited research conducted in controlled studies fails to support the effectiveness of behavioral strategies in preventing or treating aggression, ultimately resulting in clinical practice continuing to be based on empirical evidence [102].

1.2.2.3 The Hot Issue of Avoiding Involuntary Admissions and Coercive Measures

Involuntary admissions of people with mental disorders and consequent treatments have long provided reason for concern from an ethical point of view, although traditionally the principle of beneficence is invoked to counterbalance the violation of patients' autonomy (i.e., involuntary admission is justified in the best interest of the patients). However, the fact that mental health laws are generally discriminatory of the mentally ill, failing to respect their acknowledged medical rights to self-determination or self-governance, is seen as a consequence of an impairment of decision-making capacity which leads to refusal of treatment and a consequent need to override the same in the best interest of patients, with a view to protecting both patients and others from potential harm [103]. These assumptions are in contrast with the United Nations Convention on the Rights of Persons with Disabilities (CRPD) [104], which states that "the existence of a disability shall in no case justify a deprivation of liberty" (Article 14). Indeed, the Convention, generally interpreted as considering people with severe mental disorders as disabled, states that any involuntary detention and treatment of these people are prohibited, and accordingly substitute decision-making is also not deemed consistent with the Convention [105]. Needless to say, the Convention has given rise to considerable criticism and controversy [106–108]. The criticism relates largely to the fact that a person's ability to make a decision may not be ignored, regardless of circumstance, with controversies focusing mainly on aspects such as legal capacity, best interest, will, and preferences of disabled persons [109]. However, as the majority of countries adhering to the UN have undersigned the Convention, an extremely puzzling problem has arisen ensuant to the enforcement in numerous national laws of involuntary treatments. To ensure compliance of all countries with the UN Convention, the approval of a so-called fusion law aimed at eliminating the discrimination of the mentally ill and applying to all people irrespective of status (i.e., being mentally or physically ill) and allowing involuntary treatment only when decision-making capability for treatments is impaired, independent of the health setting and cause of impairment, and decision-making supports have failed [110] represents an interesting proposal. In recent years, attempts have been made to resort to advance directives, written documents, or oral statements issued by adults who maintain some degree of decision-making capacity, thus allowing them to express treatment preferences and/or designate substitute decision makers should they subsequently be deemed incapable of making informed choices. Unfortunately, these advance directives have proven rather difficult to implement, in particular due to a series of barriers occurring at system level (e.g., unauthorized practice of law), agency level (e.g., lack of resources, lack of staff training), and individual level (e.g., engaging clients) [111]. Moreover, a review of RCTs involving adults with severe mental illness, comparing advance directives and standard care, found no difference in hospital admissions, attendance of outpatient services, treatment compliance, and acts of self-harm and arrests, although subjects who had provided advance directives were involved to a lesser degree in violent acts and use of social services [112]. Of all forms of advance directives, joint crisis plans are viewed as the most promising practice, being highly appreciated by service users, capable of improving the therapeutic relationship, and of reducing involuntary admissions [113, 114]; the actual impact however of these plans in common clinical practice on both a national or supranational level cannot currently be evaluated due to a lack of relevant studies.

To prevent involuntary admissions (and subsequent coercive measures), several countries have adopted community treatment orders (CTOs) and legal statutes requiring those affected by a serious mental illness to adhere to a plan of treatment and supervision while living in the community. CTOs have been one of the most widely debated issues in recent years, with different opinions and interpretation of research data. The first meta-analysis of published controlled trials, based only on three relatively small, possibly biased trials, with low- to moderate-quality evidence, found no significant differences between coercive community treatments and voluntary treatment in any of the main outcome measures (service use, readmission to hospital, service use, compliance with medication, social functioning, being arrested, homelessness, satisfaction with care, and perceived coercion), although people under CTOs were less likely to be victims of violent or nonviolent crime; it was unclear whether the latter advantage could be due to the intensity of treatment or its compulsory nature [115]. The most recent systematic study and meta-analysis of RCTs and non-randomized controlled studies found no apparent effect of CTOs on hospital readmissions and inpatient stays, a moderate increase in use of community services, and a nonsignificant increase in treatment adherence; moreover, the effect on use of community services was only nonsignificant when taking into account RTCs alone. In the same meta-analysis, on taking into account pre-post studies only, all outcomes evaluated were significantly better in the case of CTOs, although this evidence was not considered reliable by the authors of the study due to intrinsic methodological problems in pre-post studies (vulnerability to regression to the mean and temporal effects) [116]. Interestingly, other authors, applying the same argument used to criticize the appropriateness of RTCs in evaluating the effectiveness of long-acting injections of antipsychotics (LAI), i.e., generally conducted on samples of better adherent patients, thus resulting in false-negative findings for LAI, maintain that pre-post studies represent the best means of evaluating CTOs, reaching conflicting conclusions with regard to the data emerging from the above-cited study [117]. When considering the issue of CTOs, their significance for patients should be considered, particularly in the light of studies demonstrating how they give rise to intense feelings of coercion and control in a highly ambivalent context [118]. Moreover, some authors have pointed out how decision makers frequently hold a very different point of view compared to patients in considering CTOs as a useful means of ensuring control, continuity, and follow-up, based on a varied knowledge of patient's everyday life and a limited attention to patients' experiences of coercion, suggesting that decision makers should focus more carefully on the negative consequences experienced by patients who opt for a CTO [119].

A markedly different approach in reducing the risk of involuntary admission has focused on the use of intensive care programs such as assertive community treatment (ACT), as suggested by recent studies. Data from a Danish study revealed how over a 5-year period a decrease in admission trends compared to standard care was observed in patients with severe mental illnesses allocated to ACT, accompanied by a significant difference in trends relating to both voluntary and involuntary admissions based on a criterion of dangerousness, and a decreased number of contacts with the psychiatric emergency room; ACT was moreover deemed the preferred option by both staff members and patients [120]. The access study relating to an integrated care plan, including assertive community treatment, to be offered to patients with psychotic disorders, among other results, reported a decrease in involuntary admissions from 35% over the 2 years prior to the study to 8% over 4 years [121].

1.3 Violence as a Forensic Problem

1.3.1 Challenges and Difficulties in Forensic Psychiatry Assessment

Forensic psychiatrists are nominated by the relevant authorities to assess subjects with mental disorders who have been charged with homicide or other forms of violence against persons. In such cases the forensic psychiatric assessment plays a fundamental role in the judicial process, considering that all subsequent decisions on the sentence, detention, placement, or treatment will take into account this assessment [122]. Moreover, forensic psychiatrists may be required to evaluate the competence of a person to make decisions throughout all stages of the judiciary procedures, including competence to stand trial, to plead guilty, to be sentenced, to waive appeal, and to be executed [123]. Independent of the huge variation in legal frameworks in different countries, a basic common assumption is that a mental disorder may significantly affect the person's ability to exercise "free will" and control his/her actions [124]. The forensic psychiatrist is generally asked to determine whether or not the accused has a mental disorder, specifying whether the latter affects discernment and control of actions at the time of offense; according to local laws, the expert may also be required to assess the degree of influence of the altered mental state on discernment and control, an evaluation upon which the criminal responsibility of the defendant is decided, and which may justify a complete non-imputability or a "partial imputability." The intrinsic difficulties and largely subjective nature of a similarly "quantitative" evaluation are among the main reasons underlying the frequently large variations in forensic assessments and controversies during trials. Moreover, differences between experts appear to focus mainly on forensic interpretation, with particular regard to the relationship between pathology and offense, with disagreements seemingly more related primarily to personal ideologies or different schools of thought than to other factors [125]. Forensic psychiatrists are often engaged in violence risk assessments related to decisions concerning the detention and release of offenders, an extremely challenging task taking into account the wide diffusion of stereotypes of dangerousness of the mentally ill and the increasing expectations of "protection" in the public opinion. As mentioned previously, structured instruments developed for the purpose of risk assessment may allow subjects to be classified according to the probability of their becoming violent, and are generally deemed superior over clinical judgement. Although these tools are increasingly used in the context of forensic psychiatry, relevant, reliable, and unbiased data on their predictive accuracy have been reported to still be somewhat limited, highlighting how an excess of reliance on and improper use of these instruments may negatively prejudice the risks of discrimination and further stigmatization [126]. The performance of currently used instruments beyond the first days of admission to forensic institutes is considered variable, with some evidence of the utility of certain tools only in the case of imminent violence [127]. Moreover, on considering the high levels of comorbidity in forensic populations between personality disorders and other disorders (psychotic, mood, and/or substance-use disorders) [128], it is remarkable how the predictive capacity of structured tools was found to be poor or no better than chance for people with antisocial personality disorders, with no instrument being considered better than chance in the case of psychopathy, a relatively infrequent disorder among the general population, but with a much higher impact on violence and recidivism than any other psychiatric disorder [129].

1.3.2 The Challenging Task of Treating Forensic Patients

The treatment of mentally ill offenders is largely provided worldwide in forensic hospital/wards, and a trend towards an increasing number of beds in these institutions has been reported [130]. Evaluation of psychiatric care in forensic settings is limited by the paucity of research, as emerged from a recent overview of systematic reviews focused on research activities in several practice-relevant areas of forensic psychiatry (diagnosis/risk assessment, pharmacologic interventions, psychological interventions, psychosocial interventions/rehabilitation, restraint interventions). This overview highlighted the presence in all domains of more or less pronounced "knowledge gaps" (i.e., lack of sufficient scientific evidence), with some domains burdened by severe gaps such as psychosocial interventions and rehabilitation, and an overall "urgent need" for further studies [131]. Indeed, the picture described by the recent literature is not encouraging. A national study shows how following hospital discharge (mean follow-up approx. 16 years), 30% of patients had died (n = 1949), approx. 70% had been readmitted, and 40% had repeated a violent offense within 4 years of discharge [132].

Fazel et al. [133] recently published a systematic review and meta-analysis of adverse outcomes after discharge in forensic psychiatric patients, comparing the results obtained with rates from other clinical and forensic groups; a very high mortality of discharged patients was observed in both absolute and relative terms, comparable to the mortality generally found among psychotic patients in general. The same review reported equally high readmission rates, although difficulties were encountered in identifying data for comparison from other observational studies of non-forensic samples; finally, reoffence rates were found to vary between 0 and 24,244 per 100,000 patient-years, a huge heterogeneity that the authors were unable to explain. However, patients discharged from forensic hospitals were characterized by lower offending outcomes than comparative groups of general prisoners, a finding explained by the marked difference in characteristics of the sample confronted, with forensic patients representing a more selected sample (e.g., in terms of criminal career, psychopathology, treatments received). The general system based on the use of forensic psychiatric hospitals was adopted in Italy for more than a century; however in 2014, following the passing of Law n.81, the responsibility for treating mentally ill patients deemed non-responsible for their actions and socially "dangerous," passed from the Department of Justice to the Department of Health, with high-security forensic psychiatric hospitals (OPGs) being closed and treatments delivered in a network of small regional community facilities with no more than 20 beds, the so-called REMS (Residences for the Execution of Security Measures) [134, 135]. In this way, the radical change in mental health care that had started in Italy in 1978 with the psychiatric reform law, marking a transition from a hospital-based system of care to a model of community mental health care [49], was completed. The implementation of Law n.81 is expected to progressively increase the quality of mental health care for subjects affected by mental disorders who have committed crimes, paying due respect to human rights [136]. The reform may have the potential to change the landscape in this area of psychiatry, providing a potential blueprint to be followed by other countries [137, 138]. However, by closing its high-security hospitals and moving to an overt community mental health system, Italy was "entering uncharted waters," with considerable concern being raised as to the effectiveness of the new model [138]. Outcome studies should therefore be set up to monitor and evaluate this changing landscape to ascertain whether it truly meets those treatment needs which had previously remained unmet by the traditional system of forensic psychiatric hospitals, promoting an effective recovery of patients, without exposing the public to undue risks [137–139].

1.4 Conclusions

Psychopathology-related violence is probably among the most controversial topic in psychiatry. In fact, not only violence largely determines the stigmatization of those who suffer from a mental disorder, but it also contributes to the stigmatization of the discipline itself. Frequently the field of psychiatry is thought to perpetrate, probably the only case among all branches of medicine, in disregard of human rights and to neglect the dignity of the person, due to the use of treatments without consent and coercive measures. This scenario also depends on the difficulty of making the public opinion and the other stakeholders fully aware of the complexity of those human conditions we call mental disorders as well as of the influence that these have, at a given time in each individual life, on self-awareness, on mental status, and consequently voluntary adhesion to care. Similarly, it remains difficult to explain another specificity of psychiatry, which consists of the difficult and undesirable role of "social defense," with which this discipline has to, however, come to terms, looking for, in each single case, a problematic balance between the divergent needs posed by the respect of the individual and collective rights. Optimal options for the prevention of violence in at-risk cases should be based on a strong and assertive handling by community services as well as on the diffusion of clinical care projects, including joint crisis intervention plans. These approaches might limit and hopefully avoid the implementation of coercive measures, which, we believe, no psychiatrist takes lightly and without a painful awareness of their consequences, and certainly with the clear conviction that these should be the last resort only when any other attempt has failed.

References

1. World Health Organization. World Health Assembly Resolution 49.25: Prevention of violence: a public health priority. 1996. https://www.who.int/violence_injury_prevention/resources/publications/en/WHA4925_eng.pdf
2. WHO Global Consultation on Violence and Health. Violence: a public health priority. Geneva: World Health Organization; 1996 (document WHO/EHA/SPI.POA.2).
3. Krug EG, Dahlberg LL, Mercy JA, Zwi AB, Lozano R, editors. World report on violence and health. Geneva: World Health Organization; 2002.
4. Krug EG, Mercy JA, Dahlberg LA, Zwi AB. The world report on violence and health. Lancet. 2002;360:1083–8.

5. World Health Organization. Global status report on violence prevention. Geneva: World Health Organization; 2014.
6. Wolf A, Gray R, Fazel S. Violence as a public health problem: an ecological study of 169 countries. Soc Sci Med. 2014;104:220–7.
7. Harris A, Lurigio AJ. Mental illness and violence: a brief review of research and assessment strategies. Aggress Viol Behav. 2007;12:542–51.
8. Choe JY, Teplin LA, Abram KM. Perpetration of violence, violent victimization and severe mental illness: balancing public health concerns. Psychiatr Serv. 2008;59:153–64.
9. Osea SS, Lilleengb S, Pettersen I, Ruudd T, van Weeghelf J. Risk of violence among patients in psychiatric treatment: results from a national census. Nord J Psychiatry. 2017;71:551–60.
10. Swanson JW, McGinty EE, Fazel S, Mays VM. Mental illness and reduction of gun violence and suicide: bringing epidemiologic research to policy. Ann Epidemiol. 2014;25:366–76.
11. Hanzawa S, Bae JK, Bae YJ, Chae MH, Tanaka H, Nakane H, Ohta Y, Zhao X, Iizuka H, Nakane Y. Psychological impact on caregivers traumatized by the violent behavior of a family member with schizophrenia. Asian J Psychiatr. 2013;6:46–51.
12. Solomon P, Cavanaugh M, Gelles R. Family violence among adults and severe mental illness: a neglected area of research. Trauma Violence Abuse. 2006;6:40–54.
13. Bowman S, Alvarez-Jimenez M, Wade D, Howie L, McGorry P. The impact of first episode psychosis on sibling quality of life. Soc Psychiatry Psychiatric Epidemiol. 2014;49:1071–81.
14. Silver E, Teasdale B. Mental disorder and violence: an examination of stressful life events and impaired social support. Soc Probl. 2005;52:62–78.
15. Swanson JW. Alcohol abuse, mental disorder, and violent behavior: an epidemiologic inquiry. Alcohol Health Res World. 1993;17:123–32.
16. Swanson JW, Holzer CE, Ganju VK, Jono RT. Violence and psychiatric disorder in the community: evidence from the Epidemiologic Catchment Area surveys. Hosp Community Psychiatry. 1990;41:761–70.
17. Corrigan PW, Watson AC. Findings from the National Comorbidity Survey on the frequency of violent behavior in individuals with psychiatric disorders. Psychiatry Res. 2005;136:153–62.
18. Pinna F, Tusconi M, Dessì C, Pittaluga G, Fiorillo A, Carpiniello B. Violence and mental disorders. A retrospective study of people in charge of a community mental health center. Int J Psychiatry Law. 2016;47:122–8.
19. Walsh E, Buchanan A, Fahy T. Violence and schizophrenia: examining the evidence. Br J Psychiatry. 2002;180:490–5.
20. Van Dorn R, Volavka J, Johnson N. Mental disorder and violence: is there a relationship beyond substance use? Soc Psychiatry Psychiatric Epidemiol. 2012;47:487–503.
21. Markowitz FE. Mental illness, crime and violence: risk, context and social control. Aggress Viol Behav. 2011;16:36–44.
22. Elbogen EB, Johnson SC. The intricate link between violence and mental disorder: results from the National Epidemiologic Survey on Alcohol and Related Conditions. Arch Gen Psychiatry. 2009;66:152–61.
23. Maniglio R. Severe mental illness and criminal victimization: a systematic review. Acta Psychiatr Scand. 2009;119:180–91.
24. Khalifeh H. Violence against people with severe mental illness in Europe. Acta Psychiatr Scand. 2009;119:414.
25. Brekke JS, Prindle C, Bae SW, Long JD. Risks for individuals with schizophrenia who are living in the community. Psychiatr Serv. 2001;52:1358–66.
26. Khalifeh H, Oram S, Osborn D, Howard LM, Johnson S. Recent physical and sexual violence against adults with severe mental illness: a systematic review and meta-analysis. Int Rev Psychiatry. 2016;28:433–51.
27. Oram S, Trevillion K, Feder G, Howard LM. Prevalence of experiences of domestic violence among psychiatric patients: systematic review. Br J Psychiatry. 2013;202:94–9.
28. Schomerus G, Schwann C, Holzinger A, Corrigan PW, Grabe HJ, Carta MG, Angermeyer MC. Evolution of public attitudes about mental illness: a systematic review and meta-analysis. Acta Psychiatr Scand. 2012;125:440–52.

29. Faruqui R. Mental illness and moral panic: a qualitative study of perceptions of a link between violent crime and mental illness. Eur Psychiatry. 2011;26:529.
30. Carpiniello B, Girau R, Orrù MG. Mass-media, violence and mental illness. Evidence from some Italian newspapers. Epidemiol Psichiatr Soc. 2007;16:251–5.
31. Wehring HJ, Carpenter WT. Violence and schizophrenia. Schizophr Bull. 2011;37:877–8.
32. Pescosolido BA, Medina TR, Martin JK, Long JS. The "backbone" of stigma: identifying the global core of public prejudice associated with mental illness. Am J Public Health. 2013;103:853–60.
33. Maiorano A, Lasalvia A, Sampogna G, Pocai B, Ruggeri M, Henderson C. Reducing stigma in media professionals: is there room for improvement? Results from a systematic review. Can J Psychiatry. 2017;62:702–15.
34. Rhydderch D, Krooupa AM, Ahefer G, Goulden R, Williams P, Thornicroft A, Rose D, Thornicroft G, Henderson C. Changes in newspapers coverage of mental illness from 2008 to 2014 in England. Acta Psychiatr Scand. 2016;134(Suppl 446):45–52.
35. Pingani L, Sampogna G, Borghi G, Nasi A, Coriani S, Luciano L, Galeazzi GM, Evans-Lacko S, Fiorillo A. How the use of the term "schizo" has changed in an Italian newspaper from 2001 to 2015: findings from a descriptive analysis. Psychiatry Res. 2018;270:792–800.
36. Murphy NA, Fatoye F, Wibberley C. The changing face of newspapers representations of the mentally ill. J Ment Health. 2013;22:271–82.
37. Whitley R, Wang G. Good news? A longitudinal analysis of newspaper portrayals of mental illness in Canada 2005 to 2015. Can J Psychiatry. 2017;62:278–85.
38. Whitley R, Wang J. Television coverage of mental illness in Canada: 2013–2015. Soc Psychiatry Psychiatric Epidemiol. 2017;52:241–4.
39. Editorial. Truth versus myth on mental illness, suicide, and crime. Lancet. 2013;382:1309.
40. Torrey EF. The association of stigma with violence. Am J Psychiatry. 2011;168:325.
41. Torrey EF. Stigma and violence: isn't it time to connect the dots? Schizophr Bull. 2011;37:892–6.
42. Jüriloo A, Pesonen L, Lauerma H. Knocking on prison's door: a 10-fold rise in the number of psychotic prisoners in Finland during the years 2005–2016. Nord J Psychiatry. 2017;71:543–8.
43. Kramp P, Gabrielsen G. The organization of the psychiatric service and criminality committed by the mentally ill. Eur Psychiatry. 2009;24:401–11.
44. Kalapos MP. Penrose's law: methodological challenges and call for data. Int J Law Psychiatry. 2016;49:1–9.
45. Hartvig P, Kjelsberg E. Penrose's Law revisited: the relationship between mental institution beds, prison population and crime rate. Nord J Psychiatry. 2009;63:51–6.
46. Prins SJ. Does transinstitutionalization explain the overrepresentation of people with serious mental illnesses in the criminal justice system? Community Ment Health J. 2011;47:716–22.
47. Priebe S, Frottier P, Gaddini A, Kilian R, Lauber C, Martínez-Leal R, Munk-Jørgensen P, Walsh D, Wiersma D, Wright D. Mental health care institutions in nine European countries, 2002 to 2006. Psychiatr Serv. 2008;59:570–3.
48. Salize HJ, Schanda H, Dressing H. From the hospital into the community and back again—a trend towards re-institutionalisation in mental health care? Int Rev Psychiatry. 2008;20:527–34.
49. Barbui C, Papola D, Saraceno B. Forty years without mental hospitals in Italy. Int J Ment Heal Syst. 2018;12:43.
50. Morzycka-Markowska M, Drozdowicz E, Nasierowski T. Deinstitutionalization in Italian psychiatry—the course and consequences. Part II. The consequences of deinstitutionalization. Psychiatr Pol. 2015;49:403–12.
51. Taylor PJ, Gunn J. Homicides by people with mental illness: myth and reality. Br J Psychiatry. 1999;174:9–14.
52. Large M, Smith G, Swinson N, Shaw J, Nielssen O. Homicide due to mental disorder in England and Wales over 50 years. Br J Psychiatry. 2008;193:130–3.

53. Simpson AI, McKenna B, Moskowitz A, Skipworth J, Walsh JB. Homicide and mental illness in New Zealand, 1970–2000. Br J Psychiatry. 2004;185:394–8.
54. Eurostat. Crime statistics in Europe. https://ec.europa.eu/eurostat/statistics-explained/index. php/Crime_statistics
55. Greenberg J, Kim H, Greenley J. Factors associated with subjective burden in siblings of adults with severe mental illness. Am J Orthopsychiatry. 1997;67:231–41.
56. Bowman S, Alvarez-Jimenez M, Wade D, Howie L, McGorry P. The impact of first-episode psychosis on the sibling relationship. Psychiatry. 2015;78:141–55.
57. Smith M, Greenberg J. Factors contributing to the quality of sibling relationships for adults with schizophrenia. Psychiatr Serv. 2008;59:57–62.
58. Bowman S, Alvarez-Jimenez M, Wade D, Howie L, McGorry P. The positive and negative experiences of caregiving for siblings of young people with first episode psychosis. Front Psychol. 8:730. https://doi.org/10.3389/fpsyg.2017.00730.
59. Hanzawa S, Bae J, Bae Y, Chae M, Tanaka H, Nakane H, Ohta Y, Zhao X, Iizuka H, Nakane Y. Psychological impact on caregivers traumatized by the violent behaviour of a family member with schizophrenia. Asian J Psychiatr. 2013;6:46–51.
60. Lora A, Cosentino U, Rossini MS, Lanzara D. A cluster analysis of patients with schizophrenia in community care. Psychiatr Serv. 2001;52:682–4.
61. Fazel S, Gulati G, Linsell L, Geddes JR, Grann M. Schizophrenia and violence: systematic review and meta-analysis. PLoS Med. 2009;6(8):e1000120. https://doi.org/10.1371/journal. pmed.1000120.
62. Fazel S, Lichtenstein P, Grann M, Goodwin GM, Långström N. Bipolar disorder and violent crime: new evidence from population-based longitudinal studies and systematic review. Arch Gen Psychiatry. 2010;67:931–8.
63. Fountoulakis KN, Leucht S, Kaprinis GS. Personality disorders and violence. Curr Opin Psychiatry. 2008;21:84–92.
64. Taylor PJ. When symptoms of psychosis drive serious violence. Soc Psychiatry Psychiatric Epidemiol. 1998;33(Suppl 1):S47–54.
65. Bo S, Abu-Akel A, Kongerslev M, Haahr UH, Simonsen E. Risk factors for violence among patients with schizophrenia. Clin Psychol Rev. 2011;31:711–26.
66. Lamsma J, Harte JM. Violence in psychosis: conceptualizing its causal relations with risk factors. Aggress Violent Behav. 2015;24:75–82.
67. Beech DR, Harvey PD, Dill J. Neuropsychological and symptom predictors of aggression on the psychiatric inpatient service. J Clin Exp Neuropsychol. 2008;30:700–9.
68. Reinharth J, Reynolds G, Dill G, Serper M. Cognitive predictors of violence in schizophrenia: a meta-analytic review. Schizophrenia Res Cognition. 2014;1:101–11.
69. Sedgwick O, Susan Young S, Baumeister D, Greer B, Das M, Kumari V. Neuropsychology and emotion processing in violent individuals with antisocial personality disorder or schizophrenia: the same or different? A systematic review and meta-analysis. Aust NZ J Psychiatry. 2017;51:1178–97.
70. Ahmed AO, Richardson J, Buckner A, Romanoff S, Feder M, Oragunye N, Ilnicki A, Bhat I, Hoptman MJ, Lindenmayer JP. Do cognitive deficits predict negative emotionality and aggression in schizophrenia? Psychiatry Res. 2018;259:350–7.
71. Nielssen N, Large M. Rates of homicide during the first episode of psychosis and after treatment: a systematic review and meta-analysis. Schizophr Bull. 2010;36:702–12.
72. Langeveld J, Bjørkly S, Auestad B, Barder H, Evensen J, ten Velden Hegelstad W, Joa J, Johannessen JO, Larsen TK, Melle I, Opjordsmoen S, Røssberg JI, Rund BR, Simonsen E, Vaglum P, McGlashan T, Friis S. Treatment and violent behavior in persons with first episode psychosis during a 10-year prospective follow up study. Schizophr Res. 2014;156:271–6.
73. Latalova K. Violence and duration of untreated psychosis in first-episode patients. Int J Clin Practice. 2014;68:330–5.
74. González RA, Kallis C, Ullrich S, Barnicot K, Keers R, Coid JW. Childhood maltreatment and violence: mediation through psychiatric morbidity. Child Abuse Negl. 2016;52:70–84.

75. Monahan J, Vesselinov R, Clark Robbins P, Appelbaum PS. Violence to others, violent self-victimization, and violent victimization by others among persons with a mental illness. Psychiatr Serv. 2017;68:516–9.
76. Sariaslan A, Lichtenstein P, Larsson H, Fazel S. Triggers for violent criminality in patients with psychotic disorders. JAMA Psychiat. 2016;73:796–803.
77. Winsper C, Singh P, Marwaha S, Amos T, Lester H, Everard L, Jones P, Fowler D, Marshall M, Lewis S, Sharma W, Freemantle N, Birchwood M. Pathways to violent behaviours during first psychotic episode. A report from the UK National EDEN Study. JAMA Psychiat. 2013;70:1287–93.
78. Kumar S, Simpson AIF. Application of risk assessment for violence methods to general adult psychiatry: a selective literature review. Aust NZ J Psychiatry. 2005;39:328–35.
79. Fazel S, Sigh YP, Doll H, Grann M. Use of risk assessment instruments to predict violence and antisocial behaviour in 73 samples involving 24827 people: systematic review and meta-analysis. BMJ. 2012;345:e4692.
80. Singh YP, Serper M, Reinhart F, Fazel S. Structured assessment of violence risk in schizophrenia and other psychiatric disorders: a systematic review of the validity, reliability, and item content of 10 available instruments. Schizophr Bull. 2011;37:899–912.
81. Viljoen J, McLachlan K, Vincent G. Assessing violence risk and psychopathy in juvenile and adult offenders: a survey of clinical practices. Assessment. 2010;17:377–95.
82. Szmukler G. Violence risk prediction in practice. Br J Psychiatry. 2001;178:84–5.
83. Fazel S, Wolf A, Larsson H, Lichtenstein P, Mallett S, Fanshawe TR. Identification of low risk of violent crime in severe mental illness with a clinical prediction tool (Oxford Mental Illness and Violence tool [OxMIV]): a derivation and validation study. Lancet Psychiatry. 2017;4:461–8.
84. Colasanti A, Natoli A, Moliterno D, Rossattini M, De Gaspari IF, Mauri MC. Psychiatric diagnosis and aggression before acute hospitalisation. Eur Psychiatry. 2008;23:441–8.
85. Amore M, Menchetti M, Tonti C, Scarlatti F, Lundgren E, Esposito W, Berardi D. Predictors of violent behavior among acute psychiatric patients: clinical study. Psychiatry Clin Neurosci. 2008;62:247–25.
86. Marty S, Jaeger M, Moetteli S, Theodoridou A, Seifritz E, Hotzy F. Characteristics of psychiatric emergency situations and the decision-making process leading to involuntary admission. Front Psych. 2019;9:760. https://doi.org/10.3389/fpsyt.2018.00760.
87. Canova Moselea PH, Chervenski Figueirac G, Bertuol Filhob AA, Reis Ferreira de Limac JA, Crestani Calegarod V. Involuntary psychiatric hospitalization and its relationship to psychopathology and aggression. Psychiatry Res. 2018;265:13–8.
88. Dressing H, Salize HJ. Compulsory admission of mentally ill patients in European Union Member States. Soc Psychiatry Psychiatric Epidemiol. 2004;39:797–803.
89. Dazzan P, Bhugra D, Carta MG, Carpiniello B. Decision making process for compulsory admission: study of a group of psychiatrists of Sardinia, Italy. Epidemiol Psichiatr Soc. 2001;10:37–45.
90. Feiring E, Ugstad KN. Interpretations of legal criteria for involuntary psychiatric admission: a qualitative analysis. BMC Health Serv Res. 2014;14:500. https://doi.org/10.1186/s12913-014-0500-x.
91. Jacobsen TB. Involuntary treatment in Europe: different countries, different practices. Curr Opin Psychiatry. 2012;25:307–10.
92. Kallert TW, Glöckner M, Schützwohl M. Involuntary vs. voluntary hospital admission. A systematic literature review on outcome diversity. Eur Arch Psychiatry Clin Neurosci. 2008;258:195–209.
93. Cornaggia CM, Beghi M, Pavone F, Barale F. Aggression in psychiatry wards: a systematic review. Psychiatry Res. 2011;189:10–20.
94. d'Ettorre G, Pellicani V. Workplace violence toward mental healthcare workers employed in psychiatric wards. Saf Health Work. 2017;8:337–42.
95. Catanesi R, Carabellese F, Candelli C, Valerio A, Martinelli D. Violent patients. What Italian psychiatrists feel and how this could change their patient care. Int J Offender Ther Comp Criminol. 2010;54:441–7.

96. Raboch J, Kalisová L, Nawka A, Kitzlerová E, Onchev G, Karastergiou A, Magliano L, Dembinskas A, Kiejna A, Torres-Gonzales F, Kjellin L, Priebe S, Kallert TW. Use of coercive measures during involuntary hospitalization: findings from ten European countries. Psychiatr Serv. 2010;61:1012–7.

97. Kalisova L, Raboch J, Nawka A, Sampogna G, Cihal L, Kallert TW, Onchev G, Karastergiou A, Del Vecchio V, Kiejna A, Adamowski T, Torres-Gonzales F, Cervilla JA, Priebe S, Giacco D, Kjellin L, Dembinskas A, Fiorillo A. Do patient and ward-related characteristics influence the use of coercive measures? Results from the EUNOMIA international study. Soc Psychiatry Psychiatric Epidemiol. 2014;49:1619–29.

98. Luciano M, De Rosa C, Sampogna G, Del Vecchio V, Giallonardo V, Fabrazzo M, Catapano F, Onchev G, Raboch J, Mastrogianni A, Solomon Z, Dembinskas A, Nawka P, Kiejna A, Torres-Gonzales F, Kjellin L, Kallert T, Fiorillo A. How to improve clinical practice on forced medication in psychiatric practice: suggestions from the EUNOMIA European multicentre study. Eur Psychiatry. 2018;54:35–40.

99. McLaughlin P, Giacco D, Priebe S. Use of coercive measures during involuntary psychiatric admission and treatment outcomes: data from a prospective study across 10 European countries. PLoS One. 2018;11(12):e0168720.

100. Tingleff EB, Bradley SK, Gildberg FA, Munksgaard G, Hounsgaard L. "Treat me with respect". A systematic review and thematic analysis of psychiatric patients' reported perceptions of the situations associated with the process of coercion. J Psychiatry Mental Health Nurs. 2017;24:681–98.

101. Hallett N, Huber JW, Dickens GL. Violence prevention in inpatient psychiatric settings: systematic review of studies about the perceptions of care staff and patients. Aggress Violent Behav. 2014;19:502–14.

102. Muralidharan S, Fenton M. Containment strategies for people with serious mental illness. Cochrane Database Syst Rev. 2006;(3):CD002084.

103. Szmuckler G. Compulsion and "coercion" in mental health care. World Psychiatry. 2015;14:259–62.

104. United Nations Committee on the Rights of Persons with Disabilities. Guidelines on Article 14 of the Convention on the Rights of Persons with Disabilities: the right to liberty and security of persons with disabilities. 2015.

105. Szmukler G. The UN convention on the rights of persons with disabilities: 'Rights, will and preferences' in relation to mental health disabilities. Int J Law Psychiatry. 2017;54:90–7.

106. Appelbaum PS. Saving the UN convention on the rights of persons with disabilities from itself. World Psychiatry. 2019;18:1–2.

107. Calda de Almeida JM. The CRPD article 12, the limits of reductionist approaches to complex issues and the necessary search for compromise. World Psychiatry. 2019;1:46–7.

108. Galderisi S. The UN convention on the rights of persons with disabilities: great opportunities and dangerous interpretations. World Psychiatry. 2019;1:47–8.

109. Szmukler G. "Capacity", "best interests", "will and preferences" and the UN convention on the rights of persons with disabilities. World Psychiatry. 2019;18:34–41.

110. Szmukler G, Daw R, Callard F. Mental health law and the UN convention on the rights of persons with disabilities. Int J Law Psychiatry. 2014;37:245–52.

111. Zelle H, Kemp K, Bonnie RJ. Advance directives in mental health care: evidence, challenges and promise. World Psychiatry. 2015;14:278–80.

112. Campbell LA, Kisely SR. Advance treatment directives for people with severe mental illness. Cochrane Database Syst Rev. 2009;21(1):CD005963.

113. Maître E, Debien C, Nicaise P, Wyngaerden F, Le Galudec M, Genest P, Ducrocq F, Delamillieure P, Lavoisy B, Walter M, Dubois V, Vaiva G. Advanced directives in psychiatry: a review of the qualitative literature, a state-of-the-art and viewpoints. Encéphale. 2013;39:244–51.

114. Henderson C, Farrelly S, Moran P, Borschmann R, Thornicroft G, Birchwood M, Crimson T, Joshua; Study Groups. Joint crisis planning in mental health care: the challenge of implementation in randomized trials and in routine care. World Psychiatry. 2015;14:281–3.

115. Kisely SR, Campbell LA, O'Reilly R. Compulsory community and involuntary outpatient treatment for people with severe mental disorders. Cochrane Database Syst Rev. 2017;17(3):CD004408.
116. Barnett P, Matthews H, Lloyd-Evans B, Mackay E, Pilling S, Johnson S. Compulsory community treatment to reduce readmission to hospital and increase engagement with community care in people with mental illness: a systematic review and meta-analysis. Lancet Psychiatry. 2018;12:1013–22.
117. Feras AM. Compulsory community treatment: beyond randomised controlled trials. Lancet Psychiatry. 2018;5:949–50.
118. Corring D, O'Reilly R, Sommerdyk C. A systematic review of the views and experiences of subjects of community treatment orders. Int J Law Psychiatry. 2017;52:74–80.
119. Riley H, Lorem GF, Høyer G. Community treatment orders. What are the views of decision makers? J Ment Health. 2018;27:97–102.
120. Aagaard J, Tuszewski B, Kølbæk P. Does assertive community treatment reduce the use of compulsory admissions? Arch Psychiatr Nurs. 2017;31:641–6.
121. Schöttle D, Schimmelmann BG, Ruppelt F, Bussopulos A, Frieling M, Nika E, Nawara LA, Golks D, Kerstan A, Lange M, Schödlbauer M, Daubmann A, Wegscheider K, Rohenkohl A, Sarikaya G, Sengutta M, Luedecke D, Wittmann L, Ohm G, Meigel-Schleiff C, Gallinat J, Wiedemann K, Bock T, Karow A, Lambert M. Effectiveness of integrated care including therapeutic assertive community treatment in severe schizophrenia-spectrum and bipolar I disorders: four-year follow-up of the ACCESS II study. PLoS One. 2018;13(2):e0192929. https://doi.org/10.1371/journal.pone.0192929. eCollection 2018
122. Dressing H, Salize HJ. Forensic psychiatric assessment in European Union member states. Acta Psychiatr Scand. 2006;114:282–9.
123. Sher L. Forensic psychiatric evaluations: an overview of methods, ethical issues, and criminal and civil assessments. Int J Adolesc Med Health. 2015;27:109–15.
124. Dressing H, Salize HJ, Gordon H. Legal frameworks and key concepts regulating diversion and treatment of mentally disordered offenders in European Union member states. Eur Psychiatry. 2007;22:427–32.
125. Guivarch J, Piercecchi-Marti MD, Glezer D, Chabannes JM. Differences in psychiatric expertise of responsibility: assessment and initial hypotheses through a review of literature. Encéphale. 2015;41:244–50.
126. Douglas T, Pugh J, Singh I, Savulescu J, Fazel S. Risk assessment tools in criminal justice and forensic psychiatry: the need for better data. Eur Psychiatry. 2017;42:134–7.
127. Ramesha T, Igoumenoub A, Vazquez Montesc M, Fazel S. Use of risk assessment instruments to predict violence in forensic psychiatric hospitals: a systematic review and meta-analysis. Eur Psychiatry. 2018;52:47–53.
128. Žarkovic Palijan T, Mužinić L, Radeljak S. Psychiatric comorbidity in Forensic Psychiatry. Psychiatr Danub. 2009;21:429–36.
129. Coid JW, Ullrich S, Kallis C. Predicting future violence among individuals with psychopathy. Br J Psychiatry. 2013;203:387–8.
130. Chow WS, Priebe S. How has the extent of institutional mental health care changed in Western Europe? Analysis of data since 1990. BMJ Open. 2016;6(4):e010188.
131. Owner K, Andiné P, Bertilsson G, Hultcrantz M, Lindström E, Mowafi F, Snellman A, Hofvander B. Mapping systematic reviews on forensic psychiatric care: a systematic review identifying knowledge gaps. Front Psych. 2018;9:452. https://doi.org/10.3389/fpsyt.2018.00452.
132. Fazel S, Wolf A, Fimińska Z, Larsson H. Mortality, rehospitalisation and violent crime in forensic psychiatric patients discharged from hospital: rates and risk factors. PLoS One. 2016;11(5):e0155906. https://doi.org/10.1371/journal.pone.0155906.
133. Fazel S, Fimińska Z, Cocks C, Coid J. Patient outcomes following discharge from secure psychiatric hospitals: systematic review and meta-analysis. Br J Psychiatry. 2016;208:17–25.

134. Casacchia M, Malavolta M, Bianchini V, Giusti L, Di Michele V, Giosuè P, Ruggeri M, Biondi M, Roncone R. Closing forensic psychiatric hospitals in Italy: a new deal for mental health care? Riv Psichiatr. 2015;50:199–209.
135. Di Lorito C, Castelletti L, Lega I, Gualco B, Scarpa F, Völlm B. The closing of forensic psychiatric hospitals in Italy: determinants, current status and future perspectives. A scoping review. Int J Law Psychiatry. 2017;55:54–63.
136. Barbui B, Saraceno B. Closing forensic psychiatric hospitals in Italy: a new revolution begins? Br J Psychiatry. 2015;206:445–6.
137. Hopkin G, Messina E, Thornicroft G, Ruggeri M. Reform of Italian forensic mental health care. Challenges and opportunities following Law 81/2014. Int J Prison Health. 2018;14:1–3.
138. Carabellese F, Felthous AR. Closing Italian Forensic Psychiatry Hospitals in favor of treating insanity acquittees in the community. Behav Sci Law. 2016;34:444–59.
139. Traverso S, Traverso GB. Revolutionary reform in psychiatric care in Italy: the abolition of forensic mental hospitals. Crim Behav Mental Health. 2017;27:107–11.

Neurobiology of Violence

2

Mirko Manchia, Linda Booij, Federica Pinna, Janice Wong,
Florian Zepf, and Stefano Comai

M. Manchia (✉)
Department of Medical Sciences and Public Health, University of Cagliari, Cagliari, Italy

Department of Pharmacology, Dalhousie University, Halifax, NS, Canada
e-mail: mirkomanchia@unica.it

L. Booij
Department of Psychology, Concordia University, Montreal, QC, Canada

CHU Sainte-Justine Hospital Research Centre, Montreal, QC, Canada

Department of Psychiatry, McGill University, Montreal, QC, Canada
e-mail: linda.booij@umontreal.ca

F. Pinna
Department of Medical Sciences and Public Health, University of Cagliari, Cagliari, Italy

J. Wong
Centre & Discipline of Child and Adolescent Psychiatry, Psychosomatics and Psychotherapy,
The University of Western Australia, Perth, WA, Australia

Telethon Kids Institute, Perth, WA, Australia

Department of Health, Child and Adolescent Health Service—Mental Health,
Perth, WA, Australia
e-mail: Janice.Wong@telethonkids.org.au

F. Zepf
Department of Child and Adolescent Psychiatry, Psychosomatic Medicine and Psychotherapy,
Jena University Hospital, Jena, Germany
e-mail: Florian.Zepf@med.uni-jena.de

S. Comai
Department of Psychiatry, McGill University, Montreal, QC, Canada

San Raffaele Scientific Institute and Vita-Salute University, Milan, Italy
e-mail: comai.stefano@hsr.it

© Springer Nature Switzerland AG 2020
B. Carpiniello et al. (eds.), *Violence and Mental Disorders*, Comprehensive
Approach to Psychiatry 1, https://doi.org/10.1007/978-3-030-33188-7_2

2.1   Introduction

Violence is generally defined as an overt physical aggressive behaviour against another human being [1]. These behaviours are characterised by several different executional forms (e.g. verbal, physical), often serve a functional purpose (e.g. to protect, goal motivated) and may be with or without intent (e.g. proactive or reactive violent behaviour). Paralleling the advancement in the delineation of the role of clinical predictors and environmental precipitating factors in modulating the liability toward violence, significant research advancements in the recent years have shed light on the neurobiological underpinnings of this disruptive behaviour. Indeed, there is now a vast consensus that an altered function in the main neurochemical pathways underlies the manifestation of violence [2]. For instance, disruption in dopaminergic and serotonergic signalling is considered to confer a substantial liability toward the manifestation of violent behaviour [2, 3]. However, there is still uncertainty about the temporal manifestations of these pathological changes. The delineation of the developmental trajectory of violence shows that in a proportion of cases these behaviours decline in adulthood, with only a small subset of the population continuing to commit violent acts [4, 5]. For instance, a longitudinal study of serious adolescent offenders showed that violent offending in adolescence is a poor predictor of violent criminal behaviour throughout the life course [4]. Furthermore, it appears that the developmental trajectory of violence acquires a distinct pattern according to biological sex [6]. Indeed, the longitudinal analysis of patterns of violent behaviour across 7 years among 172 females and 172 matched males with age from 15 to 24 years showed a significantly lower rate of females persisting in violence (25%) than males (46%) [6]. Clearly, the intra-individual heterogeneity in the propensity toward violence, with at least two high-risk peaks in early childhood and middle to late adolescence [5], has motivated researchers to focus on a neurodevelopmental perspective. There is consistent evidence, for instance, that exposure to violence in early years of life leads to persistent neurobiological changes that, while adaptive for survival in violent contexts, become maladaptive in other environments, conferring life-long risk for psychopathology [7].

The absence of stability in the propensity toward violent behaviour during the life course has rendered difficult the identification of reliable biological signatures (biomarkers) of violence. Certainly, a clearer depiction of the neurobiology of violence will serve the search for diagnostic (i.e. whether the subject has a substantial risk of committing violent acts) or prognostic (i.e. whether the subject has a substantial risk of persisting in a trajectory of violent behaviour over time). So far, however, the added value of biomarkers in the prediction of violent behaviour remains limited compared to the information accessible through accurate clinical characterisation.

A final introductory remark should be made. It should be noted that neurobiological factors represent one facet of the complex multifactorial manifestation of violent behaviour. As described by Loeber and Pardini [5], the underlying factors and behavioural manifestations of violence are the result of neurobiological, social, individual, economic and environmental causes. The calculation of a prediction index using the cumulative risk determined by the 11 strongest determinants of violence identified through a systematic review of the literature (truancy, low school motivation, onset of delinquency before age 10, cruelty to people, depressed mood, physical aggression, callous–unemotional behaviour, low family socioeconomic status, family on welfare, high parental stress and disadvantaged neighbourhood) showed that the higher individuals scored on the index, the higher was the risk of committing violent acts. In this context, the delineation of the risk conferred by the neurobiological make-up of each individual should be considered in light of the eventual presence of concomitant risk factors. Importantly, these same factors, often of environmental nature, can, in turn, modulate the neurobiological liability, acting on the epigenetic machinery.

In this chapter, we aim to summarise the main advancements in the comprehension of the neurobiological underpinnings of violent behaviour, starting from neurochemical imbalances and describing then the current knowledge on neuroimaging and genetic/epigenetics of violent behaviour. A brief description of the potential role of metabolomics in violence will follow.

2.2 Neurochemistry of Violence

Several decades of preclinical and clinical research have demonstrated a central role for different neurotransmitters and neuromodulators in the neurobiology of violence. Biogenic amines including serotonin (5-HT), norepinephrine (NE), dopamine (DA), glutamate and GABA, as well as neuropeptides such as substance P, vasopressin and oxytocin, all appear to play a key modulating function in violent behaviour. These neurotransmitters pertain to those biochemical pathways involved in the development, modulation, regulation and patterning of brain circuits that appear to be disrupted in individuals with a high propensity toward violent behaviour (please see the next section for details on these circuits). A depiction of these neurobiological pathways is presented in Fig. 2.1. In this section, we summarise the current knowledge on the neurobiological involvement of these neurotransmitters in the pathophysiology of violence. From a historical point of view, the monoaminergic neurotransmitters

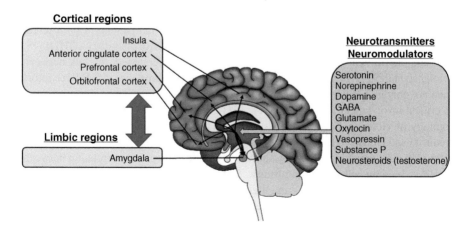

Fig. 2.1 Brain circuits and neurotransmitters/neuromodulators involved in the neurobiology of violence

5-HT and NE have been the most studied and characterised, with the first evidence in rodents dating back to the mid-1960s [8–10].

2.2.1 Serotonin

Preclinical and clinical research consistently points to a general reduction in the activity of the 5-HT system in the brain of violent individuals. However, this neurobiological relationship is still not yet completely elucidated and seems to be not only an issue of low 5-HT levels [11]. Indeed, research on this topic remains very active as evidenced by the high number (339) of publications in PubMed during the last 5 years (search performed using the generic terms "serotonin" and "violence" or "aggressive behaviour" on June 14, 2019). A 5-HT deficiency seems mostly related to the impulsive forms of violence and not to the premeditated forms. Importantly, the relationship between 5-HT and violence should be seen in the context not only of 5-HT levels but more in general of changes occurring in distinct elements constituting the 5-HT system, including the expression of the different 5-HT receptor subtypes at presynaptic and postsynaptic levels and in different brain regions implicated in the control of emotions and behaviour [2, 12]. In humans, indirect measures of brain 5-HT activity such as cerebrospinal fluid (CSF) levels of its metabolite 5-hydroxyindoleacetic acid (5-HIAA) or plasma/serum levels of its precursor tryptophan (Trp) have been measured in violent individuals with different underlying psychiatric disorders, but also in non-psychiatric violent individuals. For a detailed overview of the studies examining 5-HT biomarkers of aggressive behaviour, please see a recent review by Manchia et al. [12]. Although some contrasting findings have been reported, there is now consensus that impulsive violent individuals display lower CSF 5-HIAA levels [13, 14] or lower serum Trp levels [15] than non-impulsive violent individuals. This finding has also been replicated in children and adolescents with disruptive behavioural disorders [16]. The concept of a reduced 5-HT activity as an etiological factor for violent behaviour has been supported by neuroendocrine challenge studies using the 5-HT releaser and uptake inhibitor fenfluramine or tryptophan depletion studies in both healthy individuals [17] and patients with different psychiatric disorders including attention-deficit/hyperactivity disorder (ADHD) [18, 19] and intermittent explosive disorder (IED) [20]. As mentioned, the link between violence and 5-HT might involve also changes in the expression of 5-HT receptors and not only in 5-HT levels. Indeed, both preclinical and clinical studies have shown a critical involvement of 5-HT_{1A}, 5-HT_2 [21] and 5-HT_3 [22] receptors in the neurobiology of violence. Further, 5-HT_{1A} and 5-HT_{1B} receptors knockout mice display reduced and enhanced levels of aggression, respectively [23]. In humans, a positron-emission tomography (PET) study showed a significant negative correlation between 5-HT_{1A} binding of the high-affinity 5-HT_{1A} antagonist [carbonyl-C-11]WAY-100635 in several brain regions and lifetime aggression [24]. Impaired 5-HT_{1A} receptor functioning associated with increased aggressive behaviour has also been shown following the neuroendocrine responses to the selective 5-HT_{1A} receptor partial agonist ipsapirone [25]. Similarly, dysfunction in other elements of the 5-HT system including the rate-limiting enzyme in the 5-HT synthesis, the tryptophan hydroxylase, or in the degradation of 5-HT, the monoamine oxidase A (MAO-A) enzyme, as well as the serotonin transporter (5-HTT) involved in the synaptic re-uptake of the neurotransmitter, has been related to the neurobiology of violence by several studies. Interestingly, MAO-A knockout male mice with enhanced 5-HT levels in the brain display increased aggressive behaviour in the resident intruder test, a preclinical test to study aggression [26]. In antisocial individuals who have enhanced violent behaviour, there is a significant hypermethylation of the MAO-A gene promoter that is associated with increased circulating levels of 5-HT [27]. Finally, variants within the gene encoding for the TPH-2 (the isoform mostly expressed in the brain) were associated to violent behaviour in both mice [28] and humans [29].

2.2.2 Norepinephrine

From a physiological point of view, the activation of the NE system at both central and peripheral level is linked to the so-called flight or fight response. In the brain, the NE system is strongly involved in controlling behavioural arousal, and overactivity of this system has been observed in anxiety, irritability and emotional instability, but also in highly arousing activities including violent behaviour. However, as we recently reviewed [30], no biomarker of the NE system has demonstrated yet to have an adequate sensitivity and specificity to predict violent behaviour. The CSF levels of 3-methoxy-5-hydroxyphenylglycol (MHPG), the main metabolite of NE in the brain, have been positively correlated to violent behaviour [31–34], although not all studies confirmed this relationship [35–37]. However, at preclinical level, pharmacological manipulations aimed at reducing NE neurotransmission (for example with 6-hydroxydopa) led to increased fighting of the rodents [38, 39]. Similarly to 5-HT, the relationship between NE and violence should account for changes occurring within the NE system and not only to NE levels. Indeed, α_2 receptor knockout mice attack faster than wild-type controls in the resident-intruder paradigm [40], and activation of α_2 receptors with clonidine has been used to treat agitated and violent patients [41]. Moreover, also β-blockers have clinically been used to treat violent individuals although they have certain limitations in their efficacy [42, 43].

2.2.3 Dopamine

The link between violence and DA has not yet been clarified although for some authors DA is necessary for the motivational aspects of violent behaviour given the modulating role of DA in the mesocorticolimbic system [44, 45]. However, insight into the role of DA in violent behaviour is derived by the clinical evidence that the most effective drugs to treat violent behaviour are first- and second-generation antipsychotics which act on D_1 and D_2 receptors (for a review see [46]).

2.2.4 GABA

It is known that the GABAergic system is the major inhibitory player in the CNS. GABA, by binding to the GABA-A receptor, increases the influx of chloride ions into the neuron, thus hyperpolarising the postsynaptic membrane and making the postsynaptic neuron less prone to excitation. However, the link between GABA and violence shows opposing patterns since benzodiazepines, GABA-A receptor-positive modulators, may either enhance or reduce violence in both animals and humans. Indeed, in rats, low doses of chlordiazepoxide increase aggression whereas high doses decrease aggression [47]. Similarly, in humans, benzodiazepines are largely used for their sedative/anxiolytic properties in violent individuals but may also enhance violent responses [48]. Similarly, other neurochemicals including neurosteroids (e.g. testosterone) by acting on the allosteric binding site on the GABA-A receptor may also be involved in violent behaviour. Few studies have investigated the relationship between GABA levels and violence showing either positive [49], negative [50] or absence [51] of correlation.

2.2.5 Glutamate

Glutamate is the main excitatory neurotransmitter in the mammalian CNS by acting on the synaptic but also non-synaptic ionotropic (NMDA, AMPA and kainate) and metabotropic (mGlu) receptors. Among the different neurotransmitters here discussed for their role in violence, glutamate is historically the less studied, and evidence mostly derives from preclinical studies manipulating glutamate levels or NMDA receptors. For example, injection of glutamate into the hypothalamic attack area raised the aggressive responses of cats [52], and into the dorsal raphe of male mice increased the number of bites toward an intruder in a dose-dependent manner [53]. Interestingly, the authors also reported enhanced glutamate release during an aggressive encounter [53]. Concerning the role of glutamate receptors in violence, pharmacological studies using selective ligands have mainly focused on the NMDA [54] and on mGlu1 receptor subtypes [55], indicating that antagonists of these receptors inhibit violent behaviour in mice. Although only few studies investigated the levels of glutamate in violent individuals, overall, they tend to corroborate the preclinical findings showing a positive relationship between glutamate levels/activity and violence [56–58].

2.2.6 Testosterone

In nature, males tend to exert higher levels of violence than females. This is partly explained by the evidence of higher levels of testosterone in males than in females. Indeed, administration of testosterone has been shown to increase violent behaviour in both animals and humans [59]. However, a recent study in humans suggests that testosterone may enhance violence only in individuals with dominant or impulsive personality styles implying that only specific subgroups of individuals, those with a specific personality profile, might be impacted by the effects of this hormone [60]. In particular, it seems that testosterone affects neural circuits implicated in social aggression, including the amygdala, the hypothalamus and the orbitofrontal cortex, by enhancing their responsiveness following exposure to social challenges [61]. This specific role of testosterone in the neurocircuitry of violence may thus likely explain decades of inconsistent research examining the relationship between violence and testosterone levels. Indeed, although a large number of studies have indicated a positive association, many others failed to find any significant association (for a detailed review see [30]).

2.2.7 Oxytocin

The neuropeptide oxytocin, synthesised in the hypothalamus, is known to influence affectivity, stress response and prosocial behaviour [62]. As a consequence, the administration of oxytocin has been studied to promote prosocial behaviour in individuals displaying antisocial behaviours such as violence. Campbell and Hausmann [63] showed that nasal administration of oxytocin reduced reactive aggression in women with high-state anxiety but not with low-state anxiety, whereas Alcorn et al. [64] in a preliminary study in six males with antisocial personality disorder (APD) observed that oxytocin modulated violent behaviour, but the direction and magnitude of the effects were not uniform (with either increase or decrease). Similarly, a subsequent study in healthy adult males did not find a main effect of oxytocin on aggressive behaviour measured with the Point Subtraction Aggression Paradigm due to the large individual differences in the response to oxytocin [65]. Again, either increase or decrease of violent behaviour was reported depending on the individual personality traits. However, a very recent and larger sample size study in healthy young males ($N = 57$), using the same paradigm, showed that oxytocin reduced aggressive behaviour [66]. Interestingly, increased endogenous urinary oxytocin levels were associated with a decrease in aggressive responses [66].

The link between oxytocin and violence has been further demonstrated in oxytocin knockout mice that display exaggerated aggressive behaviour compared with wild-type controls [67], and in medication-free individuals with and without a DSM-IV diagnosis of personality disorder who show lumbar CSF oxytocin levels inversely correlated with life history of aggression [68].

2.2.8 Substance P

The neuropeptide substance P is an excitatory neurotransmitter and neuromodulator that acts by activating NK1 receptors. It is present in both the central and the peripheral nervous system, and it has been involved in the induction of animal rage and aggressive behaviour [69, 70]. Indeed, substance P and NK1 receptors are highly expressed in brain regions implicated in the regulation of emotions among which are the hypothalamic attack area and the periaqueductal area [71]. Knockout mice for NK1 receptors display significantly less aggressive behaviour than their wild-type controls [72], and while the NK1 antagonist L-703,606 lowers violent behaviour [73], the NK1 agonist GR73632 enhances violent behaviour [74]. A clinical study also confirmed the relationship between substance P and violence [75]. Coccaro and collaborators found a positive correlation between CSF substance P-like immunoreactivity levels and aggressive behaviour in subjects with personality disorder [75]. However, there is evidence indicating that the relationship between substance P and violence could be more complex than expected. For instance, File [76] reported enhanced aggressive response in the social interaction test following treatment with the NK1 receptor antagonist NKP608, but at doses higher than those inducing anxiolytic effects. Conversely, two studies conducted in the 1970s showed that peripheral injection of substance P reduced aggressive response [77, 78].

2.2.9 Vasopressin

Preclinical and clinical studies have highlighted the role of the arginine vasopressin system in the neurobiology of violence. During an aggressive encounter in the maternal aggression paradigm, an increased release of vasopressin in the amygdala has been reported [79]. As a consequence, local microinjection of a vasopressin V1a receptor antagonist inhibited the maternal aggressive behaviour [79]. Also in males, exposure to an aggressive encounter was associated with increased activation in vasopressin-containing neurons in the nucleus circularis and in the medial division of the supraoptic nucleus [80]. Accordingly, hypothalamic injection of vasopressin increased aggressive responses [81, 82]. Of interest, reduced levels of aggression were observed in knockout mice for vasopressin V1b receptors [83], but not in those for vasopressin V1a receptors [84]. In humans, arginine vasopressin levels in the lumbar CSF of individuals with a personality disorder were positively correlated with lifetime history of violent behaviour [85].

In summary, there is consistent evidence associating neurochemical imbalances with the manifestation of violent behaviour. These pathological changes appear to be more prominent in patients affected by severe mental disorders but to extend, to some extent, also to unaffected individuals. Although impacted by the heterogeneity of this complex behaviour, neurochemical fingerprints of violence will likely become more reliable in the future, with potential for clinical implementation.

2.3   Brain Circuitry in Violence: Insights from Neuroimaging Studies

As previously mentioned, human violence is a complex behaviour that might often manifest with a childhood onset [86]. Research relating to violence from a neuroimaging perspective can provide insight into areas of the brain implicated in its pathophysiology, and may also shed light on its putatively associated neurochemical projections.

2.3.1 Brain Regions Implicated in Aggression

The so-called corticolimbic network has been suggested to play an important role in aggression and violence [3]. This network represents the connection between brain areas in the cortical region, such as the anterior cingulate cortex (ACC), the prefrontal cortex (PFC) and the insula, and the limbic region, such as the amygdala [87]. The literature proposes that violence is a response to interpretation of environmental stimuli and threat, a response that is also influenced by the social, biological and environmental context of the individual. Within the corticolimbic structure, the amygdala plays a key role in perceiving and interpreting threat stimuli in the surrounding environment [3, 87]. Central nervous 5-HT has been studied using challenge techniques; such techniques have been demonstrated to alter amygdala activity in response to threatening stimuli, or stimuli that may elicit violence [88]. Responses from the amygdala then activate or dampen activity in the surrounding cortices; however, such responses differ, depending on the type of violence being exhibited [3, 89]. Two major forms of violent behaviour that are typically described, and are also different in terms of the underlying biology, are reactive and proactive (or instrumental) aggression [89, 90]. Underlying both forms of violent behaviour are different types of impaired executive functions that reflect activity in the surrounding corticolimbic network and are further discussed below.

2.3.2 Regions Implicated in Reactive Aggression

Reactive aggression is a form of violent behaviour that is characterised by impulsivity, reacting to a perceived trigger, and is often not goal directed or planned [90, 91]. The major brain regions that have been associated with reactive aggression include the amygdala and the orbitofrontal cortex (OFC). In human studies, amygdala atrophy due to encephalitis has been associated with an increase in reactive aggressive behaviours [92]. In patient groups, such as individuals with IED (in which a key diagnostic symptom is reactive aggression), and also individuals with BPD, the magnitude of activity in the amygdala in response to affective stimuli (e.g. the presentation of faces showing different emotions) is significantly different from that of healthy control groups [93].

The information received by the amygdala is then processed by surrounding brain areas, including the PFC, the temporal cortex and the parietal cortex. These cortices play a key role in information processing, including assigning the stimuli meaning, reality testing and emotion regulation. In a review by Siever [3], this information is supplemented by processing of additional stimuli, such as visual and auditory information in the surrounding environment. Combined, the meanings derived from the stimuli may lead to a response characterised by reactive aggression. In healthy populations, the OFC and the anterior ACC are responsible for inhibiting behaviours that are associated with negative consequences. Therefore, it has been hypothesised that reactive aggression is the result of either an impairment in the OFC or the ACC in inhibiting impulsive aggressive responses that are generated by areas responsible for emotion regulation such as the PFC, or heightened sensitivity of the amygdala and surrounding cortices in information processing [3]. Notably, sensitivities to different environmental or affective stimuli may contribute to the presentation of different psychiatric disorders. Specifically, numerous studies have observed that individuals with BPD have increased sensitivities to angry faces, individuals with IED may be particularly sensitive to stimuli with negative affect and individuals with anxiety may have increased sensitivity to threatening stimuli [3, 93]. Further support of the above theory of reactive aggression comes from studies investigating the functional and structural connectivity of the aforementioned brain regions. In healthy individuals, central nervous 5-HT challenges (e.g. acute tryptophan depletion, ATD) are used to mimic the reduced central nervous 5-HT that is typically associated with aggression. Using the ATD technique, Passamonti et al. found that ATD impacted the connectivity between the amygdala and prefrontal cortices, including the ACC and the ventrolateral PFC compared to connectivity observed under placebo conditions [94]. In a study that investigated the functional connectivity between the amygdala and the OFC in individuals with IED compared to healthy controls, results showed the absence of connectivity between the amygdala and the OFC, which contrasted findings for the healthy control group [93].

In summary, the amygdala and the corticolimbic network are implicated in reactive aggression, with possible substantial disruption of their connectivity. However, there is still debate on the magnitude of this disruption and on the direction of its impact.

2.3.3 Regions Implicated in Proactive Aggression

Proactive aggression, otherwise known as instrumental aggression, is goal directed. For proactive aggression, the amygdala has also been strongly implicated. A review by Sterzer and Stadler suggested that reduced activity in the amygdala may be observed in proactive aggression, indicating impaired ability to detect and interpret distress in others, as well as an impairment in the processing of affective information [89]. Additionally, a reduction in amygdala activity may also indicate altered or poor empathic ability [95].

The major difference between brain functions in proactive and reactive aggression is the brain regions that are more or less activated following receipt of information by the amygdala. Unlike reactive aggression, there has been minimal evidence to suggest that proactive aggression is due to deficits in executive functioning processes [96], although there is some evidence to suggest that youths who exhibit callous unemotional traits are more likely to have high executive control [97]. In proactive aggression, activation of the ventromedial PFC has also been observed. Sterzer and Stadler summarised that the role of the ventromedial PFC is to monitor types of expected or unexpected reinforcement. Increased activity in the ventromedial PFC may indicate poor learning of rules leading to an increased risk for frustration [89]. It has been posited that this increased risk may therefore impact subsequent aggression [89] via increased likelihood of emotional dysregulation. Functional connectivity studies investigating connectivity between brain regions in proactive aggression have typically found decreased connectivity between the amygdala and the prefrontal cortices [89], and this has been observed in patient groups [98]. Diminished activity between the amygdala and other brain regions has also been observed. For example, in a study that investigated functional amygdala connectivity in healthy adult males, results showed diminished functional amygdala connectivity to the bilateral supramarginal gyrus (SMG) following ATD, compared to the placebo condition during exposure to playing a violent video game [88]. Klasen and colleagues also found amygdala connectivity to other regions including the bilateral SMG, bilateral anterior insula, dorsal ACC, left middle frontal gyrus and somatosensory cortex under the placebo condition [88]. With regard to examining associations between resting-state functional connectivity (i.e. rsFC; functional connectivity of brain regions when the brain is at rest) and proactive aggression, studies have been limited. Kolla and colleagues found a correlation between proactive aggression and rsFC between the ventral striatum and angular gyrus [99], a region associated with moral reasoning [95].

When considering the currently available evidence relating to the brain regions implicated in aggression and violence, several factors should be taken into account. As stated previously, and noted by reviews [86], incidents of violence typically decrease over development, coinciding with maturation of the brain and the prefrontal cortex. The impact of the social and environmental context of individuals also contributes to individual development. Noting these factors, it may be important to consider whether there may be differences in the function of brain regions and also changes in functional connectivity between regions that are implicated with aggression and impulsive behaviours over development. Other limitations of neuroimaging research in the area of aggression include the significant number of tasks that are used to elicit "aggressive behaviour" for measurement purposes, as well as typically smaller sample sizes that are utilised.

2.4 Genetics and Epigenetics of Violence

2.4.1 Genetic Factors in Relation to Violence

Behavioural genetic studies suggest that violence is heritable. Meta-analyses of twin and adaption studies report heritability rates of antisocial and/or aggressive behaviour between 32 and 65% [100]. Although very few studies focus specifically on violence, it has been suggested that heritability rates of aggressive behaviours are highest when presented as severe violent behaviour [101].

Various studies used candidate gene and genome-wide approaches with the aim to identify specific genes involved in violence and associated behavioural phenotypes as detailed in the extensive reviews and meta-analyses on the genetics of aggression [2, 100, 102, 103]. Here, we highlight some of the findings most relevant to violence.

Quantitative data synthesis has explored the role of the monoamine oxidase A (MAOA) gene in violence. One meta-analysis showed that the low-expression variant of the MAOA gene is associated with various forms of antisocial behaviour in clinical and community samples (OR = 1.14) [104]. Another meta-analysis, including 22 studies, did not find a statistically significant association between the variation of the MAOA gene and aggressive and violent behaviour [102]. However, when focusing on violence only (three studies), a significant association was observed for MAOA promoter 30 bpVNTR polymorphism in males with a history of violence (OR = 0.63) [102]. A more recent study published after this meta-analysis by Tiihonen and colleagues [105] investigated MAOA gene variation in association with various levels of violent behaviours in two independent cohorts of Finnish prisoners. Participants were 538 violent offenders, 84 extreme violent offenders and 215 non-violent offenders in the discovery cohort, as well as 114 violent offenders who had committed at least one homicide in the replication cohort. The low-activity MAOA genotype was associated with violent offending (OR = 1.7 in the discovery cohort and OR = 1.5 in the replication cohort), and the association was strongest in the most extreme violent cases (OR = 2.66) [105]. Notably, while various studies in community samples point to greater levels of antisocial behaviours in carriers of the low-activity MAOA allele only in those who were exposed to childhood maltreatment [103], the latter study in violent offenders did not find a moderating role of childhood adversity [105].

In addition to childhood environment, a possible important element to consider, often overlooked in current genetic research, is the impact of age. While longitudinal twin studies have shown that genetic contributions to aggression may be developmentally dynamic [106, 107], with different genes contributing to aggression at different stages in development, genetic association studies, including those related to the MAOA gene, differ largely in age of the participants. Pingault and colleagues [108] investigated the impact of MAOA gene variants on the developmental course of physical aggression in boys rated yearly on physical aggression between 6 and 12 years. Several SNPs (rs5906957, rs5953385 and rs2283725) were found to have age-dependent effects. For instance, while physical aggression levels significantly decreased with age in the C carriers of the rs5906957 MAOA gene polymorphism, in the T carriers these levels remained relatively stable over time [108]. These findings suggest that MAOA gene may not affect physical aggression in a static manner; but rather its effects become more apparent later in life [108]. Whether such findings can be generalised to violent behaviours remains to be seen.

Perhaps the most widely studied gene variant in the field of the mental health is the 5-HTTLPR polymorphism of the 5-HTT gene, and its short allele, also known as an "s" allele (coding for lowered functioning of the serotonin transporter [109]). The s allele variant has been linked to various psychopathologies and behavioural traits, including violence, aggression and associated mental disorders. While one meta-analysis (18 studies) found an association between antisocial behaviours and the s allele of the 5-HTTLPR (OR = 1.53) [104], another meta-analysis, focusing on aggression and violence (19 studies), did not find such association [102]. In both meta-analyses, the number of studies that investigated gene-environment interactions was too small to produce reliable results. Yet, in a study conducted in 184 violent offenders, the s allele was predictive of violent behaviours, but only in those who were exposed to childhood adversity [110].

Various other candidate gene studies reported associations between antisocial and aggressive behaviours and polymorphic variation in other genes, such as the *HTR2A, HTR1B, TPH1* and *TPH2, DRD4, SLC6A3, OXTR, COMT*, arginine vasopressin receptor 1B (*AVPR1B*), *CHRR1* and *BDNF* genes [100, 102, 103]. However, these were generally small-scale non-replicated studies and/or not focusing explicitly on violence.

In recent years, various genome-wide association studies (GWAS) on aggression/antisocial behaviour have been published (for more detailed reviews, see [100, 103]). So far, the results of the genome-wide studies focusing on aggressive have been inconclusive, at best [100]. Findings of a single GWAS study, focusing specifically on violence, indicated that extreme violent behaviour (characterised by ten or more violent crimes) was associated with polymorphism rs11649622 on chromosome 16q23.3 inside the intron of a gene coding for a neural adhesion protein cadherin 13 (*CDH13*) [105]. Replication studies in individuals with violent behaviours are needed to further confirm these findings. Importantly, GWAS studies did not identify significant associations for the genes that are generally being investigated in candidate gene studies [100].

2.4.2 Epigenetic Processes in Relation to Violence

In addition to examining the genome, an increasing number of studies in the field focused on epigenetic modifications. Epigenetic changes involve alterations in gene expression without affecting the structure of the DNA itself. DNA methylation is the most studied epigenetic modification in the context of human aggression. Various GWAS and candidate gene DNA methylation studies have pointed toward alterations in DNA methylation in genes involved in immune and inflammatory function, serotonin function and stress response in individuals with chronic aggressive behaviours [111–115]. Of particular relevance here is a candidate gene methylation study showing that incarcerated individuals with APD had greater MAOA gene methylation (indicative of reduced MAOA gene expression) relative to a healthy non-incarcerated control population [27]. In a recent candidate gene study, child sexual offenders showed greater methylation in the androgen receptor gene than healthy controls, and the number of sexual offenses correlated positively with androgen receptor methylation [116]. In addition, there was an interaction effect on DNA methylation levels between offense status and androgen receptor functionality [116]. Lastly, results of a recent epigenome-wide study indicated that, relative to healthy controls, individuals with IED displayed differential DNA methylation patterns in genes involved in inflammatory/immune system, endocrine system and neuronal differentiation, albeit these results did not reach genome-wide statistical significance [117].

2.4.3 Genetics and Epigenetic Processes and the Violent Human Brain

Molecular imaging studies (combining MRI with genetic assessments) have identified neural differences as a function of genotypes relevant for violent behaviours. Most research has been done in relation to the MAOA gene. A seminal study by Meyer-Lindenberg et al. [118] showed that healthy individuals with lowered expression MAOA genotype had limbic volume reductions as well as increased amygdala reactivity during emotional arousal and diminished reactivity of regulatory prefrontal regions, relative to those with the high expression allele. Several molecular imaging studies have elaborated on these findings [119–121]. While most of the molecular imaging studies were done in healthy volunteers, a recent MRI study examined brain morphometry as a function of MAOA genotype in APD individuals with a history of violent offending, and healthy controls [122]. Relative to controls with the low-expression MAOA gene variant, violent offenders carrying the low-expression variant had decreased subcortical surface area in the right basolateral amygdala and increased right anterior cortical amygdaloid surface area, while there were no differences between violent offenders and controls with high-expression variant [122]. These findings suggest that the deficits in emotion regulation that contribute to violent behaviours might be (at least in part) under the control of the MAOA gene [122].

Hence, various studies suggest that violent behaviour has a relatively strong genetic basis. However, findings of both GWAS and candidate gene studies are still inconclusive. Although most support was found for the MAOA gene, studies focusing specifically on violence are scarce. Furthermore, findings of GWAS and candidate gene studies do not overlap. Likewise, DNA methylation studies focusing specifically on violence are lacking.

Notwithstanding the limited evidence for specific clinically relevant gene markers for violent behaviours, the notion of genetic contributions fits well with the recent hypothesis that chronic adult violence has strong neurodevelopmental origins [101]. In addition to genetic factors, adverse exposures during the prenatal period and in the early postnatal years of life might disrupt normal brain development, which, in turn, may predispose individuals to violent behaviours [101].

Among the various neurodevelopmental mechanisms that may play a role in predisposing to violence, 5-HT may be an important contributor due to its major role in shaping early brain development [123]. Different serotonergic components (e.g. *SLC6A4, MAOA*) appear to have a unique pattern of development, expression and function, with some being developed early in life and others not stabilising before adulthood, and each of them having potential specific functions in brain development [123]. The expression of these molecules is modulated by genetic and environmental factors, and it could be speculated that DNA methylation may be an underlying physiological mechanism explaining how these genetic factors and environment interact in predisposing individuals to violence [115]. Whether violent behaviour (rather than other emotional dysregulation problems) may actually emerge likely depends on various factors such as (but not limited to) the type of adverse exposures, timing of adverse experiences as well as specific genetic make-up.

2.5   Metabolomics of Violence

Metabolomics exerts a crucial role in the identification of short-term changes and subtle modifications in the biological pathways in various physiological conditions and in aberrant processes [124]. This approach consists of the measurement of the metabolome, i.e. the complete set of metabolites representing the intermediates and products of cellular metabolism (of less than 1 kDa in size) within a biological sample [125]. This approach can be targeted (directed to specific molecules) or untargeted (without an a priori hypothesis on the pathway involved). Metabolomics has proven useful in the detection of risk signatures for many complex diseases, including psychiatric disorders such as major depression [126], schizophrenia [127] and autism spectrum disorder (ASD) [128, 129], but has still a limited application in behavioural science. Recently, Hagenbeek and co-authors have performed a review of biochemical markers whose levels were altered in relation to violent behaviour [130]. Given the heterogeneity of findings, showing changes in the concentrations of inflammatory markers, neurotransmitters, lipoproteins and hormones, the authors highlight the importance of applying a holistic approach such as that provided by metabolomics [130]. The literature, indeed, lacks a systematic investigation of metabolomics signatures of aggression in humans. Thus, here we decide to focus on a severe psychiatric disorder, ASD, that appears to be associated with an increased risk violence [131] and that can serve as a phenotypic proxy of this disruptive behaviour. Most of the findings on metabolomics of ASD come from urinary samples. Patients with ASD show an increased urinary excretion of N-methyl-2-pyridone-5-carboxamide, N-methyl nicotinic acid and N-methyl nicotinamide (indicating a perturbation in the tryptophan-nicotinic acid metabolic pathway) and altered levels of taurine and glutamate, NAG and succinate compared to controls [132]. Further, patients with ASD, in comparison to healthy controls, have significant perturbations of amino acid, oxidative and mammalian microbial metabolism [133]. Interesting, in terms of diagnostic validity, is the ability of metabolomic signatures in urine to discriminate effectively patients with ASD from healthy controls [134–139]. Another set of studies performed metabolomics profiling in peripheral plasma [129, 140] and serum [128]. Again, all these studies found metabolomics fingerprints that were able to discriminate with adequate sensitivity and specificity patients with ASD from healthy controls. Specifically, West et al. found decreased citric acid and increased succinic acid, decreased fatty acids, increased 3-aminoisobutyric acid and decreased creatinine in patients with ASD [129]. Wang et al. reported that ASD was consistently associated with two particular metabolites: sphingosine 1-phosphate and docosahexaenoic acid [128]. Finally, a recent study found a substantial perturbation of the amino acid metabolism with combination of glutamine, glycine and ornithine amino acid metabotypes detectable with a specificity of 96.3% and a positive predictive value of 93.5% within ASD patients [140]. In summary, findings in ASD patients show that metabolomics might have sufficient accuracy in discriminating affected subjects from healthy controls. It remains to be seen whether this validity will extend to violent behaviour.

2.6 Conclusions

The burden exacted by violent behaviour at a global level has led to progresses in the comprehension of its neurobiological underpinnings. The current amount of knowledge, however, has still not translated to the identification of reliable biomarkers that, in conjunction with reliable phenotypic information (particularly about the longitudinal developmental trajectory in at-risk subjects), could lead to the implementation of valid predictive models. Multidisciplinary longitudinal research in well-characterised clinical and community samples, combining genetic and epigenetic measures with behavioural-cognitive, brain imaging and metabolomics signatures, is needed to further identify mechanisms of predisposition to violence and importantly under which conditions these risk factors will lead to actual violent behaviours.

References

1. Volavka J. The neurobiology of violence. J Neuropsychiatry Clin Neurosci. 1999; 11(3):307–14.
2. Rosell DR, Siever LJ. The neurobiology of aggression and violence. CNS Spectr. 2015;20(03):254–79.
3. Siever LJ. Neurobiology of aggression and violence. Am J Psychiatry. 2008;165(4):429–42.
4. Cardwell SM, Piquero AR. Does violence in adolescence differentially predict offending patterns in early adulthood? Int J Offender Ther Comp Criminol. 2018;62(6):1603–28.
5. Loeber R, Pardini D. Neurobiology and the development of violence: common assumptions and controversies. Philos Trans R Soc Lond Ser B Biol Sci. 2008;363(1503):2491–503.
6. Cauffman E, Fine A, Thomas AG, Monahan KC. Trajectories of violent behavior among females and males. Child Dev. 2017;88(1):41–54.
7. Mead HK, Beauchaine TP, Shannon KE. Neurobiological adaptations to violence across development. Dev Psychopathol. 2010;22(1):1–22.
8. Karli P, Vergnes M. Role of the rhinencephalon in the control of interspecies rat-mouse aggressive behavior. J Physiol Paris. 1963;55:272–3.
9. Consolo S, Garattini S, Valzelli L. Sensitivity of aggressive mice to centrally acting drugs. J Pharm Pharmacol. 1965;17(9):594.
10. Garattini S, Giacalone E, Valzelli L. Isolation, aggressiveness and brain 5-hydroxytryptamine turnover. J Pharm Pharmacol. 1967;19(5):338–9.
11. Pisanu C, Congiu D, Costa M, Sestu M, Chillotti C, Ardau R, et al. No association of endocannabinoid genes with bipolar disorder or lithium response in a Sardinian sample. Psychiatry Res. 2013;210(3):887–90.
12. Manchia M, Carpiniello B, Valtorta F, Comai S. Serotonin dysfunction, aggressive behavior, and mental illness: exploring the link using a dimensional approach. ACS Chem Neurosci. 2017;8(5):961.
13. Linnoila M, Virkkunen M, Scheinin M, Nuutila A, Rimon R, Goodwin FK. Low cerebrospinal fluid 5-hydroxyindoleacetic acid concentration differentiates impulsive from nonimpulsive violent behavior. Life Sci. 1983;33(26):2609–14.
14. Virkkunen M, Goldman D, Nielsen DA, Linnoila M. Low brain serotonin turnover rate (low CSF 5-HIAA) and impulsive violence. J Psychiatry Neurosci. 1995;20(4):271–5.
15. Comai S, Bertazzo A, Vachon J, Daigle M, Toupin J, Côté G, et al. Tryptophan via serotonin/kynurenine pathways abnormalities in a large cohort of aggressive inmates: markers for aggression. Prog Neuro-Psychopharmacol Biol Psychiatry. 2016;70:8–16.

16. Kruesi MJ, Rapoport JL, Hamburger S, Hibbs E, Potter WZ, Lenane M, et al. Cerebrospinal fluid monoamine metabolites, aggression, and impulsivity in disruptive behavior disorders of children and adolescents. Arch Gen Psychiatry. 1990;47(5):419–26.
17. Moeller FG, Dougherty DM, Swann AC, Collins D, Davis CM, Cherek DR. Tryptophan depletion and aggressive responding in healthy males. Psychopharmacology. 1996;126(2):97–103.
18. Kötting WF, Bubenzer S, Helmbold K, Eisert A, Gaber TJ, Zepf FD. Effects of tryptophan depletion on reactive aggression and aggressive decision-making in young people with ADHD. Acta Psychiatr Scand. 2013;128(2):114–23.
19. Zimmermann M, Grabemann M, Mette C, Abdel-Hamid M, Uekermann J, Ueckermann J, et al. The effects of acute tryptophan depletion on reactive aggression in adults with attention-deficit/hyperactivity disorder (ADHD) and healthy controls. Guillemin GJ, editor. PLoS One. 2012;7(3):e32023.
20. McCloskey MS, Phan KL, Angstadt M, Fettich KC, Keedy S, Coccaro EF. Amygdala hyper-activation to angry faces in intermittent explosive disorder. J Psychiatr Res. 2016;79:34–41.
21. Rosell DR, Thompson JL, Slifstein M, Xu X, Frankle WG, New AS, et al. Increased serotonin 2A receptor availability in the orbitofrontal cortex of physically aggressive personality disordered patients. Biol Psychiatry. 2010;67(12):1154–62.
22. Cervantes MC, Biggs EA, Delville Y. Differential responses to serotonin receptor ligands in an impulsive-aggressive phenotype. Behav Neurosci. 2010;124(4):455–69.
23. Zhuang X, Gross C, Santarelli L, Compan V, Trillat AC, Hen R. Altered emotional states in knockout mice lacking 5-HT1A or 5-HT1B receptors. Neuropsychopharmacology. 1999;21(2 Suppl):52S–60S.
24. Parsey RV, Oquendo MA, Simpson NR, Ogden RT, Van Heertum R, Arango V, et al. Effects of sex, age, and aggressive traits in man on brain serotonin 5-HT1A receptor binding potential measured by PET using [C-11]WAY-100635. Brain Res. 2002;954(2):173–82.
25. Cleare AJ, Bond AJ. Ipsapirone challenge in aggressive men shows an inverse correlation between 5-HT1A receptor function and aggression. Psychopharmacology. 2000;148(4):344–9.
26. Cases O, Seif I, Grimsby J, Gaspar P, Chen K, Pournin S, et al. Aggressive behavior and altered amounts of brain serotonin and norepinephrine in mice lacking MAOA. Science. 1995;268(5218):1763–6.
27. Checknita D, Maussion G, Labonté B, Comai S, Tremblay RE, Vitaro F, et al. Monoamine oxidase A gene promoter methylation and transcriptional downregulation in an offender population with antisocial personality disorder. Br J Psychiatry. 2015;206(3):216–22.
28. Alenina N, Kikic D, Todiras M, Mosienko V, Qadri F, Plehm R, et al. Growth retardation and altered autonomic control in mice lacking brain serotonin. Proc Natl Acad Sci U S A. 2009;106(25):10332–7.
29. Laas K, Kiive E, Mäestu J, Vaht M, Veidebaum T, Harro J. Nice guys: homozygosity for the TPH2-703G/T (rs4570625) minor allele promotes low aggressiveness and low anxiety. J Affect Disord. 2017;215:230–6.
30. Manchia M, Comai S, Pinna F, Pinna M, Fanos V, Denovan-Wright EM, et al. Biomarkers in aggression. Adv Clin Chem. 2019;
31. Brown GL, Goodwin FK, Ballenger JC, Goyer PF, Major LF. Aggression in humans correlates with cerebrospinal fluid amine metabolites. Psychiatry Res. 1979;1(2):131–9.
32. Castellanos FX, Elia J, Kruesi MJP, Gulotta CS, Mefford IN, Potte WZ, et al. Cerebrospinal fluid monoamine metabolites in boys with attention-deficit hyperactivity disorder. Psychiatry Res. 1994;52(3):305–16.
33. Placidi GP, Oquendo MA, Malone KM, Huang YY, Ellis SP, Mann JJ. Aggressivity, suicide attempts, and depression: relationship to cerebrospinal fluid monoamine metabolite levels. Biol Psychiatry. 2001;50(10):783–91.
34. Prochazka H, Agren H. Self-rated aggression and cerebral monoaminergic turnover. Sex differences in patients with persistent depressive disorder. Eur Arch Psychiatry Clin Neurosci. 2003;253(4):185–92.
35. Soderstrom H, Blennow K, Manhem A, Forsman A. CSF studies in violent offenders I. 5-HIAA as a negative and HVA as a positive predictor of psychopathy. J Neural Transm. 2001;108(7):869–78.

36. Møller SE, Mortensen EL, Breum L, Alling C, Larsen OG, Bøge-Rasmussen T, et al. Aggression and personality: association with amino acids and monoamine metabolites. Psychol Med. 1996;26(2):323–31.
37. Limson R, Goldman D, Roy A, Lamparski D, Ravitz B, Adinoff B, et al. Personality and cerebrospinal fluid monoamine metabolites in alcoholics and controls. Arch Gen Psychiatry. 1991;48(5):437–41.
38. Crawley JN, Contrera JF. Intraventricular 6-hydroxydopamine lowers isolation-induced fighting behavior in male mice. Pharmacol Biochem Behav. 1976;4(4):381–4.
39. Kantak KM, Hegstrand LR, Eichelman B. Facilitation of shock-induced fighting following intraventricular 5,7-dihydroxytryptamine and 6-hydroxydopa. Psychopharmacology. 1981;74(2):157–60.
40. Sallinen J, Haapalinna A, Viitamaa T, Kobilka BK, Scheinin M. Adrenergic alpha(2C)-receptors modulate the acoustic startle reflex, prepulse inhibition, and aggression in mice. J Neurosci. 1998;18(8):3035–42.
41. Fava M. Psychopharmacologic treatment of pathologic aggression. Psychiatr Clin North Am. 1997;20(2):427–51.
42. Volavka J. Can aggressive behavior in humans be modified by beta blockers? Postgrad Med. 1988;Spec No:163–8.
43. Comai S, Tau M, Gobbi G. The psychopharmacology of aggressive behavior: a translational approach: part 1: neurobiology. J Clin Psychopharmacol. 2012;32:1.
44. de Almeida RM, Ferrari PF, Parmigiani S, Miczek KA. Escalated aggressive behavior: dopamine, serotonin and GABA. Eur J Pharmacol. 2005;526(1–3):51–64.
45. Nelson RJ, Chiavegatto S. Molecular basis of aggression. Trends Neurosci. 2001; 24(12):713–9.
46. Comai S, Tau M, Pavlovic Z, Gobbi G. The psychopharmacology of aggressive behavior: a translational approach: part 2: clinical studies using atypical antipsychotics, anticonvulsants, and lithium. J Clin Psychopharmacol. 2012;32:2.
47. Miczek KA. Intraspecies aggression in rats: effects of d-amphetamine and chlordiazepoxide. Psychopharmacologia. 1974;39(4):275–301.
48. Albrecht B, Staiger PK, Hall K, Miller P, Best D, Lubman DI. Benzodiazepine use and aggressive behaviour: a systematic review. Aust N Z J Psychiatry. 2014;48(12):1096–114.
49. Gulsun M, Oznur T, Aydemir E, Ozcelik F, Erdem M, Zincir S, et al. Possible relationship between amino acids, aggression and psychopathy. Int J Psychiatry Clin Pract. 2016;20(2):91–100.
50. Bjork JM, Moeller FG, Kramer GL, Kram M, Suris A, Rush AJ, et al. Plasma GABA levels correlate with aggressiveness in relatives of patients with unipolar depressive disorder. Psychiatry Res. 2001;101(2):131–6.
51. Lee R, Petty F, Coccaro EF. Cerebrospinal fluid GABA concentration: relationship with impulsivity and history of suicidal behavior, but not aggression, in human subjects. J Psychiatr Res. 2009;43(4):353–9.
52. Brody JF, DeFeudis PA, DeFeudis FV. Effects of micro-injections of L-glutamate into the hypothalamus on attack and flight behaviour in cats. Nature. 1969;224(5226):1330.
53. Takahashi A, Lee RX, Iwasato T, Itohara S, Arima H, Bettler B, et al. Glutamate input in the dorsal raphe nucleus as a determinant of escalated aggression in male mice. J Neurosci. 2015;35(16):6452–63.
54. Belozertseva I, Bespalov A, Gmiro E, Danysz W, Zvartau E. Effects of NMDA receptor channel blockade on aggression in isolated male mice. Aggress Behav. 1999;25(1):48–9.
55. Navarro JF, De Castro V, Martín-López M. JNJ16259685, a selective mGlu1 antagonist, suppresses isolation-induced aggression in male mice. Eur J Pharmacol. 2008;586(1–3):217–20.
56. Coccaro EF, Lee R, Vezina P. Cerebrospinal fluid glutamate concentration correlates with impulsive aggression in human subjects. J Psychiatr Res. 2013;47(9):1247–53.
57. McGale EH, Pye IF, Stonier C, Hutchinson EC, Aber GM. Studies of the inter-relationship between cerebrospinal fluid and plasma amino acid concentrations in normal individuals. J Neurochem. 1977;29(2):291–7.

58. Alfredsson G, Wiesel FA, Tylec A. Relationships between glutamate and monoamine metabolites in cerebrospinal fluid and serum in healthy volunteers. Biol Psychiatry. 1988;23(7):689–97.
59. Giammanco M, Tabacchi G, Giammanco S, Di Majo D, La Guardia M. Testosterone and aggressiveness. Med Sci Monit. 2005;11(4):RA136–45.
60. Carré JM, Geniole SN, Ortiz TL, Bird BM, Videto A, Bonin PL. Exogenous testosterone rapidly increases aggressive behavior in dominant and impulsive men. Biol Psychiatry. 2017;82(4):249–56.
61. Hermans EJ, Ramsey NF, van Honk J. Exogenous testosterone enhances responsiveness to social threat in the neural circuitry of social aggression in humans. Biol Psychiatry. 2008;63(3):263–70.
62. Heinrichs M, von Dawans B, Domes G. Oxytocin, vasopressin, and human social behavior. Front Neuroendocrinol. 2009;30(4):548–57.
63. Campbell A, Hausmann M. Effects of oxytocin on women's aggression depend on state anxiety. Aggress Behav. 2013;39(4):316–22.
64. Alcorn JL, Rathnayaka N, Swann AC, Moeller FG, Lane SD. Effects of intranasal oxytocin on aggressive responding in antisocial personality disorder. Psychol Rec. 2015;65(4):691–703.
65. Alcorn JL, Green CE, Schmitz J, Lane SD. Effects of oxytocin on aggressive responding in healthy adult men. Behav Pharmacol 2015;26(8 Spec No):798–804.
66. Berends YR, Tulen JHM, Wierdsma AI, van Pelt J, Feldman R, Zagoory-Sharon O, et al. Intranasal administration of oxytocin decreases task-related aggressive responses in healthy young males. Psychoneuroendocrinology. 2019;106:147–54.
67. Ragnauth AK, Devidze N, Moy V, Finley K, Goodwillie A, Kow L-M, et al. Female oxytocin gene-knockout mice, in a semi-natural environment, display exaggerated aggressive behavior. Genes Brain Behav. 2005;4(4):229–39.
68. Lee R, Ferris C, Van de Kar LD, Coccaro EF. Cerebrospinal fluid oxytocin, life history of aggression, and personality disorder. Psychoneuroendocrinology. 2009;34(10):1567–73.
69. Bhatt S, Gregg TR, Siegel A. NK1 receptors in the medial hypothalamus potentiate defensive rage behavior elicited from the midbrain periaqueductal gray of the cat. Brain Res. 2003;966(1):54–64.
70. Han Y, Shaikh MB, Siegel A. Medial amygdaloid suppression of predatory attack behavior in the cat: I role of a substance P pathway from the medial amygdala to the medial hypothalamus. Brain Res. 1996;716(1–2):59–71.
71. Katsouni E, Sakkas P, Zarros A, Skandali N, Liapi C. The involvement of substance P in the induction of aggressive behavior. Peptides. 2009;30(8):1586–91.
72. De Felipe C, Herrero JF, O'Brien JA, Palmer JA, Doyle CA, Smith AJH, et al. Altered nociception, analgesia and aggression in mice lacking the receptor for substance P. Nature. 1998;392(6674):394–7.
73. Halasz J, Toth M, Mikics E, Hrabovszky E, Barsy B, Barsvari B, et al. The effect of neurokinin1 receptor blockade on territorial aggression and in a model of violent aggression. Biol Psychiatry. 2008;63(3):271–8.
74. Gregg TR, Siegel A. Differential effects of NK1 receptors in the midbrain periaqueductal gray upon defensive rage and predatory attack in the cat. Brain Res. 2003;994(1):55–66.
75. Coccaro EF, Lee R, Owens MJ, Kinkead B, Nemeroff CB. Cerebrospinal fluid substance P-like immunoreactivity correlates with aggression in personality disordered subjects. Biol Psychiatry. 2012;72(3):238–43.
76. File SE. NKP608, an NK1 receptor antagonist, has an anxiolytic action in the social interaction test in rats. Psychopharmacology. 2000;152(1):105–9.
77. Uyeno ET, Chang D, Folkers K. Substance P found to lower body temperature and aggression. Biochem Biophys Res Commun. 1979;86(3):837–42.
78. Stern P, Hadzović J. Pharmacological analysis of central actions of synthetic substance P. Arch Int Pharmacodyn Ther. 1973;202(2):259–62.
79. Bosch OJ, Neumann ID. Vasopressin released within the central amygdala promotes maternal aggression. Eur J Neurosci. 2010;31(5):883–91.

80. Delville Y, De Vries GJ, Ferris CF. Neural connections of the anterior hypothalamus and agonistic behavior in golden hamsters. Brain Behav Evol. 2000;55(2):53–76.
81. Delville Y, Mansour KM, Ferris CF. Serotonin blocks vasopressin-facilitated offensive aggression: interactions within the ventrolateral hypothalamus of golden hamsters. Physiol Behav. 1996;59(4–5):813–6.
82. Ferris CF, Melloni RH, Koppel G, Perry KW, Fuller RW, Delville Y. Vasopressin/serotonin interactions in the anterior hypothalamus control aggressive behavior in golden hamsters. J Neurosci. 1997;17(11):4331–40.
83. Wersinger SR, Ginns EI, O'Carroll A-M, Lolait SJ, Young WS. Vasopressin V1b receptor knockout reduces aggressive behavior in male mice. Mol Psychiatry. 2002;7(9):975–84.
84. Wersinger SR, Caldwell HK, Martinez L, Gold P, Hu S-B, Young WS. Vasopressin 1a receptor knockout mice have a subtle olfactory deficit but normal aggression. Genes Brain Behav. 2007;6(6):540–51.
85. Coccaro EF, Kavoussi RJ, Hauger RL, Cooper TB, Ferris CF. Cerebrospinal fluid vasopressin levels: correlates with aggression and serotonin function in personality-disordered subjects. Arch Gen Psychiatry. 1998;55(8):708–14.
86. Runions KC, Morandini HAE, Rao P, Wong JWY, Kolla NJ, Pace G, et al. Serotonin and aggressive behaviour in children and adolescents: a systematic review. Acta Psychiatr Scand. 2019;139(2):117–44.
87. Coccaro EF, Sripada CS, Yanowitch RN, Phan KL. Corticolimbic function in impulsive aggressive behavior. Biol Psychiatry. 2011;69(12):1153–9.
88. Klasen M, Wolf D, Eisner PD, Eggermann T, Zerres K, Zepf FD, et al. Serotonergic contributions to human brain aggression networks. Front Neurosci. 2019;13:42.
89. Sterzer P, Stadler C. Neuroimaging of aggressive and violent behaviour in children and adolescents. Front Behav Neurosci. 2009;3:35.
90. Kempes M, Matthys W, De Vries H, Van Engeland H. Reactive and proactive aggression in children: a review of theory, findings and the relevance for child and adolescent psychiatry. Eur Child Adolesc Psychiatry. 2005;14(1):11–9.
91. Sturmey P, Allen JJ, Anderson CA. Aggression and violence: definitions and distinctions. In: The Wiley handbook of violence and aggression. West Sussex: John Wiley & Sons Ltd; 2017. p. 1–14.
92. van Elst LT, Woermann FG, Lemieux L, Thompson PJ, Trimble MR. Affective aggression in patients with temporal lobe epilepsy: a quantitative MRI study of the amygdala. Brain. 2000;123(Pt 2):234–43.
93. Coccaro EF, McCloskey MS, Fitzgerald DA, Phan KL. Amygdala and orbitofrontal reactivity to social threat in individuals with impulsive aggression. Biol Psychiatry. 2007;62(2):168–78.
94. Passamonti L, Crockett MJ, Apergis-Schoute AM, Clark L, Rowe JB, Calder AJ, et al. Effects of acute tryptophan depletion on prefrontal-amygdala connectivity while viewing facial signals of aggression. Biol Psychiatry. 2012;71(1):36–43.
95. Romero-Martinez A, Gonzalez M, Lila M, Gracia E, Marti-Bonmati L, Alberich-Bayarri A, et al. The brain resting-state functional connectivity underlying violence proneness: is it a reliable marker for neurocriminology? A systematic review. Behav Sci (Basel, Switzerland). 2019;9(1)
96. Ellis ML, Weiss B, Lochman JE. Executive functions in children: associations with aggressive behavior and appraisal processing. J Abnorm Child Psychol. 2009;37(7):945–56.
97. Baskin-Sommers AR, Waller R, Fish AM, Hyde LW. Callous-unemotional traits trajectories interact with earlier conduct problems and executive control to predict violence and substance use among high risk male adolescents. J Abnorm Child Psychol. 2015;43(8):1529–41.
98. Marsh AA, Finger EC, Mitchell DGV, Reid ME, Sims C, Kosson DS, et al. Reduced amygdala response to fearful expressions in children and adolescents with callous-unemotional traits and disruptive behavior disorders. Am J Psychiatry. 2008;165(6):712–20.

99. Kolla NJ, Dunlop K, Meyer JH, Downar J. Corticostriatal connectivity in antisocial personality disorder by MAO-A genotype and its relationship to aggressive behavior. Int J Neuropsychopharmacol. 2018;

100. Tuvblad C, Sild M, Frogner C, Booij L. Behavioral genetics of aggression and intermittent explosive disorder. In: Coccaro EF, editor. Intermittent explosive disorder. Amsterdam: Elsevier; 2019. p. 17–35.

101. Raine A. A neurodevelopmental perspective on male violence. Infant Ment Health J. 2019;40(1):84–97.

102. Vassos E, Collier DA, Fazel S. Systematic meta-analyses and field synopsis of genetic association studies of violence and aggression. Mol Psychiatry. 2014;19(4):471–7.

103. Waltes R, Chiocchetti AG, Freitag CM. The neurobiological basis of human aggression: a review on genetic and epigenetic mechanisms. Am J Med Genet B Neuropsychiatr Genet. 2016;171(5):650–75.

104. Ficks CA, Waldman ID. Candidate genes for aggression and antisocial behavior: a meta-analysis of association studies of the 5HTTLPR and MAOA-uVNTR. Behav Genet. 2014;44(5):427–44.

105. Tiihonen J, Rautiainen M-R, Ollila HM, Repo-Tiihonen E, Virkkunen M, Palotie A, et al. Genetic background of extreme violent behavior. Mol Psychiatry. 2015;20(6):786–92.

106. Lacourse E, Boivin M, Brendgen M, Petitclerc A, Girard A, Vitaro F, et al. A longitudinal twin study of physical aggression during early childhood: evidence for a developmentally dynamic genome. Psychol Med. 2014;44(12):2617–27.

107. Pingault J-B, Rijsdijk F, Zheng Y, Plomin R, Viding E. Developmentally dynamic genome: evidence of genetic influences on increases and decreases in conduct problems from early childhood to adolescence. Sci Rep. 2015;5(1):10053.

108. Pingault JB, Côté SM, Booij L, Ouellet-Morin I, Castellanos-Ryan N, Vitaro F, et al. Age-dependent effect of the MAOA gene on childhood physical aggression. Mol Psychiatry. 2013;18(11):1151–2.

109. Lesch KP, Bengel D, Heils A, Sabol SZ, Greenberg BD, Petri S, et al. Association of anxiety-related traits with a polymorphism in the serotonin transporter gene regulatory region. Science. 1996;274(5292):1527–31.

110. Reif A, Rösler M, Freitag CM, Schneider M, Eujen A, Kissling C, et al. Nature and nurture predispose to violent behavior: serotonergic genes and adverse childhood environment. Neuropsychopharmacology. 2007;32(11):2375–83.

111. Provençal N, Suderman MJ, Vitaro F, Szyf M, Tremblay RE, Provencal N, et al. Childhood chronic physical aggression associates with adult cytokine levels in plasma. PLoS One. 2013;8(7):e69481.

112. Wang D, Szyf M, Benkelfat C, Provençal N, Turecki G, Caramaschi D, et al. Peripheral SLC6A4 DNA methylation is associated with in vivo measures of human brain serotonin synthesis and childhood physical aggression. PLoS One. 2012;7(6):e39501.

113. Guillemin C, Provençal N, Suderman M, Côté SM, Vitaro F, Hallett M, et al. DNA methylation signature of childhood chronic physical aggression in T cells of both men and women. PLoS One. 2014;9(1):e86822.

114. Gescher DM, Kahl KG, Hillemacher T, Frieling H, Kuhn J, Frodl T. Epigenetics in personality disorders: today's insights. Front Psych. 2018;9:579.

115. Provençal N, Booij L, Tremblay RE. The developmental origins of chronic physical aggression: biological pathways triggered by early life adversity. J Exp Biol. 2015;218(Pt 1):123–33.

116. Kruger THC, Sinke C, Kneer J, Tenbergen G, Khan AQ, Burkert A, et al. Child sexual offenders show prenatal and epigenetic alterations of the androgen system. Transl Psychiatry. 2019;9(1):28.

117. Montalvo-Ortiz JL, Zhang H, Chen C, Liu C, Coccaro EF. Genome-wide DNA methylation changes associated with intermittent explosive disorder: a gene-based functional enrichment analysis. Int J Neuropsychopharmacol. 2018;21(1):12–20.

118. Meyer-Lindenberg A, Buckholtz JW, Kolachana B, Hariri AR, Pezawas L, Blasi G, et al. Neural mechanisms of genetic risk for impulsivity and violence in humans. Proc Natl Acad Sci U S A. 2006;103(16):6269–74.
119. Klasen M, Wolf D, Eisner PD, Habel U, Repple J, Vernaleken I, et al. Neural networks underlying trait aggression depend on MAOA gene alleles. Brain Struct Funct. 2018;223(2):873–81.
120. Denson TF, Dobson-Stone C, Ronay R, von Hippel W, Schira MM. A functional polymorphism of the MAOA gene is associated with neural responses to induced anger control. J Cogn Neurosci. 2014;26(7):1418–27.
121. Clemens B, Voß B, Pawliczek C, Mingoia G, Weyer D, Repple J, et al. Effect of MAOA genotype on resting-state networks in healthy participants. Cereb Cortex. 2015;25(7):1771–81.
122. Kolla NJ, Patel R, Meyer JH, Chakravarty MM. Association of monoamine oxidase-A genetic variants and amygdala morphology in violent offenders with antisocial personality disorder and high psychopathic traits. Sci Rep. 2017;7(1):9607.
123. Gaspar P, Cases O, Maroteaux L. The developmental role of serotonin: news from mouse molecular genetics. Nat Rev Neurosci. 2003;4(12):1002–12.
124. Johnson CH, Ivanisevic J, Siuzdak G. Metabolomics: beyond biomarkers and towards mechanisms. Nat Rev Mol Cell Biol. 2016;17(7):451–9.
125. Riekeberg E, Powers R. New frontiers in metabolomics: from measurement to insight. F1000Res. 2017;6:1148.
126. Czysz AH, South C, Gadad BS, Arning E, Soyombo A, Bottiglieri T, et al. Can targeted metabolomics predict depression recovery? Results from the CO-MED trial. Transl Psychiatry. 2019;9(1):11.
127. Tasic L, Pontes JGM, Carvalho MS, Cruz G, Dal Mas C, Sethi S, et al. Metabolomics and lipidomics analyses by 1H nuclear magnetic resonance of schizophrenia patient serum reveal potential peripheral biomarkers for diagnosis. Schizophr Res. 2017;185:182–9.
128. Wang H, Liang S, Wang M, Gao J, Sun C, Wang J, et al. Potential serum biomarkers from a metabolomics study of autism. J Psychiatry Neurosci. 2016;41(1):27–37.
129. West PR, Amaral DG, Bais P, Smith AM, Egnash LA, Ross ME, et al. Metabolomics as a tool for discovery of biomarkers of autism spectrum disorder in the blood plasma of children. PLoS One. 2014;9(11):e112445.
130. Hagenbeek FA, Kluft C, Hankemeier T, Bartels M, Draisma HHM, Middeldorp CM, et al. Discovery of biochemical biomarkers for aggression: a role for metabolomics in psychiatry. Am J Med Genet B Neuropsychiatr Genet. 2016;171(5):719–32.
131. Im DS. Template to perpetrate: an update on violence in autism spectrum disorder. Harv Rev Psychiatry. 2016;24(1):14–35.
132. Yap IKS, Angley M, Veselkov KA, Holmes E, Lindon JC, Nicholson JK. Urinary metabolic phenotyping differentiates children with autism from their unaffected siblings and age-matched controls. J Proteome Res. 2010;9(6):2996–3004.
133. Ming X, Stein TP, Barnes V, Rhodes N, Guo L. Metabolic perturbance in autism spectrum disorders: a metabolomics study. J Proteome Res. 2012;11(12):5856–62.
134. Mavel S, Nadal-Desbarats L, Blasco H, Bonnet-Brilhault F, Barthélémy C, Montigny F, et al. 1H-13C NMR-based urine metabolic profiling in autism spectrum disorders. Talanta. 2013;114:95–102.
135. Emond P, Mavel S, Aïdoud N, Nadal-Desbarats L, Montigny F, Bonnet-Brilhault F, et al. GC-MS-based urine metabolic profiling of autism spectrum disorders. Anal Bioanal Chem. 2013;405(15):5291–300.
136. Cozzolino R, De Magistris L, Saggese P, Stocchero M, Martignetti A, Di Stasio M, et al. Use of solid-phase microextraction coupled to gas chromatography-mass spectrometry for determination of urinary volatile organic compounds in autistic children compared with healthy controls. Anal Bioanal Chem. 2014;406(19):4649–62.

137. Noto A, Fanos V, Barberini L, Grapov D, Fattuoni C, Zaffanello M, et al. The urinary metabolomics profile of an Italian autistic children population and their unaffected siblings. J Matern Neonatal Med. 2014;27(suppl 2):46–52.
138. Nadal-Desbarats L, Aïdoud N, Emond P, Blasco H, Filipiak I, Sarda P, et al. Combined ^{1}H-NMR and ^{1}H–^{13}C HSQC-NMR to improve urinary screening in autism spectrum disorders. Analyst. 2014;139(13):3460–8.
139. Diémé B, Mavel S, Blasco H, Tripi G, Bonnet-Brilhault F, Malvy J, et al. Metabolomics study of urine in autism spectrum disorders using a multiplatform analytical methodology. J Proteome Res. 2015;14(12):5273–82.
140. Smith AM, King JJ, West PR, Ludwig MA, Donley ELR, Burrier RE, et al. Amino acid dysregulation metabotypes: potential biomarkers for diagnosis and individualized treatment for subtypes of autism spectrum disorder. Biol Psychiatry. 2019;85(4):345–54.

Epidemiology and Risk Factors for Violence in People with Mental Disorders

3

Daniel Whiting and Seena Fazel

3.1 Introduction

It has long been thought that there is some relationship between offending behaviour and mental illness [1]. For example, there have been hospitals providing psychiatric treatment to people with mental health problems who have criminally offended since the mid-nineteenth century [2]. In the latter part of the twentieth century, however, researchers had very contrasting views on the nature and magnitude of the relationship [3]. A prevailing expert view, reinforced by patient advocacy groups, was that controlling for demographic and life history factors dissipated the reported increased links with violence and crime [4], and studies in the early 1990s demonstrating increased risks were criticised on methodological grounds, by questioning violence outcome measurement and use of non-representative populations [5].

An influential study which sought to address some of these issues was the MacArthur Violence Risk Assessment study, the first findings of which were published in 1998 [6]. In a diagnostically heterogeneous group of 951 patients discharged from three US acute inpatient facilities, community violent outcomes were triangulated from three sources (self-report, collateral informants, and police and health records) and compared with rates in the general population living in the same residential areas. The widely cited primary finding was that prevalence of violence in discharged patients without substance misuse did not differ from other individuals in the same neighbourhood without substance misuse. However, links were found with violent outcomes when for example considering diagnostic groups separately, and this study has been subject to subsequent debate and further analysis [7].

In recent years, through longitudinal use of population registers that provide more precision and allow new ways to account for confounding, a more robust and nuanced understanding has emerged. This has been supported by meta-analyses. That is, many

D. Whiting · S. Fazel (✉)
Department of Psychiatry, Warneford Hospital, University of Oxford, Oxford, UK
e-mail: daniel.whiting@psych.ox.ac.uk; seena.fazel@psych.ox.ac.uk

© Springer Nature Switzerland AG 2020
B. Carpiniello et al. (eds.), *Violence and Mental Disorders*, Comprehensive Approach to Psychiatry 1, https://doi.org/10.1007/978-3-030-33188-7_3

mental disorders are associated with a small but increased risk of violence compared with the general population, which is partly explained by comorbid substance misuse. Whilst most individuals with mental illness are not violent, the risks in both relative and absolute terms, and the implications of violence for patients themselves and those affected by it, mean that assessing and reducing this risk is an important aspect of clinical psychiatric practice. Public perception of dangerousness remains central to stigma in mental illness [8], and so it is imperative that these risks are not overstated, and that context is provided—such as that individuals with mental illness are also at increased risk of crime victimisation [9] and the majority of people with mental illness will not be violent towards others. It is also increasingly appreciated however that reducing violence risk with effective treatment should form part of anti-stigma strategy [10], and being transparent about the evidence of a link is necessary for patient benefit [11].

3.2 Current Understanding of Violence Epidemiology in Mental Disorders

3.2.1 Schizophrenia Spectrum Disorders

A substantial proportion of the studies examining violence in mental illness have focussed on psychotic illnesses. A 2009 systematic review pooled results from 20 primary studies conducted between 1980 and 2009, incorporating data from 18,423 individuals with schizophrenia and related disorders compared with 1.7 million controls [12]. Overall, odds ratios in individual studies for the risk of any violent outcome in people with psychosis compared with the general population ranged from 1 to 7 in men and 4 to 29 in women. For individuals without substance use comorbidity, the presence of a psychotic illness was associated with a twofold increased risk of violence compared to the general population (pooled odds ratio [OR] 2.1, 95% confidence interval [CI] 1.7–2.7). When including comorbid substance misuse, the pooled OR rose to 8.9 (95% CI 5.4–14.7), and when considering only homicide, the pooled OR was 19.5 (95% CI 14.7–25.8). Homicide is a rare outcome however; the absolute risk in this review was 0.3%, and in a UK national clinical survey less than 6% of all homicides were by individuals with schizophrenia and other delusional disorders (326 of 5699 homicides over 10 years) [13].

Large individual studies have since supported the findings from the review. A study that used national registries to longitudinally examine post-illness-onset offending in a random sample of 25% of the total Danish population (over ½ million individuals) found a similar magnitude of association when adjusted for age, socio-economic factors and substance misuse [14]. Rates of violent offending were also examined in a Swedish population sample of 24,297 individuals with schizophrenia and related disorders followed up for 38 years, in a study that addressed confounding by matching to both general population and unaffected sibling controls [15]. The OR for offending in patients versus their sibling controls, adjusted for low family income and being born abroad, was 4.2 (95% CI 3.8–4.5). In this Swedish sample, the absolute rates of violent offending within the first 5 years following diagnosis were 11% in men and 3% in women.

The first episode of a psychotic illness in particular is a potentially high-risk phase, with pooled evidence suggesting that a quarter of patients perpetrate some violence before treatment is initiated [16]. Longitudinally, a rate of 14% was found for the 12 months after service engagement in a UK cohort of 670 individuals with first-episode psychosis [17]. Specialist psychiatric services for individuals presenting with first-episode psychosis, typically modelled as 'early intervention' services, are now well established internationally and deliver a range of individually tailored interventions. This may be an important setting in which to identify higher risk subgroups at an early stage of illness, in order to target preventative approaches and reduce downstream violence and other adverse outcomes [18].

3.2.2 Mood Disorders

Alongside other adverse outcomes such as attempted and completed suicide, bipolar disorder has been clearly associated with violent crime [19]. A systematic review of nine studies between 1990 and 2010 ($N = 6383$ individuals with bipolar disorder, compared with 112,944 controls) found a pooled OR for violence of 4.6 (95% CI 3.9–5.4) compared to the general population [20, 21]. A subsequent longitudinal study of 15,337 individuals with bipolar disorder using Swedish registers found a threefold increased risk of violent crime compared to the general population after adjustment for sociodemographic factors and substance use (adjusted risk ratio 2.8, 95% CI 2.5–3.1) [19]. In this cohort, 7.9% of men and 1.8% of women were convicted for a violent crime following diagnosis, largely in the first 5 years.

The risk of violence in unipolar depression has been less studied than the psychoses. Early results were inconsistent, with some studies finding no significant relationship or weak associations that disappeared on controlling for confounders or comorbidity [22]. However, the MacArthur risk assessment study for example found that 10.3% of patients with depression without substance use were violent compared with 4.6% of the community comparison sample [23]. More recently, a study of 47,158 Swedish psychiatric outpatients with depression found a threefold increased risk of violence compared to the general population (adjusted OR 3.0, 95% CI 2.8–3.3). The absolute rates of violence in this population (3.7% in men and 0.5% in women compared to 1.2% of men and 0.2% of women in the general population) were clearly below that seen in bipolar disorder and schizophrenia. Highlighting these differences between relative and absolute risk remains important when communicating the findings of such studies.

3.2.3 Substance and Alcohol Misuse

There are challenges in understanding the relationship between drug and alcohol misuse and risk of violent offending. These include high rates of psychiatric comorbidity [24], heterogeneity in criteria defining substance misuse and considerable overlap between consumption of different drugs and alcohol [25]. The manner in which use may relate to violence is also complex, and has been broadly considered in terms of the potential effects of acute intoxication as well as the social, environmental and lifestyle factors associated with misuse [26]. Despite these issues, many studies have replicated that there is some overall significant relationship [27].

A recent umbrella review incorporated 22 existing meta-analyses of risk factors for interpersonal violence, and of these found substance misuse to have the greatest effect size (pooled OR 7.4, 95% CI 4.3–12.7), with a population attributable risk fraction of 14.8% (95% CI 9.0–21.6%) [28]. Another meta-review included 30 meta-analyses of the effect of alcohol and illicit drug use on violence published in 1985–2014, and found a significant relationship that was held across variations in study population, type of substance, and definition of violence [29]. The overall weighted estimate for standardised mean difference (effect size, where values between 0.35 and 0.65 are regarded as 'medium' and values above 0.65 as 'large') for alcohol and illicit drugs combined was 0.49 (95% CI 0.34–0.63). Such syntheses of previously published meta-analyses are helpful to provide a broad view of the relationship in an area with considerable volume and variation in research design.

There is additional strong evidence for the link between alcohol use and risk of violence. Among 292,420 men and 193,520 women who were general population controls in a Swedish total population study, the hazard ratio (HR) for violent offending for alcohol-use disorders was 9.0 for men (95% CI 8.2–9.9) and 19.8 for women (95% CI 14.6–26.7) [15]. These findings are consistent with earlier smaller longitudinal studies, such as data from a New Zealand birth cohort of 1265 individuals followed up over 30 years [30]. Based on periodic interviews, this cohort found having five or more symptoms of alcohol misuse or dependence in the prior 12 months was associated with an incidence rate ratio (IRR) for violent offending compared to those with no symptoms of 8.0 in men (95% CI 6.4–10.1) and 15.4 in women (95% CI 11.4–20.8). Increased risk has also been demonstrated in general population surveys [31, 32].

Drug-use disorders, when taken as a group separately to alcohol-use disorders, have also been clearly linked to violence risk, including in survey data [27], pooled data from 13 individual studies (random effects OR 7.4, 95% CI 4.3–12.7) [12], and Swedish population data (HR for violent offending in men of 16.2 [95% CI 14.6–17.9] and in women of 36.0 [95% CI 27.0–48.0]) [15]. Evidence is more uncertain for individual substances. A 2016 systematic review included 17 relevant longitudinal studies [33]. Findings were mixed and hampered by the low quality of primary studies. The most frequently examined substance was marijuana, with 12 measures of association from 8 studies, of which 5 showed an increased risk of interpersonal violence, 2 showed mixed results and 5 showed no association. Other subsequent studies have similarly produced inconclusive results, such as a Swedish general population survey of anabolic steroid use in men, which found a significant association with violent conviction (OR 5.0, 95% CI 2.7–9.3) that reduced when controlling for other substance misuse (OR 1.6, 95% CI 0.8–3.3) [34]. A similar decrease in association when controlling for other lifetime substance use and alcohol misuse/dependence was found for the other five non-steroid substances considered in this investigation (Rohypnol, other benzodiazepines, amphetamines, cocaine and cannabis), although the relationship remained significant for Rohypnol (OR 2.1, 95% CI 1.2–3.7), amphetamines (OR 2.7, 95% CI 1.9–4.0) and cannabis (OR 1.8, 95% CI 1.5–2.3) [34].

New synthetic agents, such as synthetic cannabinoids, have caused considerable concern including that their higher potency is associated with more adverse effects [35], particularly acutely, which may include aggression and violence. The 2015 version of the Youth Risk Behaviour Survey ($N = 15,624$), a cross-sectional survey of US schools, included for the first time a measure of synthetic cannabinoid use [36]. Although one of the violent outcomes, 'engaged in a physical fight', was significantly more likely to occur among students who ever used synthetic cannabinoids compared with students who ever used marijuana only, over 98% of those who had ever used synthetic cannabinoids had also used marijuana making it not possible to isolate any specific effects.

3.2.4 Personality Disorders

As well as being an important comorbidity in psychiatric and forensic populations, personality disorder as a diagnostic group has been widely demonstrated to be associated with an increased risk of violence. A study of 49,398 Swedish men assessed at military conscription and followed up in national crime registers found an increased risk of future violent conviction, OR 2.7 (95% CI 2.2–3.2) [37], and research using Danish population data has reported an adjusted IRR for violent offending of 4.1 in men (95% CI 3.5–4.7) and 5.0 in women (95% CI 3.8–6.7) [14].

A 2012 meta-analysis included 14 studies and over 10,000 individuals with personality disorder compared with 12 million general population controls [38]. The pooled OR for violent outcomes for personality disorders combined versus general population controls was 3.0 (95% CI 2.6–3.5). Antisocial personality disorder (ASPD) contributed substantially; 14% of those with ASPD had a violent outcome, and when considering only studies of ASPD (excluding one outlier) the pooled OR was 10.4 (95% CI 7.3–14.0). Differential effects of different categories were further examined in a cross-sectional survey of 8397 UK adults, where ASPD was also most strongly related to violence, although paranoid, narcissistic and obsessive-compulsive also made smaller independent contributions [39]. Borderline personality disorder has also been individually considered; a systematic review did not find evidence for an independent association with violence [40], and more recent survey data found an association only with intimate partner violence [41]. Comorbidity with substance misuse and ASPD was thought to be more relevant to risk.

3.2.5 Neurodevelopmental Disorders

The over-representation of attention-deficit hyperactivity disorder (ADHD) in custodial settings has been reported [42, 43], and pooled data from longitudinal studies including over 15,000 individuals with childhood ADHD showed a significant association with future incarceration (which can be taken as a proxy of violent offending), with a relative risk of 2.9 (95% CI 1.9–4.3) [44]. A longitudinal study of 1366 children diagnosed with ADHD in Stockholm looked specifically at violent offending and similarly found odds of 2.7 (95% CI 2.0–3.8) when adjusted for confounders including substance use comorbidity [45].

The epidemiological literature examining the relationship between autistic spectrum disorders (ASD) and violence is limited. A 2014 systematic review found only two studies with unbiased samples, which were too small to draw meaningful conclusions [46]. More informative has been a longitudinal study of children in Stockholm, which included 954 individuals with ASD compared with 33,910 population controls. No significant association with violent offending was found in the unadjusted model (OR 1.3, 95% CI 0.9–2.0), and the association reduced further when adjusted for parental factors and comorbidity including psychoses, substance misuse and conduct disorder (adjusted OR 1.1, 95% CI 0.6–1.9) [45]. This finding has been replicated more recently in a Swedish population-based cohort study including 5739 individuals with ASD, where a small association with violent offending was attenuated after controlling for comorbidity, particularly ADHD and conduct disorder [47].

3.3   Risk Factors for Violence in Mental Illness

In addition to gaining understanding of the associations between the standard diagnostic categories of mental disorder and risk of violence, research has also examined specific factors that may contribute to any increased risk of violence. These factors can either be static (historical or unchangeable, such as a past criminal conviction) or dynamic (modifiable or changing over time, such as substance misuse or psychotic symptoms). Such understanding is important in order to assess risk in a more individualised manner, and, where possible, consider strategies to reduce risk.

A meta-analysis of risk factors for violence in psychotic illness considered 110 studies including 45,533 individuals diagnosed with schizophrenia (88%) bipolar disorder and other psychoses [48]. The overall prevalence of violence, defined by a variety of measures (including in 42 studies by register-based sources), was 18.5%. The review identified several important dynamic risk factors associated with violence risk, including hostile behaviour (random-effects pooled OR 2.8, 95% CI 1.8–4.2), poor impulse control (OR 3.3, 95% CI 1.5–7.2), lack of insight (OR 2.7, 95% CI 1.4–5.2), recent alcohol and/or drug misuse (OR 2.9, 95% CI 1.3–6.3), non-adherence with psychological therapies (OR 6.7, 95% CI 2.4–19.2) and non-adherence with medication (OR 2.0, 95% CI 1.0–3.7) [48]. Static factors relating to past criminal history were robustly associated with violence, such as a history of violent conviction (OR 4.2, 95% CI 2.2–9.1) and history of imprisonment for any offence (OR 4.5, 95% CI 2.7–7.7). Other important demographic features were a history of homelessness (OR 2.3, 95% CI 1.5–3.4) and male gender (OR 1.6, 95% CI 1.2–2.1).

In this review, negative symptoms were not linked with violence (OR 1.0, 95% CI 0.9–1.2). This has been a relatively consistent finding, including in previous reviews [49], surveys [50] and prospective studies [51]. Positive symptoms were significantly associated with violence, although less strongly than other combined risk factor domains. Certain positive symptoms that have been regarded as clinically relevant [52, 53] were not demonstrated in this review to be significantly associated with violence, such as command hallucinations (OR 1.0, 95% CI 0.5–2.0) and threat/control override delusions (OR 1.2, 95% CI 0.9–1.7). Other work has explored alternatives—for example, potential pathways to violence from delusional beliefs that imply threat (such as persecution or being spied on), mediated by anger related to the beliefs, were demonstrated in re-analysis of data from the MacArthur Study [54] and in a survey of 458 patients with first-episode psychosis in London [55].

Some of the factors most strongly associated with violence in this review were victimisation—whether this was violent victimisation during adulthood (OR 6.1, 95% CI 4.0–9.1), physical abuse during childhood (OR 2.2, 95% CI 1.5–3.1) or sexual abuse during childhood (OR 1.9, 95% CI 1.5–2.4). The overlap between violence victimisation and perpetration has been widely demonstrated both in individuals with mental disorders [9] and in the general population [56], and is suggested to arise partly from shared risk factors for the two outcomes, such as comorbidity and volatile social relationships [57]. Victimisation was shown to mediate the association between depressive symptoms and violent behaviour in adolescence in a longitudinal study of 682 Dutch adolescents [58]. Violent victimisation has also been shown to be a strong predictive trigger event for violent offending in psychotic illness in a Swedish registry study of individuals with schizophrenia spectrum or bipolar disorders [59]. This study used a within-individual design to compare the risk of an individual behaving violently following exposure to a trigger with risk for that same individual in earlier time periods of equivalent length. All of the triggers examined (exposure to violence, parental bereavement, self-harm, traumatic brain injury, unintentional injuries, and substance intoxication) increased risk in the following week, and this was strongest for exposure to violence (OR for schizophrenia spectrum disorders 12.7 [95% CI 8.2–19.6], OR for bipolar disorder 7.6 [95% CI 4.0–14.4]). These findings are potentially highly relevant to dynamic risk management in clinical practice.

The relative strengths of association between various static and dynamic risk factors and a violent crime conviction in the subsequent year have also been examined in a cohort of 58,771 individuals with schizophrenia spectrum or bipolar disorder in a Swedish national cohort [60]. The strongest association was for previous violent crime (adjusted OR 5.03, 95% CI 4.23–5.98). Significant links were also seen for example for previous alcohol-use disorder (adjusted OR 1.75, 95% CI 1.47–2.09) and being an inpatient at the time of episode (adjusted OR 1.37, 95% CI 1.18–1.59). Recent treatment with antipsychotic medication was associated with a reduced risk (adjusted OR 0.62, 95% CI 0.51–0.77).

3.4   Translating Epidemiology to Clinical Practice

3.4.1   Clinical Assessment

In general psychiatric practice, the prevalence of violence as an adverse outcome across a range of disorders should be carefully considered, at least as one component of a general assessment of risk, and this is partly reflected in international clinical guidelines for bipolar disorder [61], schizophrenia [62] and depression [63]. The emphasis placed on violence risk assessment will vary to some extent between diagnoses, based on the differences in relative and absolute risk; for example, consideration of violence risk should be a prominent aspect of the management of individuals with antisocial personality disorder, whereas an increased risk of violent offending has not been demonstrated in some neurodevelopmental disorders. The empirical evidence already discussed in this chapter provides some direction to the aspects of history taking and clinical examination that are most relevant to any assessment of violence risk.

Clinical history should focus on previous violence, including its severity (injuries inflicted, use of a weapon, whether resulted in criminal conviction or incarceration) and circumstances surrounding previous incidents (including relevant triggers, active dynamic factors such as substance misuse, symptoms of mental illness, engagement with supervision and treatment from health services or other agencies, and social circumstances). A thorough drug and alcohol use history is essential, with a focus on temporal relevance to previous incidents of violence and deteriorations in mental state, and the wider context of any use such as its impact on stability of accommodation, violent victimisation, conflicted social relationships, and behaviours associated with funding substance use. Past psychiatric history should include enquiry about past self-harm, inpatient hospital admission, and indications of impulsivity or comorbid antisocial personality, as well as exploring previous response to treatment. Background history should explore educational level, elicit any family history of violent crime or substance misuse [60], and inquire about previous traumatic brain injury [64], past victimisation and abuse. A current social history should include housing and financial circumstances, and importantly identify whether any specific individuals are at risk. Wherever possible, collateral history from those close to the individual should be sought in order to identify any such concerns.

On mental state examination, general features such as irritability and hostility should be observed. The theme and content of any delusional beliefs should be explored fully, including whether beliefs relate to a particular person with whom the individual may have contact, and noting the relevance to risk of persecutory belief systems that involve feeling threatened and paranoid. The level of distress, preoccupation and presence of any affective component to these beliefs should be examined, and the extent to which behaviour has been modified in the context of these beliefs should be probed—for example, whether the individual has taken any steps to protect themselves from a perceived threat. More generally the overall burden of positive psychotic symptoms is relevant [48]. Finally, assessment of the level of insight and likely engagement with mental health services and treatment will be integral to the immediate plans to manage any identified risks.

3.4.2 Treatment

One of the key purposes of understanding and assessing the risk of violence in mental illness, such as Oxford Mental Illness and Violence tool (OxMIV) is to reduce this risk. Effective treatment of several of the dynamic risk factors that are associated with violence has indeed been shown to lead to reduced rates of violence.

Due to the strength of association, targeting substance misuse (whether as a comorbidity or primary disorder) will be an important aspect of reducing risk. This may include treatment with medication. Four such medications (acamprosate, naltrexone, methadone and buprenorphine) were examined in 21,281 individuals who had been prescribed at least one of these [65]. Within-individual comparisons demonstrated decreased risks of arrest for violent crime for the opioid substitutes buprenorphine (hazard ratio [HR] 0.65, 95% CI 0.50–0.84) and methadone (HR 0.84, 95% CI 0.73–0.96). In a study of Swedish released prisoners with schizophrenia spectrum disorders or bipolar disorder, treatment of co-occurring addiction disorders with medication was also shown to be associated with a substantial reduction in subsequent violent offending (HR 0.13, 95% CI 0.02–0.95), equating to a risk difference in number of violent re-offences per 1000 person years of −104.5 (95% CI −118.4 to −5.7), although caution is warranted as confidence intervals were large [66].

Appropriately treating core symptoms of mental illness with medication has also been shown to reduce the risk of violence. A Swedish population study of pre-scribed antipsychotics and mood stabilisers over 4 years found a 45% reduction in violent crime when individuals were prescribed antipsychotic medication compared with when they were not (hazard ratio [HR] 0.55, 95% CI 0.47–0.64), and a 24% reduction with mood-stabilising medication (HR 0.76, 95% CI 0.62–0.93) [67]. Importantly, when separated by diagnosis, the reduction in violence with mood-stabilising medication was only found in those with a diagnosis of bipolar disorder. Clozapine has been specifically linked to an anti-aggressive effect that may go beyond improved symptom control alone [68]. In a study of individuals with a psy-chotic or schizoaffective disorder, prescription of clozapine was associated with a lower rate of violent offending compared with the period before treatment (rate ratio 0.13, 95% CI 0.05–0.34, $N = 1004$ individuals treated with clozapine for longer than 8 weeks), and had a significantly greater rate reduction effect on violent offences than olanzapine prescription [69].

Such findings support the view that effective treatment by psychiatric services can help reduce risks of violence. There is however a need for more evidence-based preventative interventions to specifically target this important adverse outcome in psychiatric populations [70]. This may be particularly relevant in certain settings and patient groups, one example being individuals presenting with first-episode psychosis (as discussed above). Here, factors such as premorbid antisocial behav-iours have been shown to increase the risk of future violence independent of psychosis-related factors, and so prevention may need to go further than symptom control alone and specifically target such behaviours [17].

3.4.3   Risk Assessment Tools

Whilst epidemiology can help frame risk assessments broadly around those factors most empirically related to violence, one challenge for clinicians is translating this evidence more directly into clinical assessment. This will involve weighing up the relative importance of different risk factors in order to reach some quantifiable and communicable judgement of the magnitude of the risk, both in absolute terms and relative to thresholds. This may lead to identifying a need for more intensive provi-sion of support and treatment.

Part of the gap between epidemiology and the clinical world can be bridged through the use of risk assessment tools. Many tools facilitate a 'structured clinical judgement' approach, prompting clinicians to consider certain factors as a basis for their judgement of risk. However, these tools are resource intensive [71] to the extent that their practical utility outside of forensic psychiatric settings is highly doubtful, and furthermore they offer limited predictive accuracy in such settings [72]. A more effective approach may be the use of prediction models that statistically combine information about different risk factors to give an overall prediction of the risk of a particular outcome (such as a violent offence) over a particular time period. The key to the utility of such models is their translation into simple, scalable clinical tools that can then potentially act as adjuncts to clinical assessment.

Risk prediction models and tools are already integral to clinical practice in other areas of medicine, such as guiding the primary prevention of cardiovascular disease or decisions about adjuvant therapy in cancer, and are regarded as central to the advancement of healthcare delivery by data science [73]. There is promise that such models and tools may also have clinical utility for the prediction of violence in mental illness, such as Oxford Mental Illness and Violence tool (OxMIV) [60], which would facilitate a more stratified approach—in which the updated evidence is directly and accurately incorporated into the process of assessing risk. In turn, this should lead to linked interventions, particularly non-harmful ones with good evidence in support. Use of a supportive tool can introduce transparency and consistency that may be lacking from unstructured clinical assessments of risk [74]. In addition, for some services, screening out individuals accurately who are at low risk using risk tools will be clinically useful.

3.5   Summary

Whilst risks should not be overstated, violence risk is increased in a range of mental disorders. Large population-level datasets have clarified these associations by accounting for the temporality of disease onset and outcome, and they have provided more information on confounding factors. Among individuals with mental illness, criminal history and substance misuse factors are strongly related to increased risk, and treating modifiable factors has been shown to reduce risks. In the future, risk prediction models and tools will enable a stratified and precise approach to violence prevention in psychiatry.

References

1. Monahan J. Mental disorder and violent behavior. Perceptions and evidence. Am Psychol. 1992;47(4):511–21.
2. Stevens M. Broadmoor revealed: Victorian crime and the lunatic asylum. Barnsley: Pen and Sword Social History; 2013.
3. Coid JW. Dangerous patients with mental illness: increased risks warrant new policies, adequate resources, and appropriate legislation. BMJ. 1996;312(7036):965–6.

4. Monahan J, Steadman HJ. Crime and mental disorder: an epidemiological approach. Crime Justice. 1983;4:145–89.
5. Lindqvist P, Allebeck P. Schizophrenia and crime: a longitudinal follow-up of 644 schizophrenics in Stockholm. Br J Psychiatry. 1990;157(3):345–50.
6. Steadman HJ, Mulvey EP, Monahan J, Robbins PC, Appelbaum PS, Grisso T, et al. Violence by people discharged from acute psychiatric inpatient facilities and by others in the same neighborhoods. Arch Gen Psychiatry. 1998;55(5):393–401.
7. Torrey EF, Stanley J, Monahan J, Steadman HJ. The MacArthur violence risk assessment study revisited: two views ten years after its initial publication. Psychiatr Serv. 2008;59(2):147–52.
8. Seeman N, Tang S, Brown AD, Ing A. World survey of mental illness stigma. J Affect Disord. 2016;190:115–21.
9. Dean K, Laursen TM, Pedersen CB, Webb RT, Mortensen PB, Agerbo E. Risk of being subjected to crime, including violent crime, after onset of mental illness: a Danish national registry study using police data. JAMA Psychiat. 2018;75(7):689–96.
10. Torrey EF. Stigma and violence: isn't it time to connect the dots? Schizophr Bull. 2011;37(5):892–6.
11. Mullen PE. Facing up to unpalatable evidence for the sake of our patients. PLoS Med. 2009;6(8):e1000112.
12. Fazel S, Gulati G, Linsell L, Geddes JR, Grann M. Schizophrenia and violence: systematic review and meta-analysis. PLoS Med. 2009;6(8):e1000120.
13. The National Confidential Inquiry into Suicide and Safety in Mental Health. Annual report: England NI, Scotland, Wales. University of Manchester; 2018.
14. Stevens H, Laursen TM, Mortensen PB, Agerbo E, Dean K. Post-illness-onset risk of offending across the full spectrum of psychiatric disorders. Psychol Med. 2015;45(11):2447–57.
15. Fazel S, Wolf A, Palm C, Lichtenstein P. Violent crime, suicide, and premature mortality in patients with schizophrenia and related disorders: a 38-year total population study in Sweden. Lancet Psychiatry. 2014;1(1):44–54.
16. Winsper C, Ganapathy R, Marwaha S, Large M, Birchwood M, Singh SP. A systematic review and meta-regression analysis of aggression during the first episode of psychosis. Acta Psychiatr Scand. 2013;128(6):413–21.
17. Winsper C, Singh SP, Marwaha S, et al. Pathways to violent behavior during first-episode psychosis: a report from the UK national EDEN study. JAMA Psychiat. 2013;70(12):1287–93.
18. Brewer WJ, Lambert TJ, Witt K, Dileo J, Duff C, Crlenjak C, et al. Intensive case management for high-risk patients with first-episode psychosis: service model and outcomes. Lancet Psychiatry. 2015;2(1):29–37.
19. Webb RT, Lichtenstein P, Larsson H, Geddes JR, Fazel S. Suicide, hospital-presenting suicide attempts, and criminality in bipolar disorder: examination of risk for multiple adverse outcomes. J Clin Psychiatry. 2014;75(8):e809–16.
20. Fazel S, Lichtenstein P, Grann M, Goodwin GM, Langstrom N. Bipolar disorder and violent crime: new evidence from population-based longitudinal studies and systematic review. Arch Gen Psychiatry. 2010;67(9):931–8.
21. Fazel S, Lichtenstein P, Frisell T, Grann M, Goodwin G, Langstrom N. Bipolar disorder and violent crime: time at risk reanalysis. Arch Gen Psychiatry. 2010;67(12):1325–6.
22. Arseneault L, Moffitt TE, Caspi A, Taylor PJ, Silva PA. Mental disorders and violence in a total birth cohort: results from the Dunedin study. Arch Gen Psychiatry. 2000;57(10):979–86.
23. Monahan J. Reducing violence risk: diagnostically based clues from the MacArthur violent risk assessment study. In: Hodgins S, editor. Effective prevention of crime and violence among the mentally ill. Amsterdam: Kluwer; 2000. p. 19–34.
24. Goldstein RB, Dawson DA, Chou SP, Grant BF. Sex differences in prevalence and comorbidity of alcohol and drug use disorders: results from wave 2 of the National Epidemiologic Survey on Alcohol and Related Conditions. J Stud Alcohol Drugs. 2012;73(6):938–50.

25. Falk D, Yi HY, Hiller-Sturmhofel S. An epidemiologic analysis of co-occurring alcohol and drug use and disorders: findings from the National Epidemiologic Survey of Alcohol and Related Conditions (NESARC). Alcohol Res Health. 2008;31(2):100–10.
26. Boles SM, Miotto K. Substance abuse and violence: a review of the literature. Aggress Viol Behav. 2003;8(2):155–74.
27. Van Dorn R, Volavka J, Johnson N. Mental disorder and violence: is there a relationship beyond substance use? Soc Psychiatry Psychiatr Epidemiol. 2012;47(3):487–503.
28. Fazel S, Smith EN, Chang Z, Geddes JR. Risk factors for interpersonal violence: an umbrella review of meta-analyses. Br J Psychiatry. 2018;213(4):609–14.
29. Duke AA, Smith KM, Oberleitner LM, Westphal A, McKee SA. Alcohol, drugs, and violence: a meta-meta-analysis. Psychol Violence. 2018;8(2):238–49.
30. Boden JM, Fergusson DM, Horwood L. Alcohol misuse and violent behavior: findings from a 30-year longitudinal study. Drug Alcohol Depend. 2012;122(1–2):135–41.
31. Coker KL, Smith PH, Westphal A, Zonana HV, McKee SA. Crime and psychiatric disorders among youth in the US population: an analysis of the National Comorbidity Survey-Adolescent Supplement. J Am Acad Child Adolesc Psychiatry. 2014;53(8):888–98, 898.e1–2
32. Harford TC, Yi HY, Freeman RC. A typology of violence against self and others and its associations with drinking and other drug use among high school students in a U.S. general population survey. J Child Adolesc Subst Abuse. 2012;21(4):349–66.
33. McGinty EE, Choksy S, Wintemute GJ. The relationship between controlled substances and violence. Epidemiol Rev. 2016;38(1):5–31.
34. Lundholm L, Frisell T, Lichtenstein P, Langstrom N. Anabolic androgenic steroids and violent offending: confounding by polysubstance abuse among 10,365 general population men. Addiction. 2015;110(1):100–8.
35. van Amsterdam J, Brunt T, van den Brink W. The adverse health effects of synthetic cannabinoids with emphasis on psychosis-like effects. J Psychopharmacol. 2015;29(3):254–63.
36. Clayton HB, Lowry R, Ashley C, Wolkin A, Grant AM. Health risk behaviors with synthetic cannabinoids versus marijuana. Pediatrics. 2017;139(4):e20162675.
37. Moberg T, Stenbacka M, Tengstrom A, Jonsson EG, Nordstrom P, Jokinen J. Psychiatric and neurological disorders in late adolescence and risk of convictions for violent crime in men. BMC Psychiatry. 2015;15:299.
38. Yu R, Geddes JR, Fazel S. Personality disorders, violence, and antisocial behavior: a systematic review and meta-regression analysis. J Personal Disord. 2012;26(5):775–92.
39. Coid JW, Gonzalez R, Igoumenou A, Zhang T, Yang M, Bebbington P. Personality disorder and violence in the national household population of Britain. J Forens Psychiatry Psychol. 2017;28(5):620–38.
40. Allen A, Links PS. Aggression in borderline personality disorder: evidence for increased risk and clinical predictors. Curr Psychiatry Rep. 2012;14(1):62–9.
41. Gonzalez RA, Igoumenou A, Kallis C, Coid JW. Borderline personality disorder and violence in the UK population: categorical and dimensional trait assessment. BMC Psychiatry. 2016;16:180.
42. Fazel S, Doll H, Langstrom N. Mental disorders among adolescents in juvenile detention and correctional facilities: a systematic review and metaregression analysis of 25 surveys. J Am Acad Child Adolesc Psychiatry. 2008;47(9):1010–9.
43. Gaiffas A, Galera C, Mandon V, Bouvard MP. Attention-deficit/hyperactivity disorder in young French male prisoners. J Forensic Sci. 2014;59(4):1016–9.
44. Mohr-Jensen C, Steinhausen HC. A meta-analysis and systematic review of the risks associated with childhood attention-deficit hyperactivity disorder on long-term outcome of arrests, convictions, and incarcerations. Clin Psychol Rev. 2016;48:32–42.
45. Lundstrom S, Forsman M, Larsson H, Kerekes N, Serlachius E, Langstrom N, et al. Childhood neurodevelopmental disorders and violent criminality: a sibling control study. J Autism Dev Disord. 2014;44(11):2707–16.
46. King C, Murphy GH. A systematic review of people with autism spectrum disorder and the criminal justice system. J Autism Dev Disord. 2014;44(11):2717–33.

47. Heeramun R, Magnusson C, Gumpert CH, Granath S, Lundberg M, Dalman C, et al. Autism and convictions for violent crimes: population-based cohort study in Sweden. J Am Acad Child Adolesc Psychiatry. 2017;56(6):491–7.e2.
48. Witt K, van Dorn R, Fazel S. Risk factors for violence in psychosis: systematic review and meta-regression analysis of 110 studies. PLoS One. 2013;8(2):e55942.
49. Large MM, Nielssen O. Violence in first-episode psychosis: a systematic review and meta-analysis. Schizophr Res. 2011;125(2–3):209–20.
50. Swanson JW, Swartz MS, Van Dorn RA, Elbogen EB, Wagner HR, Rosenheck RA, et al. A national study of violent behavior in persons with schizophrenia. Arch Gen Psychiatry. 2006;63(5):490–9.
51. Coid JW, Kallis C, Doyle M, Shaw J, Ullrich S. Shifts in positive and negative psychotic symptoms and anger: effects on violence. Psychol Med. 2018;48(14):2428–38.
52. McNiel DE, Eisner JP, Binder RL. The relationship between command hallucinations and violence. Psychiatr Serv. 2000;51(10):1288–92.
53. Link B, Stueve A, Phelan J. Psychotic symptoms and violent behaviours: probing the components of "threat/control-override" symptoms. J Soc Psychiatry Psychiatr Epidemiol. 1998;33(Suppl 1):S55.
54. Ullrich S, Keers R, Coid JW. Delusions, anger, and serious violence: new findings from the MacArthur violence risk assessment study. Schizophr Bull. 2014;40(5):1174–81.
55. Coid JW, Ullrich S, Kallis C, Keers R, Barker D, Cowden F, et al. The relationship between delusions and violence: findings from the East London first episode psychosis study. JAMA Psychiat. 2013;70(5):465–71.
56. Jennings WG, Piquero AR, Reingle JM. On the overlap between victimization and offending: a review of the literature. Aggress Violent Behav. 2012;17(1):16–26.
57. Silver E. Mental disorder and violent victimization: the mediating role of involvement in conflicted social relationships. Criminology. 2002;40(1):191–212.
58. Yu R, Branje S, Meeus W, Koot HM, van Lier P, Fazel S. Victimization mediates the longitudinal association between depressive symptoms and violent behaviors in adolescence. J Abnorm Child Psychol. 2018;46(4):839–48.
59. Sariaslan A, Lichtenstein P, Larsson H, Fazel S. Triggers for violent criminality in patients with psychotic disorders. JAMA Psychiat. 2016;73(8):796–803.
60. Fazel S, Wolf A, Larsson H, Lichtenstein P, Mallett S, Fanshawe TR. Identification of low risk of violent crime in severe mental illness with a clinical prediction tool (Oxford Mental Illness and Violence tool [OxMIV]): a derivation and validation study. Lancet Psychiatry. 2017;4(6):461–8.
61. American Psychiatric Association (APA). Practice guideline for the treatment of patients with bipolar disorder. 2nd ed. Washington, DC: American Psychiatric Association Publishing; 2010.
62. National Institute for Health and Care Excellence. Psychosis and schizophrenia in adults: prevention and management [CG178]. London: NICE; 2014.
63. American Psychiatric Association (APA). Practice guideline for the treatment of patients with major depressive disorder. 3rd ed. Washington, DC: American Psychiatric Association Publishing; 2010.
64. Fazel S, Lichtenstein P, Grann M, Långström N. Risk of violent crime in individuals with epilepsy and traumatic brain injury: a 35-year Swedish population study. PLoS Med. 2011;8(12):e1001150.
65. Molero Y, Zetterqvist J, Binswanger IA, Hellner C, Larsson H, Fazel S. Medications for alcohol and opioid use disorders and risk of suicidal behavior, accidental overdoses, and crime. Am J Psychiatry. 2018;175(10):970–8.
66. Chang Z, Lichtenstein P, Långström N, Larsson H, Fazel S. Association between prescription of major psychotropic medications and violent reoffending after prison release. JAMA. 2016;316(17):1798–807.
67. Fazel S, Zetterqvist J, Larsson H, Långström N, Lichtenstein P. Antipsychotics, mood stabilisers, and risk of violent crime. Lancet. 2014;384(9949):1206–14.

68. Frogley C, Taylor D, Dickens G, Picchioni M. A systematic review of the evidence of clozapine's anti-aggressive effects. Int J Neuropsychopharmacol. 2012;15(9):1351–71.
69. Bhavsar V, Kosidou K, Widman L, Orsini N, Hodsoll J, Dalman C, et al. Clozapine treatment and offending: a within-subject study of patients with psychotic disorders in Sweden. Schizophr Bull. 2019; https://doi.org/10.1093/schbul/sbz055.
70. Wolf A, Whiting D, Fazel S. Violence prevention in psychiatry: an umbrella review of interventions in general and forensic psychiatry. J Forens Psychiatry Psychol. 2017;28(5):659–73.
71. Singh JP, Serper M, Reinharth J, Fazel S. Structured assessment of violence risk in schizophrenia and other psychiatric disorders: a systematic review of the validity, reliability, and item content of 10 available instruments. Schizophr Bull. 2011;37(5):899–912.
72. Fazel S, Singh JP, Doll H, Grann M. Use of risk assessment instruments to predict violence and antisocial behaviour in 73 samples involving 24 827 people: systematic review and meta-analysis. BMJ. 2012;345:e4692.
73. The Topol Review. Preparing the healthcare workforce to deliver the digital future. Health Education England; 2019.
74. Berman NC, Stark A, Cooperman A, Wilhelm S, Cohen IG. Effect of patient and therapist factors on suicide risk assessment. Death Stud. 2015;39(7):433–41.

Part II

Risk Factors, Phenomenology and Characteristics of Violence in Mental Disorders

Violence in Major Mental Disorders

4

Mario Amore, Andrea Aguglia, Francesca Santi, and Gianluca Serafini

4.1 The Relationship Between Violence and Mental Illness: A Historical Perspective

The relationship between mental illness and violence is characterized by the difficult legacy of the past that linked these two terms in a traditional binomial that, even today, struggles to be split.

The association between mental illness and aggressive behavior had already been hypothesized in the classical era and Socrates first suggested that violent episodes were rare in Athens due to his healthy population [1]. Plato, a noted disciple of Socrates, considered mental illness as an insidious disease for both patients and society as subjects affected by psychiatric conditions may compromise the public order exposing citizens to danger as well as committing crimes. Therefore, Plato encouraged clinicians to collaborate with law in order to treat predisposed individuals in terms of physical and spiritual aspects. Those who did not have these risk factors had left to die. In order to guarantee citizens safety, Plato proposed the detention of psychiatric patients at their home. Those who showed an altered mental status were not allowed to move freely around the city. Family members were obliged to keep psychiatric patients at home; otherwise they had to pay a fine [2].

The relationship between psychopathology and violence raises several questions which involve philosophical, juridical, ethical, and institutional aspects as well as the scientific one. Indeed in a historical perspective, the relation between criminal behaviors and mental illness suggests the need to carefully verify the presence of a mental disorder in offenders.

M. Amore (✉) · A. Aguglia · F. Santi · G. Serafini
Department of Neuroscience, Rehabilitation, Ophthalmology, Genetics, Maternal and Child Health, Section of Psychiatry, University of Genoa, Genoa, Italy

IRCCS Ospedale Policlinico San Martino, Genoa, Italy
e-mail: mario.amore@unige.it; andrea.aguglia@hsanmartino.it; gianluca.serafini@unige.it

© Springer Nature Switzerland AG 2020
B. Carpiniello et al. (eds.), *Violence and Mental Disorders*, Comprehensive Approach to Psychiatry 1, https://doi.org/10.1007/978-3-030-33188-7_4

The stereotypical belief of violence associated with mental illness seems very present in general population as well [3]. The acute clinical presentation of major mental disorders, as schizophrenia and bipolar disorder (BD), provokes anxiety and fear in the healthy subjects and increases the request of restraining interventions for the altered behaviors.

The stigma against psychiatric patients as well as the mental hospital treatment at least until the middle of the twentieth century may be explained by a firmly rooted cultural and social heritage. However, literature reports that psychiatric patients do not usually commit violence, but they suffer from it as they are not correctly believed and discredited [4].

Since 1950, the cultural and social evolution as well as the development of novel and more effective pharmacological treatments changed the goal of psychiatric treatment from restrain to health and rehabilitation. This new belief led, through pilot experiences in the 1960s and 1970s, both to the end of the madhouse in Italy and to the emergence of new community psychiatric services.

4.2   First Studies on Violent Behaviors and Mental Illness: A Significant Correlation with Bipolar Disorder and Schizophrenia

Since the mid-nineteenth century, the relationship between mental illness and violent behaviors has been investigated thoroughly [5]. In 1922, Ashley reported a prevalence of imprisonment of approximately 1.7%, in 700 psychiatric patients that have been followed for 3 months after discharge [6]. In 1938, a study of patients paroled from all New York State hospitals showed a lower probability to be arrested of these subjects when compared to healthy controls [7].

These findings were confirmed by either clinical or epidemiological studies carried out between the 1940s and the 1970s [8–14], showing a reduced association between mental illness and higher risk of violence.

Taylor and Gunn in England and Gottlieb and colleagues in Denmark, respectively, were the first to find an association between specific psychiatric disorders and violent behaviors (particularly murder), emphasizing the importance of psychotic symptoms as most relevant risk factors associated with violence [15, 16].

Furthermore, Beck highlighted that delusional thoughts in schizophrenic patients were often considered as an important risk factor for violent behaviors and that their "dangerousness" could be contained by appropriate pharmacological treatment as antipsychotic medications [17]. This hypothesis was confirmed by a revision on homicides committed during psychotic illness in New South Wales from 1993 to 2002. The authors showed that more severe violent behaviors were usually associated with frightening or distressing persecutory delusional beliefs, typically associated with schizophrenia-related psychosis than mania [18]. An Italian study showed that physical aggression during hospitalization in a psychiatric ward was correlated with more severe levels of thought disorders and that higher levels of hostility were also predictive of a worsening of violent behavior [19], whereas other authors underlined the importance of number of admissions in an emergency psychiatric ward as clinical variable associated with recurrent violent behaviors in a sample of 678 outpatients [20]. Lastly, considering the frequent correlation between gun violence and mental illness, paranoid, depressive, and grandiose personality features were represented in several mass murders, even if these events were rare, accounting for less than 1% of a total of homicides [21].

Swanson and coworkers [22], evaluating data from the National Institute of Mental Health's Epidemiologic Catchment Area project, found that the prevalence of affective disorders was three times higher among respondents who were violent than those who were not. The same was true for schizophrenia or schizophreniform disorder. Recent studies conducted using the Swedish National Criminal Registry on the whole population have also highlighted important differences in terms of crime rates which were doubled in patients with schizophrenia than subjects with other diagnoses [23, 24].

Hodgins pointed out the role of gender on violent behaviors. He showed that males with major psychiatric disorders were 2.5 times more likely than males with no disorders or handicap to be registered for criminal offenses and 4 times more likely to be registered for a violent offense. Females with major disorders were 5 times more likely than females with no disorders or handicap to be registered for an offense and 27 times more likely to be registered for a violent offense [25].

The increased rate of violent offenses among recovered psychiatric patients compared to healthy control group (400 adults who lived in the same social context) emphasized the potential to explain this phenomenon as an artifact [26].

Indeed, the pathogenesis of violent behavior is caused by the combination of both static and dynamic related factors, which are closely correlated. In fact, several studies showed that family and social factors (e.g., abuse and emotional neglect, parental conflict, social support, socioeconomic status) during childhood and adolescence have a negative impact on the tendency to manifest violent behavior in adulthood. Additionally, a history of child maltreatment, particularly sexual trauma, has been related to the increased risk of suicide attempts, self-harm, and interpersonal violence [27–29].

The potential bias of the selected samples, different evaluation instruments, or confounding clinical factors such as psychiatric comorbidity, substance use, or presence of cognitive dysfunctions should be carefully considered in studies evaluating the presence of violence in psychiatric patients or the existence of mental disorder in violent offenses. The different and heterogeneous methodology of clinical studies should help the readers in careful interpretation of the findings, above all for the growing stigma on psychiatric patients.

In conclusion, although controversial, the association between increased risk of violent behavior and mental disorders has been documented by numerous epidemiological [22, 30, 31] and clinical [32, 33] studies where the risk of violence seems to be higher among inpatients and those with more severe disorders such as schizophrenia and BD.

4.3 The Impact of Violence and Aggression in Schizophrenia

Aggressive and violent behaviors are socially widespread whereas in patients affected by severe mental illnesses the nature of the association between violence and major psychiatric conditions tends to be overrepresented, is generally complex to explain, and is often linked to other clinical features such as impulsivity, irritability, and hostility. The relationship between psychiatric disorders and aggressive/violent behaviors has been investigated by both clinicians and researchers for many years [31], with several determinants which have been associated with aggression [34].

A definition of altered behaviors is needed due to the existence of different meanings; thus, the need to ameliorate the understanding among the general readership is needed. *Impulsivity* is a tendency to act on a whim, displaying behaviors which are characterized by little or no forethought, reflection, or consideration of the consequences. Impulsive actions are typically "poorly conceived, prematurely expressed, unduly risky, or inappropriate to the situation that often result in undesirable consequences. *Aggressive behavior* could be overt or covert, often harmful, usually social interactions with the intention of inflicting damage or other unpleasantness toward another individual. It may occur either reactively or without provocation. Human aggression may be classified into direct and indirect aggression; while the former is characterized by physical or verbal behavior intended to cause harm to someone, the latter is characterized by behaviors intended to harm the social relations of an individual or a group. *Violence* is defined as the use of physical force to injure, abuse, damage, or destroy. The World Health Organization (WHO) provides a less conventional definition of violence as follows: "the intentional use of physical force or power, threatened or actual, against oneself, another person, or against a group or community, which either results in or has a high likelihood of resulting in injury, death, psychological harm, maldevelopment, or deprivation." These altered behaviors represent a major concern in the clinical practice for patients with schizophrenia and other major psychoses.

Aggression in major psychoses and, in particular, schizophrenia has been widely investigated referring to several theoretical frameworks and providing different perspectives about the characterization of violent behavior in these patients. Aggression in schizophrenia is really a heterogeneous and manifold construct associated with psychological interactions. Recent brain imaging techniques focused on the existence of both structural and functional alterations of the brain underlying aggressive behavior aiming to better differentiate schizophrenia subtypes and improve long-term outcomes related to this disabling condition [35]. Evidence documented that, when compared with the general population, schizophrenia and major psychotic disorders are linked to increased risk of violent and aggressive behavior [36–38] but there is also a common stigmatizing prejudice that most or all schizophrenic patients are potentially dangerous and that their behavior may be largely unpredictable [39]. Many studies addressed the increased risk (approximately 49–68%) of violent behavior in schizophrenia when compared to the general population [36, 40, 41] but patients with schizophrenia may be even at enhanced risk of being victims of violence [42]. Violent behavior in schizophrenia is usually associated with a chronic course, altered quality of life, and impaired social and professional rehabilitation. Violent and persistent aggressive behavior in schizophrenia represents a therapeutic challenge in the clinical practice requiring novel and multifaceted interventions aimed to prevent recurrence and psychosocial impairments in schizophrenia population.

4.3.1 Epidemiology of Violence and Aggression in Schizophrenia Patients

There are multiple evidences about the prevalence of aggressive behavior in schizophrenic hospitalized patients; however, studies about this topic may be biased due to the different definitions of aggression, variable study aims and designs, settings, methods, and selection of samples, but even the variable length of follow-up making comparisons and drawing general conclusions difficult [43]. Unfortunately, most studies are single center in nature, conducted on a single ward, and may not be generalized to the whole psychiatric population.

Studies in European countries reported that the prevalence of aggression and violence in schizophrenia is approximately 10%. Specifically, an Italian study reported a prevalence of 7.5% regarding aggression in an acute psychiatric unit [44] with a similar prevalence (7.7%) which has been documented by another report in a German psychiatric hospital [45]. Higher prevalence rates are usually reported in non-European countries. In particular, a prevalence ranging from 11.3% to 15% has also been found in Australian and New Zealand hospitalized patients [46, 47], while the 6-month prevalence of any violent behavior in schizophrenia patients was 19.1% according to a US national community-based study [33]. In addition, based on a Chinese meta-analysis including 3941 schizophrenic patients, the prevalence of aggressive behavior in psychiatric wards ranged between 15.3% and 53.2% with the pooled prevalence of aggression which resulted to be 35.4% (95% CI: 29.7%, 41.4%) [48]. The authors reported that the most commonly reported significant risk factors for aggression were hostility or suspiciousness (78.9%); delusions (63.2%); past history of aggression (42.1%); disorganized behavior (26.3%); auditory hallucinations (10.5%); and involuntary admission (10.5%). Furthermore, there is a study conducted in Bahrain that reported a lower (4.4%) prevalence rate of aggression/violence in a sample of schizophrenic inpatients [49]. Factors like severity of psychotic symptoms, substance abuse, and specific sociodemographic variables (e.g., male gender, younger age) together with depression and impulsivity, antisocial personality traits, neurocognitive impairments, and involuntary admission have been all linked to aggression among inpatients with schizophrenia [45, 50–53].

4.3.2 General Risk Factors for Violence in Schizophrenia

Generally, risk factors for schizophrenia may be divided into individual biologically determined (e.g., genetic polymorphisms-COMT valine allele, DRD2 (rs1076560)1, and AKT1 (rs2494732)), environmental factors such as being the victim of physical or sexual abuse in childhood and/or adulthood, and familial (genetic and/or early environmental) risk factors. Sociodemographic (e.g., male gender, young age, stressful life events, and socioeconomic difficulties), clinical (e.g., positive psychotic symptoms such as persecutory delusions, auditory command hallucinations, and disorganization, but even subjective experiences of dissociation, impulsivity, anger, substance abuse with particular regard to alcohol and cannabis misuse, and positive history of psychiatric disorders), neurobiological (e.g., dysfunctional frontotemporal circuitry, neuroanatomical brain loss in orbitofrontal and ventrolateral prefrontal regions), and neurocognitive characteristics (e.g., executive and working memory impairments, impaired decision-making and altered problem-solving abilities, dysregulated emotional control and evaluation, difficulty in accurately recognizing emotions in the faces of others, and cognitive inflexibility) have all been identified as possible predictors of aggressive behavior in major psychoses being able to enhance the risk of committing a violent act [54]. There are either static (or historical) risk factors such as the personal history of violence, in particular criminal attitudes, developmental trauma, and former repeated exposure to violence which are unchangeable and essentially the same for ordinary individuals or dynamic risk factors such as substance-abuse comorbidity and poor treatment adherence that are usually associated with the lack of clinical insight and illness awareness [55] and may be recognized as significant predictors of violence in schizophrenia [56].

Moreover, the prevalence of violent behavior in patients with first episode of psychosis, in particular schizophrenia, is higher than that in samples of patients with different stages of the illness. Látalová reported that first-episode psychosis is associated with an increased risk of homicide with a limited effect of duration of untreated psychosis length on severe violent or aggressive behaviors [57]. Clinicians should closely monitor patients before the onset of first psychotic episode which is frequently associated with a violent behavior. In these patients, substance use [57, 58] but even comorbid personality disorders such as borderline personality disorder sharing with schizophrenia the tendency to impulsiveness, and impulsive behavior, including impulsive aggression may be considered a further additional risk factor for violence [59].

Importantly, nonadherence with antipsychotic medications remains the most relevant critical issue associated with the management of schizophrenia and other major psychoses. Nonadherence in the first year after hospitalization was associated with a higher likelihood of rehospitalizations, dramatic use of psychiatric emergency services, and substance use in the following 2 years [60]. Importantly, relapse after discontinuation of antipsychotic medications is associated with a reduction of treatment response contributing to unfavorable course and outcome of schizophrenia and major psychoses as well as a negative impact on patients, careers, health system, and the whole community, respectively.

Finally, all the mentioned risk factors have been substantially confirmed by a systematic review and meta-regression analysis including 110 studies and 45,533 analyzed individuals (87.8% diagnosed with schizophrenia, 11.8% with other psychoses, and a small percentage (0.4%) with BD), which has been conducted by Witt and colleagues [34]. Overall, the authors reported that 8439 (18.5%) patients manifested violent behaviors. This study clearly documented that schizophrenic patients with specific dynamic (or modifiable) risk factors such as hostile behavior, recent substance (in particular, alcohol) and drug misuse, nonadherence with psychological treatments and medications, and higher poor impulsivity but even specific static risk factors such as the positive history of criminal behavior were more likely to exhibit violent behaviors than other individuals. Importantly, when schizophrenia outcomes were restricted to severe violence, the mentioned associations did not significantly change.

4.4 Aggressive and Violent Behaviors in Patients with Bipolar Disorder

The existing literature suggests that patients with BD are associated with a higher prevalence of aggressive and violent behaviors. Furthermore, bipolar patients display more lifetime aggressive behaviors in both adolescence (aggression may be considered as a possible risk factor for BD onset) and adulthood while treated compared to inpatients with other psychiatric disorders. Moreover, the rate of violent crime in bipolar patients is higher than that of both unipolar depression and general population, leading to severe worsening and disruption of occupational, social, and familial functioning [61–65]. A Danish birth cohort study found that bipolar patients of male gender were twice as likely, and bipolar patients of female gender four times as likely, to be convicted of a violent offense compared to the general population [66]. Inpatient aggression not only exposes patients and staff to potential harm, but it also leads to apprehension toward aggressive patients that may reduce staff-patient contact, enhance the risk of complications, and prolong lengths of stay.

To estimate the aggressive and violent behaviors in bipolar patients, several epidemiological and clinical studies may be found in the current literature. In the NESARC community-based representative sample, 25.3% of those with BD I and 13.6% of those with BD II reported aggressive behaviors after age 15 compared to 1% of the general population [63]; in addition, rates of violence among those with BD were 5.9 times the rate of the general population [67]. The National Comorbidity Survey showed that the 12-month adult population prevalence of violent behaviors was 1–2%, which increases up to 16% if bipolar patients were considered, a rate that was eightfold higher than that which was found among healthy subjects [61]. In addition, when compared to the general population, bipolar patients are convicted for violent offenses up to four times more [68, 69]. Lastly, several studies were conducted to evaluate aggressive behaviors in bipolar patients around the world, ranging from nearly 22.2% to 32.4% [70–73].

4.4.1 Trait-Related Factors in Patients with Bipolar Disorder

Aggressive and violent behaviors in BD occur not only during manic and mixed episodes, but also in the remission phase, but unsolved questions persist regarding trait vs. state-related factors [74]. So, the most accredited hypothesis to explain aggressive and violent behavioral phenotypes in patients with BD is that environmental factors such as substance use and/or comorbid cluster B personality disorders, but even childhood trauma or poor coping strategies, as well as the characteristic state of mood (particularly manic and mixed episodes) may act as important triggers according to a well-determined biological vulnerability during the longitudinal developmental trajectory specifically from toddlerhood to adolescence.

Thus, the predisposing biological vulnerability in bipolar patients is confirmed by the presence of higher prevalence of aggressive and violent behaviors in these patients than subjects with other diagnoses by the three following studies. The first is a linkage analysis showing a suggestive linkage on chromosomal regions 1p21.1, 6p21.3, and 8q21.13 [75]; the second is a genome-wide association reporting the existence of rs17190927 in the SPTLC3 gene [76]; the latter is a gene expression study where three TNF are inversely while one TNF gene (TNFAIP3) is positively correlated with aggressive behaviors [77].

Furthermore, existing data showed a higher likelihood of impulsive, aggressive, and violent behaviors in bipolar patients even during the euthymic phase, in the absence of any current affective recurrences, when compared with patients with other diagnoses.

This could be explained by the well-known correlation between aggressive behaviors and serotonin that plays, in the central nervous system, a role in the suppression of impulsive behaviors eventually leading to aggressive behavior and suicide [78]. Serotoninergic abnormalities within prefrontal cortex (PFC)-amygdala circuits are thought to underlie several psychiatric disorders characterized by emotional dysregulation [79]. A study reported that an acute tryptophan depletion significantly modulated the connectivity between the amygdala and two prefrontal cortex regions (e.g., ventral anterior cingulate cortex and ventrolateral prefrontal cortex) [80]. Therefore, a significant role is attributed to the serotonin transporter, a key regulator of central serotonergic activity. In a recent study, Chou and coworkers recruited euthymic bipolar II patients and healthy controls and found no statistical difference with regard to serotonin transporter (SERT) availability but a significant correlation between SERT availability and total Overt Aggression Scale mean scores was reported. This study supports the idea that aggression might be a trait marker for BD [81]; this assumption was also confirmed by a meta-analysis where impulsivity levels were showed significantly higher in remitted patients with BD when compared to healthy individuals [82].

4.4.2 State-Related Factors in Patients with Bipolar Disorder

It has been hypothesized that other clinical factors (such as borderline personality disorder or cognitive dysfunctions or specific affective temperaments) might participate in this altered behavior. Carpiniello and coworkers found that the comorbidity with borderline personality disorder was also associated with higher impulsiveness and aggressiveness in euthymic patients with BD. Furthermore, the rate of attempted suicides was approximately three times higher in BD/borderline personality disorder patients and 7.6 times higher than BD/other personality disorder with respect to BD, respectively [74]. It is well known that remitted bipolar patients showed a significant worsening of cognitive functions, in particular in executive domain, verbal and visual memory, psychomotor speed, verbal fluency, and sustained attention [83, 84] with a negative impact on general functioning and behavior [85]. It is also possible that a neuropsychological dysfunction, plus the elevated trait hostility and impulsivity mentioned before, represents a predisposing factor for aggressive behaviors in bipolar patients. The prominent cyclothymic temperament has been hypothesized as a further clinical predisposing factor related to non-motor aggressive behavior in euthymic bipolar patients relative to patients with prominent hyperthymic temperament. Therefore, the authors suggested that anger and hostility might be considered as stable personological traits that endure even in remission enhancing the risk for violent behavior [86]. Lastly, a study on 58 remitted patients with BD I focused on predictive factors of sustained anger and aggressive behavior, considering three trait domains that have been shown to be elevated in BD (e.g., approach motivation, dominance-related constructs, and emotion-relevant impulsivity; the latter was related to anger, hostility, verbal and physical aggression) [87]. The authors found that, during remission, personality traits are more informative than other clinical characteristics and trauma exposure in order to understand the sources of anger and aggression among persons with BD.

To be clear, anger and aggression levels are exacerbated by symptoms within BD. Excessive anger is a cardinal DSM-5 symptom of mania and anger is a prominent manic symptom in adults. Thus, the state-related factors in mood disorders, particularly BD, should be carefully considered and are suggested by clinical observations during hospitalization in emergency psychiatric wards as well as immediately prior to.

Dervic and coworkers focused their attention on the differences among BD I and II, and unipolar depression in terms of impulsivity/aggression traits during a major depressive episode (MDE). The authors reported a higher lifetime impulsivity, aggression, and hostility scores in bipolar I and II depressed individuals. In particular, bipolar I patients had more trait impulsivity and lifetime aggression than bipolar II patients, whereas the latter had more hostility than patients with BD I [88]. These data were confirmed recently in the BRIDGE-II-MIX study, in which the authors underlined the importance of the detection of aggressive behaviors even during a MDE in a large sample ($N = 2811$). When the authors compared MDE patients with and without aggressiveness, they reported a significant association between the presence of aggressive behaviors and severity of (hypo)manic symptoms, presence of psychotic symptoms, diagnosis of BD, and comorbid borderline personality disorder but not substance abuse (although patients with MDE and aggressiveness reported recurrent alcohol and substance-related legal problems). Lastly, the authors found mixed features, according to DSM-5 diagnostic criteria, as the most important clinical variable predicting aggressive behaviors [89]. Therefore, these altered behaviors are not a rare clinical condition during MDE, and they may be particularly associated to mixed features and diagnosis of bipolar spectrum disorders.

Previous studies described how manic patients may display high levels of violence during the first days of hospitalization as well as the 2 weeks prior to admission in the community. Among clinical predictors, the authors identified involuntary admission, positive psychotic symptoms, and lack of insight. Their prevalence of violence tended to reduce in the subsequent post-admission period after receiving adequate pharmacological treatment [46, 70, 90–92]. Belete and coworkers evaluated the presence of aggressive behavior, using the Modified Overt Aggression Scale (MOAS), in a sample of 411 bipolar patients, reporting a prevalence of 29.4%. They found a significant association with previous history of aggression, presence of psychotic/manic symptoms, poor medication adherence, and social support [93]. These data were confirmed recently on a large sample of patients who were evaluated at the emergency psychiatric unit ($N = 3322$ patients). In this study, the authors reported a twofold higher risk of aggressive behaviors in bipolar patients when compared to unipolar depression. Furthermore, the authors found that a recent mixed and manic episode conferred an odds ratio of affective recurrence of 4.3 and 2.2, compared to unipolar depression, respectively [94].

More recently, it has been reported that the risk of aggressive and violence behaviors is higher not only during acute manic or mixed episode in bipolar patients, in particular when they are restrained on their behaviors in inpatients setting, but even when a comorbidity with substance-use disorders or cluster B personality disorder occurs [23, 59, 93, 95–97]. This risk even leads to have, as remarked by Verdolini et al. [89], more likely a criminal record and history of incarceration compared to other patients. As a matter of fact, some authors conducted a systematic review on the correlation between BD and violent crime, showing an increased risk for violent crime in bipolar patients compared to the general population due to substance use rather than clinical mood state [98]. This result was confirmed in two additional clinical studies on subjects with BD I and II ($n = 255$), other psychopathology ($n = 85$), and healthy controls ($n = 84$), concluding that bipolar patients showed the highest aggressive score compared to other subgroups, depending on current mood episode and psychotic features without any influence of BD subtype, severity or polarity of the current episode, and current pharmacological treatments [95, 96]. Moreover, Alniak and coworkers conducted a specific study on the impact of substance use in 100 male inpatients with BD I, who were experiencing a current mood episode, evaluating in this sample the impact of violent behaviors defined as physical aggression against others. The authors affirmed the importance of the current substance-use disorder (the most commonly abused substances were cannabis and alcohol, followed by synthetic cannabinoids), being associated with a threefold increase in violent behavior but even with the previous history of violent behavior [97].

The aggressive and violent behavior has also been reported on 216 first-psychotic-episode subjects diagnosed as BD I. The authors identified as predictors of violence as well as alcohol abuse and initial manic episode, recent suicide attempts and learning disability, putting the previous existing data literature in agreement. Therefore, these results encourage the early detection and closer management of patients with alcohol use, suicide behavior, manic symptoms, and learning problems in bipolar I patients [99]. Lastly, histories of childhood trauma may be considered as potential risk factors for affect dysregulation in pediatric and adulthood BD. A study on 59 pediatric bipolar patients showed that male gender and childhood trauma were strong determinants of irritability and aggressive/violent behavior against property and people is particularly enhanced in those with a history of emotional and sexual abuse [100].

Thus, some findings are in contrast, presumably due to the different study design, presence of other psychiatric conditions, and inclusion of forensic or inpatient populations that do not allow the generalizability of results. Another possible explanation is that most of these studies did not separate specific diagnostic subgroups of patients with BD I and II or did not account for the differential presence of comorbidity, substance abuse, suicide, or personality disorders.

4.5 Conclusion

A risk assessment of potential aggression and/or violence is crucial for clinicians when evaluating psychiatric patients in both outpatient and inpatient settings, in particular when the patient has a primary diagnosis of major mental illnesses such as schizophrenia and BD. When considering strategies to decrease these risk factors that may contribute to enhance future violence, clinicians should distinguish static from dynamic risk factors. Static factors include trait-related factors (biological vulnerability, serotonin transporter availability, cognitive dysfunctions) together with a past history of violence. Dynamic factors are subject to change with interventions and include access to weapons, acute psychotic symptoms, current substance use, a person's living setting, and mood affective recurrences in particular manic and mixed episodes.

Clinicians should organize a clinical chart that underlines known risk factors, and management and treatment strategies, in order to address dynamic risk factors. This approach will assist in the development of an aggression or violence prevention plan allowing the recognition of personalized risk factors for each patient [101].

References

1. Asnis GM, Kaplan ML. Violence and homicidal behaviors in psychiatric disorders. Psychiatric Clin North Am. 1997;20(2):405–25.
2. Platone. Politeia, III, 410 a 1. In: Turolla E, editor. I Dialoghi etc. Milano: Rizzoli; 1964, vol II. p. 185.
3. Crisp A, Gelder M, Goddard E, Meltzer H. Stigmatization of people with mental illnesses: a follow-up study within the Changing Minds campaign of the Royal College of Psychiatrists. World Psychiatry. 2005;4:106–13.
4. Pettit B, Greenhead S, Khalifeh H, Drennan V, Hart TC, Hogg J, et al. At risk, yet dismissed: the criminal victimisation of people with mental health problems. London: Mind; 2013.
5. Gray JP. Homicide in insanity. Am J Insanity. 1857;14:119–43.
6. Ashley M. Outcome of 1.000 cases paroled from the Middletown. State Hospital Quarterly. 1922;8:64–70.

7. Pollock HH. Is the paroled patient a threat to the community? Psychiatry Q. 1938;12:236–44.
8. Cohen L, Freeman H. How dangerous to the community are state hospital patients? Conn State Med J. 1945;9:697–700.
9. Brill H, Malzberg B. Statistical report based on the arrest records of 5.346 male ex-patients released from N.Y. State Mental Hospitals during the period 1946–1948. Washington, DC: American Psychiatric Association. (Mental Hospital Service Supplement 153); 1962.
10. Morrow WR, Peterson DB. Follow-up of discharged offenders "not guilty by reason of insanity" and "Criminal sexual psychopaths". J Crim Law Criminol Pol Sci. 1966;57(1):31–4.
11. Rubin B. Prediction of dangerousness in mentally ill criminals. Arch Gen Psychiatry. 1972;27(3):397–407.
12. Häfner H, Böker W. Violent acts of mental patients. A psychiatric-epidemiologic study in the German Federal Republic. Fortschr Med. 1974;92(2):50–4.
13. Guze SB, Woodruff RA Jr, Clayton PJ. Psychiatric disorders and criminality. JAMA. 1974;227(6):641–2.
14. Steadman HJ, Cocozza JJ. Psychiatry, dangerousness and the repetitively violent offender. J Crim Law Criminol. 1978;69(2):226–31.
15. Taylor PJ, Gunn J. Violence and psychosis. I. Risk of violence among psychotic men. Br Med J. 1984;288(6435):1945–9.
16. Gottlieb P, Gabrielsen G, Kramp P. Psychotic homicides in Copenhagen from 1959 to 1983. Acta Psychiatr Scand. 1987;76(3):285–92.
17. Beck JL. Mental illness and violent acts protecting the patient and public. Paper presented at the annual meeting of the American Psychiatric Association, Toronto, Ontario; 1998.
18. Nielssen OB, Westmore BD, Large MM, Hayes RA. Homicide during psychotic illness in New South Wales between 1993 and 2002. Med J Aust. 2007;186:301–4.
19. Amore M, Menchetti M, Tonti C, Scarlatti F. Predictors of violent behavior among acute psychiatric patients: clinical study. Psychiatry Clin Neurosci. 2008;62(3):247–55. https://doi.org/10.1111/j.1440-1819.2008.01790.x.
20. Pinna F, Tusconi M, Dessì C, Pittaluga G, Fiorillo A, Carpiniello B. Violence and mental disorders. A retrospective study of people in charge of a community mental health center. Int J Law Psychiatry. 2016;47:122–8. https://doi.org/10.1016/j.ijlp.2016.02.015.
21. Gold LH, Simon RI, editors. Gun violence and mental illness. Arlington, VA: American Psychiatric Association; 2016.
22. Swanson JW, Holzer CE 3rd, Ganju VK, Jono RT. Violence and psychiatric disorder in the community: evidence from the Epidemiologic Catchment Area surveys. Hosp Community Psychiatry. 1990;41:761–70.
23. Fazel S, Lichtenstein P, Frisell T, Grann M, Goodwin G, Långström N. Bipolar disorder and violent crime: time at risk reanalysis. Arch Gen Psychiatry. 2010a;67:1325–6. https://doi.org/10.1001/archgenpsychiatry.2010.171.
24. Fazel S, Wolf A, Chang Z, Larsson H, Goodwin GM, Lichtenstein P. Depression and violence: a Swedish total population study. Lancet Psychiatry. 2015;2:224–32. https://doi.org/10.1016/S2215-0366(14)00128-X.
25. Hodgins S. Mental disorder, intellectual deficiency, and crime. Evidence from a birth cohort. Arch Gen Psychiatry. 1992;49(6):476–83.
26. Link BG, Andrews HA, Cullen FT. The violent and illegal behavior of mental patients reconsidered. Am Soc Rev. 1992;57(3):275–92.
27. Leyton M. Are people with psychiatric disorders violent? J Psychiatry Neurosci. 2018;43(4):220–2. https://doi.org/10.1503/jpn.180058.
28. McMahon K, Hoertel N, Olfson M, Wall M, Wang S, Blanco C. Childhood maltreatment and impulsivity as predictors of interpersonal violence, self-injury and suicide attempts: a national study. Psychiatry Res. 2018;269:386–93. https://doi.org/10.1016/j.psychres.2018.08.059.
29. Gawęda L, Pionke R, Krężolek M, Frydecka D, Nelson B, Cechnicki A. The interplay between childhood trauma, cognitive biases, psychotic-like experiences and depression and their additive impact on predicting lifetime suicidal behavior in young adults. Psychol Med. 2019:10:1–9. https://doi.org/10.1017/S0033291718004026.

30. Brennan W. We don't have to take this: dealing with violence at work. Nurs Stand. 2000a;14(28 suppl):3–17.
31. Elbogen EB, Johnson SC. The intricate link between violence and mental disorder: results from the national epidemiologic survey on alcohol and related conditions. Arch Gen Psychiatry. 2009;66:152–61. https://doi.org/10.1001/archgenpsychiatry.2008.537.
32. Fazel S, Grann M. The population impact of severe mental illness on violent crime. Am J Psychiatry. 2006;163:1397–403. https://doi.org/10.1176/ajp.2006.163.8.1397.
33. Swanson JW, Swartz MS, Van Dorn RA, Elbogen EB, Wagner HR, Rosenheck RA, et al. A national study of violent behavior in persons with schizophrenia. Arch Gen Psychiatry. 2006;63:490–9. https://doi.org/10.1001/archpsyc.63.5.490.
34. Witt K, van Dorn R, Fazel S. Risk factors for violence in psychosis: systematic review and meta-regression analysis of 110 studies. PLoS One. 2013;8:e55942. https://doi.org/10.1371/journal.pone.0055942.
35. Leclerc MP, Regenbogen C, Hamilton RH, Habel U. Some neuroanatomical insights to impulsive aggression in schizophrenia. Schizophr Res. 2018;201:27–34. https://doi.org/10.1016/j.schres.2018.06.016.
36. Fazel S, Gulati G, Linsell L, Geddes JR, Grann M. Schizophrenia and violence: systematic review and meta-analysis. PLoS Med. 2009a;6:e1000120. https://doi.org/10.1371/journal.pmed.1000120.
37. Large MM, Nielssen O. Violence in first-episode psychosis: a systematic review and meta-analysis. Schizophr Res. 2011;125:209–20. https://doi.org/10.1016/j.schres.2010.11.026.
38. Iozzino L, Ferrari C, Large M, Nielssen O, de Girolamo G. Prevalence and risk factors of violence by psychiatric acute inpatients: a systematic review and meta-analysis. PLoS One. 2015;10:e0128536. https://doi.org/10.1371/journal.pone.0128536.
39. Mohr P, Knytl P, Voráčková V, Bravermanová A, Melicher T. Long-acting injectable antipsychotics for prevention and management of violent behavior in psychotic patients. Int J Clin Pract. 2017;71(9) https://doi.org/10.1111/ijcp.12997.
40. Dodge KA. Do social information-processing patterns mediate aggressive behaviour? New York: The Guildford Press; 2003.
41. Fazel S, Grann M, Carlstrom E, Lichtenstein P, Langstrom N. Risk factors for violent crime in Schizophrenia: a national cohort study of 13,806 patients. J Clin Psychiatry. 2009b;70:362–9.
42. Maniglio R. Severe mental illness and criminal victimization: a systematic review. Acta Psychiatr Scand. 2009;119:180–91. https://doi.org/10.1111/j.1600-0447.2008.01300.x.
43. Kraus JE, Sheitman BB. Characteristics of violent behavior in a large state psychiatric hospital. Psychiatr Serv. 2004;55:183–5. https://doi.org/10.1176/appi.ps.55.2.183.
44. Grassi L, Peron L, Marangoni C, Zanchi P, Vanni A. Characteristics of violent behaviour in acute psychiatric in-patients: a 5-year Italian study. Acta Psychiatr Scand. 2001;104:273–9.
45. Ketelsen R, Zechert C, Driessen M, Schulz M. Characteristics of aggression in a German psychiatric hospital and predictors of patients at risk. J Psychiatr Ment Health Nurs. 2007;14(1):92–9. https://doi.org/10.1111/j.1365-2850.2007.01049.x.
46. El-Badri SM, Mellsop G. Aggressive behaviour in acute general adult psychiatric unit. Psychiatr Bull. 2006;30:166–8. https://doi.org/10.1192/pb.30.5.166.
47. Carr VJ, Lewin TJ, Sly KA, Conrad AM, Tirupati S, Cohen M, et al. Adverse incidents in acute psychiatric inpatient units: rates, correlates and pressures. Aust N Z J Psychiatry. 2008;42:267–82. https://doi.org/10.1080/00048670701881520.
48. Zhou JS, Zhong BL, Xiang YT, Chen Q, Cao XL, Correll CU, et al. Prevalence of aggression in hospitalized patients with schizophrenia in China: A meta-analysis. Asia Pac Psychiatry. 2016;8(1):60–9. https://doi.org/10.1111/appy.12209.
49. Hamadeh RR, Al Alaiwat B, Al Ansari A. Assaults and nonpatient-induced injuries among psychiatric nursing staff in Bahrain. Issues Ment Health Nurs. 2003;24:409–17.
50. Serper MR, Goldberg BR, Herman KG, Richarme D, Chou J, Dill CA, et al. Predictors of aggression on the psychiatric inpatient service. Compr Psychiatry. 2005;46:121–7. https://doi.org/10.1016/j.comppsych.2004.07.031.

51. Abderhalden C, Needham I, Dassen T, Halfens R, Fischer JE, Haug HJ. Frequency and severity of aggressive incidents in acute psychiatric wards in Switzerland. Clin Pract Epidemol Ment Health. 2007;3:30.
52. Krakowski MI, Czobor P. Executive function predicts response to antiaggression treatment in schizophrenia: a randomized controlled trial. J Clin Psychiatry. 2012;73(1):74–80. https://doi.org/10.4088/JCP.11m07238.
53. Krakowski MI, Czobor P. Depression and impulsivity as pathways to violence: implications for antiaggressive treatment. Schizophr Bull. 2014;40:886–94. https://doi.org/10.1093/schbul/sbt117.
54. Silverstein SM, Del Pozzo J, Roché M, Boyle D, Miskimen T. Schizophrenia and violence: realities and recommendations. Crime Psychol Rev. 2015;1:21–42. https://doi.org/10.1080/23744006.2015.1033154.
55. Dack C, Ross J, Papadopoulos C, Stewart D, Bowers LA. Review and meta-analysis of the patient factors associated with psychiatric in-patient aggression. Acta Psychiatr Scand. 2013;127(4):255–68. https://doi.org/10.1111/acps.12053.
56. Ekinci O, Ekinci A. Association between insight, cognitive insight, positive symptoms and violence in patients with schizophrenia. Nord J Psychiatry. 2013;67(2):116–23. https://doi.org/10.3109/08039488.2012.687767.
57. Látalová K. Violence and duration of untreated psychosis in first-episode patients. Int J Clin Pract. 2014;68(3):330–5. https://doi.org/10.1111/ijcp.12327.
58. Volavka J. Violence in schizophrenia and bipolar disorder. Psychiatr Danub. 2013;25(1):24–33.
59. Volavka J. Comorbid personality disorders and violent behavior in psychotic patients. Psychiatry Q. 2014;85(1):65–78. https://doi.org/10.1007/s11126-013-9273-3.
60. Ascher-Svanum H, Faries DE, Zhu B, Ernst FR, Swartz MS, Swanson JW. Medication adherence and long-term functional outcomes in the treatment of schizophrenia in usual care. J Clin Psychiatry. 2006;67(3):453–60.
61. Corrigan PW, Watson AC. Findings from the National Comorbidity Survey on the frequency of violent behavior in individuals with psychiatric disorders. Psychiatry Res. 2005;136:153–62. https://doi.org/10.1016/j.psychres.2005.06.005.
62. Graz C, Etschel E, Schoech H, Soyka M. Criminal behaviour and violent crimes in former inpatients with affective disorder. J Affect Disord. 2009;117:98–103. https://doi.org/10.1016/j.jad.2008.12.007.
63. Latalova K. Bipolar disorder and aggression. Int J Clin Pract. 2009;63(6):889–99. https://doi.org/10.1111/j.1742-1241.2009.02001.x.
64. Perroud N, Baud P, Mouthon D, Courtet P, Malafosse A. Impulsivity, aggression and suicidal behavior in unipolar and bipolar disorders. J Affect Disord. 2011;134:112–8. https://doi.org/10.1016/j.jad.2011.05.048.
65. Comai S, Tau M, Gobbi G. The psychopharmacology of aggressive behavior: a translational approach: part 1: neurobiology. J Clin Psychopharmacol. 2012;32(1):83–94. https://doi.org/10.1097/JCP.0b013e31823f8770.
66. Brennan PA, Mednick SA, Hodgins S. Major mental disorders and criminal violence in a Danish birth cohort. Arch Gen Psychiatry. 2000b;57:494–500.
67. Van Dorn R, Volavka J, Johnson N. Mental disorder and violence: is there a relationship beyond substance use. Soc Psychiatry Psychiatr Epidemiol. 2012;47(3):487–503. https://doi.org/10.1007/s00127-011-0356-x.
68. Arseneault L, Moffitt TE, Caspi A, Taylor PJ, Silva PA. Mental disorders and violence in a total birth cohort: results from the Dunedin Study. Arch Gen Psychiatry. 2000;57(10):979–86.
69. Casiano H, Belik SL, Cox BJ, Waldman JC, Sareen J. Mental disorder and threats made by noninstitutionalized people with weapons in the national comorbidity survey replication. J Nerv Ment Dis. 2008;196(6):437–45. https://doi.org/10.1097/NMD.0b013e3181775a2a.
70. Barlow K, Grenyer B, Ilkiw-Lavalle O. Prevalence and precipitants of aggression in psychiatric inpatient units. Aust N Z J Psychiatry. 2000;34(6):967–74.

71. Bowers L, Stewart D, Papadopoulos C, Dack C, Ross J, Khanom H. Inpatient violence and aggression: a literature review. London: Health Service and Population Research—King's College London; 2011.

72. Nawka A, Rukavina TV, Nawková L, Jovanović N, Brborović O, Raboch J. Psychiatric disorders and aggression in the printed media: is there a link? A central European perspective. BMC Psychiatry. 2012;12(19) https://doi.org/10.1186/1471-244X-12-19.

73. Webb RT, Lichtenstein P, Larsson H, Geddes JR, Fazel S. Suicide, hospital presenting suicide attempts, and criminality in bipolar disorder: examination of risk for multiple adverse outcomes. J Clin Psychiatry. 2014;75(8):809–16. https://doi.org/10.4088/JCP.13m08899.

74. Carpiniello B, Lai L, Pirarba S, Sardu C, Pinna F. Impulsivity and aggressiveness in bipolar disorder with co-morbid borderline personality disorder. Psychiatry Res. 2011;188(1):40–4. https://doi.org/10.1016/j.psychres.2010.10.026.

75. Doyle AE, Biederman J, Ferreira MA, Wong P, Smoller JW, Faraone SV. Suggestive linkage of the child behavior checklist juvenile bipolar disorder phenotype to 1p21, 6p21, and 8q21. J Am Acad Child Adolesc Psychiatry. 2010;49(4):378–87.

76. Alliey-Rodriguez N, Zhang D, Badner JA, Lahey BB, Zhang X, Dinwiddie S, et al. Genome-wide association study of personality traits in bipolar patients. Psychiatr Genet. 2011;21(4):190–4. https://doi.org/10.1097/YPG.0b013e3283457a31.

77. Barzman D, Eliassen J, McNamara R, Abonia P, Mossman D, Durling M, et al. Correlations of inflammatory gene pathways, cortico-limbic functional activities, and aggression in pediatric bipolar disorder: a preliminary study. Psychiatry Res. 2014;224(2):107–11. https://doi.org/10.1016/j.pscychresns.2014.07.009.

78. Mann JJ, Currier D. A review of prospective studies of biologic predictors of suicidal behavior in mood disorders. Arch Suicide Res. 2007;11(1):3–16. https://doi.org/10.1080/13811110600993124.

79. Siever LJ. Neurobiology of aggression and violence. Am J Psychiatry. 2008;165:429–42. https://doi.org/10.1176/appi.ajp.2008.07111774.

80. Passamonti L, Crockett MJ, Apergis-Schoute AM, Clark L, Rowe JB, Calder AJ, et al. Effects of acute tryptophan depletion on prefrontal-amygdala connectivity while viewing facial signals of aggression. Biol Psychiatry. 2012;71:36–43. https://doi.org/10.1016/j.biopsych.2011.07.033.

81. Chou YH, Lin CL, Wang SJ, Lirng JF, Yang KC, Chang AC, et al. Aggression in bipolar II disorder and its relation to the serotonin transporter. J Affect Disord. 2013;147:59–63. https://doi.org/10.1016/j.jad.2012.10.007.

82. Saddichha S, Schuetz C. Is impulsivity in remitted bipolar disorder a stable trait? A meta-analytic review. Compr Psychiatry. 2014;55:1479–84. https://doi.org/10.1016/j.comppsych.2014.05.010.

83. Cullen B, Ward J, Graham NA, Deary IJ, Pell JP, Smith DJ, et al. Prevalence and correlates of cognitive impairment in euthymic adults with bipolar disorder: a systematic review. J Affect Disord. 2016;205:165–81. https://doi.org/10.1016/j.jad.2016.06.063.

84. Cardenas SA, Kassem L, Brotman MA, Leibenluft E, McMahon FJ. Neurocognitive functioning in euthymic patients with bipolar disorder and unaffected relatives: a review of the literature. Neurosci Biobehav Rev. 2016;69:193–215. https://doi.org/10.1016/j.neubiorev.2016.08.002.

85. Baune BT, Malhi GS. A review on the impact of cognitive dysfunction on social, occupational and general functional outcomes in bipolar disorder. Bipolar Disord. 2015;17 Suppl 2:41–55. https://doi.org/10.1111/bdi.12341.

86. Dolenc B, Dernovšek MZ, Sprah L, Tavcar R, Perugi G, Akiskal HS. Relationship between affective temperaments and aggression in euthymic patients with bipolar mood disorder and major depressive disorder. J Affect Disord. 2015;174:13–8. https://doi.org/10.1016/j.jad.2014.11.007.

87. Johnson SL, Carver CS. Emotion-relevant impulsivity predicts sustained anger and aggression after remission in bipolar I disorder. J Affect Disord. 2016;189:169–75. https://doi.org/10.1016/j.jad.2015.07.050.

88. Dervic K, Garcia-Amador M, Sudol K, Freed P, Brent DA, Mann JJ, et al. Bipolar I and II versus unipolar depression: clinical differences and impulsivity/aggression traits. Eur Psychiatry. 2015;30:106–13. https://doi.org/10.1016/j.eurpsy.2014.06.005.
89. Verdolini N, Perugi G, Samalin L, Murru A, Angst J, Azorin JM, et al. Aggressiveness in depression: a neglected symptom possibly associated with bipolarity and mixed features. Acta Psychiatr Scand. 2017;136:362–72. https://doi.org/10.1111/acps.12777.
90. Feldmann TB. Bipolar disorder and violence. Psychiatry Q. 2001;72(2):119–29.
91. Doyle M, Dolan M, McGovern J. The validity of North American risk assessment tools in predicting in-patients violent behaviour in England. Legal Criminol Psych. 2002;7:141–54.
92. González-Ortega I, Mosquera F, Echeburúa E, González-Pinto A. Insight, psychosis and aggressive behavior in mania. Eur J Psychiat. 2010;24(2):70–7.
93. Belete H, Mulat H, Fanta T, Yimer S, Shimelash T, Ali T, et al. Magnitude and associated factors of aggressive behaviour among patients with bipolar disorder at Amanuel Mental Specialized Hospital, outpatient department, Addis Ababa, Ethiopia: cross-sectional study. BMC Psychiatry. 2016;16(443) https://doi.org/10.1186/s12888-016-1151-8.
94. Blanco EA, Duque LM, Rachamallu V, Yuen E, Kane JM, Gallego JA. Predictors of aggression in 3.322 patients with affective disorders and schizophrenia spectrum disorders evaluated in an emergency department setting. Schizophr Res. 2018;195:136–41. https://doi.org/10.1016/j.schres.2017.10.002.
95. Ballester J, Goldstein T, Goldstein B, Obreja M, Axelson D, Monk K, et al. Is bipolar disorder specifically associated with aggression? Bipolar Disord. 2012;14:283–90. https://doi.org/10.1111/j.1399-5618.2012.01006.x.
96. Ballester J, Goldstein B, Goldstein TR, Yu H, Axelson D, Monk K, et al. Prospective longitudinal course of aggression among adults with bipolar disorder. Bipolar Disord. 2014;16:262–9. https://doi.org/10.1111/bdi.12168.
97. Alnıak I, Erkıran M, Mutlu E. Substance use is a risk factor for violent behavior in male patients with bipolar disorder. J Affect Disord. 2016;193:89–93. https://doi.org/10.1016/j.jad.2015.12.059.
98. Fazel S, Lichtenstein P, Grann M, Goodwin GM, Langstrom N. Bipolar disorder in violent crime: new evidence from population based longitudinal studies and systematic review. Arch Gen Psychiatry. 2010b;67(9):931–8. https://doi.org/10.1001/archgenpsychiatry.2010.97.
99. Khalsa HMK, Baldessarini RJ, Tohen M, Salvatore P. Aggression among 216 patients with a first-psychotic episode of bipolar I disorder. Int J Bipolar Disord. 2018;6:18. https://doi.org/10.1186/s40345-018-0126-8.
100. Cazala F, Bauer IE, Meyer TD, Spiker DE, Kazimi IF, Zeni CP, et al. Correlates of childhood trauma in children and adolescents with bipolar disorder spectrum: A preliminary study. J Affect Disord. 2019;247:114–9. https://doi.org/10.1016/j.jad.2018.12.007.
101. Scott CL, Resnick PJ. Clinical assessment of psychotic and mood disorder symptoms for risk of future violence. CNS Spectr. 2014;19:468–73.

Psychopathy, Personality Disorders, and Violence

5

Stefano Ferracuti, Gabriele Mandarelli, and
Antonio Del Casale

5.1 Introduction

The relationship between personality disorders, psychopathy, and aggression/violent crime is a central issue in forensic psychiatry and psychology. It is also relevant in clinical criminology, as it has long been demonstrated that personality factors contribute greatly to recidivism, and they can be decisive when assessing offenders for parole/probation. In this chapter, we first focus on a historical overview of the main works that led to the development of the concepts of psychopathy and personality, as well as their link to crime and violence. We then focus on the most recent evidence on DSM-5 personality disorders and violence, and their relevance for recurrence prevention.

5.2 Historical Overview of Psychopathy, Antisocial Personality, and Crime

The first formulations of personality illnesses were derived from the Pinel's concept of *"manie sans délire"* [1], which influenced most subsequent theories. In the nineteenth century, mental disorders were considered diseases of the intellect, and Pinel

S. Ferracuti (✉) · G. Mandarelli
Department of Human Neuroscience, Faculty of Medicine and Dentistry, Sapienza University, Rome, Italy

Sant'Andrea University Hospital, Rome, Italy
e-mail: stefano.ferracuti@uniroma1.it; gabriele.mandarelli@uniroma1.it

A. Del Casale
Sant'Andrea University Hospital, Rome, Italy

NESMOS (Neurosciences, Mental Health, and Sensory Organs) Department, Faculty of Medicine and Psychology, Sapienza University, Rome, Italy
e-mail: antonio.delcasale@uniroma1.it

© Springer Nature Switzerland AG 2020
B. Carpiniello et al. (eds.), *Violence and Mental Disorders*, Comprehensive
Approach to Psychiatry 1, https://doi.org/10.1007/978-3-030-33188-7_5

was among the first to affirm that some patients had no intellectual or cognitive impairments, but could manifest alterations of feelings or affections, which today we would call affective symptoms. The classification proposed by Pinel included melancholy, mania without delirium, mania with delirium, dementia, and idiocy. The description of mania without delirium included psychopathological conditions of great emotional instability and antisocial tendencies, which on some occasions were classified as epilepsy or paranoid conditions. Pinel attributed such emotional alterations to perverse constitution and inadequate education [2].

Pinel's main pupil, Esquirol [3], further developed the concept of "monomania" and subsequently proposed a classification of the mental faculties as follows:

- Comprehension
- Intellectual monomania
- Will (instinctual monomania)
- Feelings (affective monomania)

The "monomania" theorisation proved to develop circularly, to the point that a single anomalous behaviour became the only diagnostic criterion. Possible examples include pyromania, kleptomania, erotomania, and homicidal monomania. The idea of monomania underlined the concept of "irresistible impulse" of the German authors, as well as the concept of "moral madness" of the English authors [4].

Griesinger (1845–1865) thoroughly criticised the concept of monomania by stating that every fixed idea was the expression of a deeply disturbed personality, as well as an indicator of an incipient mental disorder. From the medical-legal point of view he proposed that a correct evaluation should first verify whether there was evidence of an existing mental illness, before or after the crime, and never consider the crime per se, as an expression of illness [5].

Morel's theory was based on philosophical and religious ideas and "degeneration" was considered human destiny after the Fall [6]. His theory was based on the following main concepts:

1. Degenerative changes are pathological deviations from normality.
2. Mental disorders are predominantly hereditary, with an increase in the anomaly over time, and from one generation to another.
3. Degeneration presents not only quantitative but also qualitative aspects, which give rise to new diseases.

He developed an etiological and not symptom-based taxonomy, dividing the hereditary follies according to the supposed degree of degeneration, and identified "moral fools" as persons with low intelligence, and who are eccentric, unstable, unreliable, and not respectful of the rules. His theory became the most widespread explanation of mental illness [7].

Magnan was the most eminent representative of the degeneration theory in France, yet he claimed to be a Darwinist. He developed the concept of predisposition: the superior degenerates had only affective and non-cognitive alterations, even though they behaved in an aberrant manner. He also developed the concept of short recurrent psychosis [8].

Among the anglophone authors, Rush (1746–1813), one of the fathers of the American psychiatry, and who was among the signatories of the United States Declaration of Independence, studied people with "perversion of moral faculties" and "moral alienation of the mind". He considered antisocial acts, committed without a clear reason, as manifestations of mental illnesses guided by "a form of involuntary power". Rush's ideas also influenced Cesare Lombroso [9, 10].

Prichard gave a definition that was partly based on French theories: the madness consisting of a perversion of natural feelings, affections, inclinations, temperament, moral disposition, and impulses, without the presence of evident disturbances of the ability to reason or to know and especially without hallucinations or delusions [11]. At that time, the word "moral" had different meanings:

1. It was a method of treatment that used psychological elements and environmental methods.
2. It could be used to indicate affective and volitional aspects, in opposition to intellectual ones.
3. It could be a synonym for "ethical".

Prichard followed the second meaning. He recognised various causes of moral deficit, distinguishing them from the constitutional ones, deriving from a shock or a "fever", and associated "epilepsy" with this predisposition [11].

Maudsley believed that "criminals go criminal, as the insane go mad, because they cannot help it". He also assumed that a better knowledge of crime could imply a differentiation between treating criminals and treating the insane, with possible development of a higher degree of tolerance towards criminals, derived from a better knowledge of their defective organisation. This assumption, which addressed an issue that is still relevant in modern forensic psychiatry, i.e. differentiating those doubtful cases inhabiting the borderland between insanity and crime, also implied a more indulgent approach in cases of uncertain classification [12, 13].

Maudsley focused on the importance of the evaluator's observational perspective, which influenced the decision whether the subject would be classified as a criminal or as insane. By assuming that crime is a form of junction where unresolved tendencies can find an outlet, he stated that people could become insane if they were not criminals, and they did not go mad because they are criminals. He also believed that in certain type of crimes the convulsive energy of the homicidal impulse is sometimes preceded by a strange sensation of discomfort, developed somewhere in the body and dating back to the brain, similar to the phenomenon of epileptic aura. The significance of brain mechanisms typical of epilepsy was a relevant element. Indeed, Maudsley also observed that sometimes by improving epilepsy, a moral deviation of the character was observed (a concept still alive today as "forced normalisation"). Furthermore, while he believed that epilepsy was associated with crime, he also believed that epileptics were always imputable. With respect to the idea of degeneration, he changed his mind several times. After the development of the Lombrosian perspective on crime, which he considered extremist, Maudsley stated that to say that a criminal can be a degenerate is one thing, and a real thing; yet to say that all criminals have degeneration and have the stigma of degeneration is another thing that, he believed, was false. He also supported the importance of hereditary factors, and believed that emotional factors such as frustration, being mocked or humiliated, being irritated, imitating and instigating or coercion, provocation, being illegitimate, bodily anomalies, and freakiness were psychological factors that acted organically by breaking the molecular bonds of nervous tissue and destroying its vital elasticity. At a time when most of those charged with murder were executed, Maudsley developed the theory of non-responsibility, stating that it is not necessary for the insane to act without reason, to be considered criminally irresponsible. He also argued against the social prejudice that doubted the psychiatric assessment of defendants [12, 13].

Ray was the most distinguished American forensic psychiatrist of his time, and one of the founders of the American Psychiatric Association. "A Treatise on the Medical Jurisprudence of Insanity" appeared for the first time in 1838 and was followed by five editions. Ray's discussion of moral mania was based on the assumption that even though until then mania afflicted only the intellectual faculties, it could not be denied that the propensities and feelings were also an integral part of our constitution and depend on the brain, so that a brain disease could disturb even the affective faculties. He defined moral mania as a pathological perversion of natural feelings, affections, inclinations, temperament, morals, and moral disposition, in the absence of any detectable lesion of the intellect, knowledge, or faculties of reasoning, and without manic hallucinations [14].

Ray maintained the distinction between affective and intellectual components, and included compulsive acts such as the kleptomania, pyromania, paraphilia, and homicidal madness in the category of mania. For much of the twentieth century, the English concept of psychopathy was profoundly influenced by David Henderson (1939), a pupil of Meyer (1903–1950), who considered "psychopathic states" a form of constitutional anomaly, identifying, however, the idea of "constitutional" as a sum of hereditary and environmental factors. He considered three possible types of psychopaths:

- Predominantly aggressive
- Predominantly inadequate
- Predominantly creative

The first two types have entered the conceptualisation of personality disorders and the British Mental Health Act uses the term "psychopath" in the first way. Henderson also believed that the presence of "psychopathy" was the determining prognostic factor [15].

Meyer (1903–1950) distinguished neuroses from psychopathy, indicating neurasthenia, psychasthenia, and hysteria as neuroses, to be distinguished from constitutional inferiority [16]. This terminological approach was maintained until 1920–1930. All psychodynamic theories assert that the roots of psychiatric disorders are to be identified in the early years of development. After Freud's work on character and anality, Alexander (1930) and Reich (1933–1949) proposed a concept of character neurosis, that is, a condition where the disorder was not limited to circumscribed symptoms, but to the whole character [17, 18].

Alexander used the term "character neurosis" for those cases that acted in their conflicts with impulsive behaviour. In his opinion, criminals suffer from an unconscious conflict between different parts of the ego and certainly have a superego. However, instead of presenting symptoms, they disturb others.

Reich considered the character as a defensive structure against internal impulses and external stresses. He rejected the hypothesis of symptomatic neurosis against neurosis of character, claiming that in all of them there is a neurotic character and that in these cases the perception of the symptom is lost. In this sense, neurosis of character is a progressive effort of adaptation to which a symptomatic regressive form is contrasted.

In 1930, Partridge proposed the term "sociopathy" to indicate a persistent maladjustment that could not be corrected with an ordinary education or punishment [19]. In 1969, Craft provided inclusion and exclusion criteria, introducing operational criteria for diagnosis of sociopathy. As "primary" aspects he indicated the lack of feelings towards others and impulsiveness. As "secondary" aspects he pointed to aggressiveness, lack of guilt, inability to learn from experience, and a lack of motivation. The possible co-presence of psychosis involved the exclusion of the diagnosis [20].

Karpman suggested a difference between idiopathic and symptomatic forms of psychopathy. Among the symptomatic psychopathies he gathered neurotic reactions that could be traced to intrapsychic conflicts. In his opinion, there was another group that was completely devoid of conscience and called it anetopathic [21]. Cleckley's (1941–1976) famous book, "The Mask of Sanity", contained the idea of a "semantic dementia", which described an unmotivated dissocial behaviour not due to psychosis or neurosis [22]. He listed 16 criteria for psychopathy, which then formed the basis of Hare's Psychopathy Checklist [23]. For Cleckley, psychopathy was a very serious disease [22], and McCord and McCord expressed a similar concept [24].

The work of Robins reported the observation of over 500 men, followed for a period of 30 years. The conclusion of the study stated that the degree of dissocial or aggressive behaviour in childhood and youth could be considered as the early predictor of the development of a sociopathic personality, confirming that personality traits are stable over time [25].

Among German authors, the current definition of psychopathy is attributable to Koch (1891), who theorised the "psychopathic inferiority". He divided the condition into congenital and acquired, and in each of these two categories he distinguished psychopathic predisposition, psychopathic deficit, and psychopathic degeneration. The concept subsequently evolved into a "psychopathic constitution" with the hysterical, neurasthenic, depressive, hyperthymic, paranoid, and obsessive form. The German concept was broader than the anglophone one and included other criteria besides the "dissocial" aspect [26].

Previous theories of degeneration influenced Kraepelin's concept of psychopathy, which in turn provided the basis of Schneider's model. The concept of *"die psychopathischen Zustände"* appeared in the fifth edition of his text and included compulsive, impulsive, and homosexual disorders as well as mood disorders. In the seventh edition, in a paragraph dedicated to degeneration, he dealt with personality disorders, introducing the innovative distinction between original disease conditions, in which he considered the psychopathic states, and psychopathic personalities. Kraepelin explored the psychopathic personalities with social and moral implications. He categorised the born delinquents, the unstable, liars, crooks, and pseudoquerulomaniacs. In the eighth edition, he listed the dissocial (enemies of society), the excitable, the unstable, the eccentric, liars, crooks, and quarrelsome psychopaths [27].

Kraepelin considered mild or moderate states of mood alteration as attenuated phases of manic depressive illness and not mood disorders. Kretschmer (1921–2015) suggested that there was a specific correlation between body conformation and personality, dividing people into picnics, leptosomatics, and athletics. The picnics were associated with a cyclothymic temperament. In the Kretschmer concept, the continuity between cycloid variants, normal cyclothymic character, and manic depressive psychosis was so fluid as to lie in a continuum. Leptosomal somatotypes were associated with schizotypal aspects [28].

Schneider wrote his famous monograph, "The psychopathic personalities", derived from a previous study of prostitutes, where he had already distinguished 12 types. Unlike Kraepelin, he tried not to tie his classification to social norms. He did not consider them diseases because a "disease" had to be associated with an organic alteration and was opposed to the spectrum concept of Kretschmer and Bleuer [29].

He considered them statistical deviations from the norm, which he never defined. However, the well-known definition of abnormal personality as one who "suffers and makes people suffer" is indeed Schneider's. Schneider distinguished ten clinical based types:

- Hyperthymic, depressive, insecure (in which Schneider significantly groups the patients we would describe today as obsessive-compulsive and paranoid developments on a sensitive basis)
- The fanatic, attention seeking (the personalities banally called "hysterical" or more recently "histrionic" and "narcissistic")
- Labile, explosive (which includes typologies that today we would define as "borderline")
- Affectionless, weak-willed, and asthenic (three groups, which suggest certain basic pre- or post-psychotic stages) [29]

Currently, psychopathy is considered a behavioural deviancy with specific emotional and interpersonal features [30]. Influenced by a number of prominent theorists including Karpman [21], Cleckley [22], Lykken [31, 32], and Hare [23, 33, 34], current conceptions of psychopathy include reference to features such as superficial charm, manipulativeness, egocentricity, callousness, a lack of remorse or empathy, impulsivity, and irresponsibility, along with a marked risk for violence and criminal behaviour [35]. Criminality may represent a correlate, or a consequence, of psychopathy rather than a core feature of this maladaptive personality [22, 31, 32, 35].

Research findings have consistently documented associations between psychopathy and a wide range of externalising behaviours such as crime and aggression [36, 37], criminal recidivism [38], substance use [39, 40], and sexual offending [41]. Consensus exists on the fact that psychopathy may not represent a unitary construct [42, 43]; rather, it seems to entail multiple personality traits even if the exact number of psychopathy dimensions is still controversial [34], with three dimensions being frequently reported [42, 44].

The Diagnostic and Statistical Manual of Mental Disorders—Fifth Edition [45] does not list psychopathy neither in Section II, nor in Alternative Model of Personality Disorders (AMPD). However, the DSM-5 AMPD provides the opportunity to specify if the antisocial personality disorder diagnosis is characterised by the presence of psychopathic features, defined by low levels of anxiousness and withdrawal and high levels of attention seeking. The DSM-5 AMPD provides a system of 25 dysfunctional personality traits, whose correlations are explained by five dysfunctional personality domains (negative affectivity, detachment, antagonism, disinhibition, and psychoticism), which have been shown to represent the maladaptive variants of the well-known five factor model personality traits [46]. To assess the DSM-5 AMPD dysfunctional personality traits and domains, Krueger and colleagues developed the Personality Inventory for DSM-5 (PID-5), a 220-item self-report form that yields scores for both dysfunctional personality traits and dysfunctional personality domains [47]. The PID-5 has been extensively validated across different languages [48, 49]. The PID-5 factor structure has been consistently replicated across different cultures and languages [50]. To overcome the limitations of self-report assessment (e.g. under-reporting or over-reporting of dysfunctional features) [51], Markon and colleagues proposed the PID-5-Informant Report Form (PID-5-IRF), which represents the informant-rated version of the PID-5 [52].

Considering the psychopathy construct from the perspective of dysfunctional personality may help to discern the developmental pathways leading to pathology and the possible gender differences in psychopathy phenotypic manifestations [53]. Indeed, there is a burgeoning literature trying to understand psychopathy and related conditions in women [54]. This literature highlights several similarities and differences between psychopathy manifestations between genders [54–56]. For instance, features of psychopathy are captured in a valid manner across gender by current conceptualisations and measures of psychopathy [54]. In particular, the Psychopathy Checklist-Revised (PCL-R) [33] showed strong similarity of measurement properties across genders [54].

Psychopathy may be characterised by higher levels of borderline personality disorder features/emotional dysregulation (e.g. efforts to avoid abandonment, self-harm) among women compared to men, although low levels of anxiety and high levels of impulsivity and aggression characterise both psychopathic men and women [54, 55].

5.3   Personality Disorders and Violence

Most studies failed to empirically research the individual Cluster B personality traits, and instead chose to consider diagnosis as a sole entity. As there can be many combinations of traits in order to meet the clinical cut-off for a diagnosis of each of the Cluster B PDs, there is a need to look in-depth at those traits that distinguish individuals who engage in violent behaviours from those who do not.

Borderline personality disorder (BPD). It is associated with violence towards self and others. It is characterised by difficulties with impulse control and affective dysregulation. It is unclear whether BPD contributes to the perpetration of violence or whether this is explained by comorbidity.

Harford and colleagues' large study, the National Epidemiologic Survey on Alcohol and Related Conditions-III, included 4301 patients with BPD and 19,404 for subthreshold BPD. In the study's total population, identity disturbance, impulsivity, and intense anger significantly characterised violence towards others, while avoidance of abandonment, self-mutilating behaviour, feelings of emptiness, and intense anger significantly characterised violence towards self [57].

Another study conducted on 14,753 men and women from two British national surveys of adults (≥16 years) showed that categorical diagnosis of BPD was associated only with intimate partner violence (IPV). Associations with serious violence leading to injuries and repetitive violence were better explained by comorbid substance misuse, anxiety, and antisocial personality disorder (ASPD). However, anger and impulsivity BPD items were independently associated with most violent outcomes including severity, repetition, and injury; suicidal behaviours and affective instability were not associated with violence [58].

Individuals with BPD symptoms seem to be at risk of perpetrating more severe and frequent IPV. Further, while few studies have included direct measurement and examination of potential mechanisms for this association, attachment and facial affect processing appear to be two potential mechanisms of IPV perpetration in individuals with BPD. Different data were derived from studies focused on men as perpetrators in the BPD–IPV literature, despite BPD being more frequently diagnosed in women. There was no clear sex difference in the magnitude or direction of the BPD–IPV perpetration association, but given the relatively limited research on women as IPV perpetrators and the even more limited research directly comparing men and women with borderline personality pathology who engage in IPV, additional research is needed [59].

Results suggested that BPD symptoms partially accounted for the effects of impulsive antisocial traits on self-directed violence (both self-harm and attempts) in both genders, but fully accounted for interpersonal affective factors' protective effects only in men. These findings underscore the notion that the same psychopathic trait liabilities, at least as they are currently assessed, may confer risk for different forms of behavioural maladjustment in women versus men [60].

BPD is not independently associated with increased risk of violence in the general population; rather childhood maltreatment, history of violence or criminality, and comorbid psychopathy or antisocial personality appear to be predictors of violence in patients with BPD [61].

Another aspect regards individuals with BPD symptomatology demonstrating higher rates of abuse of alcohol and prescription drugs, also in a sample of individuals convicted for perpetration of partner violence. Findings indicate the need for thorough substance abuse assessment and treatment in perpetrators of partner violence with BPD symptomatology [62]. This can be linked with the evidence that emotion dysregulation is a significant longitudinal mediator of violent behaviour among individuals with BPD, and may serve as the primary mechanism that enhances risk for violence among this population [63]. Another important predictor of violent behaviour in BPD is impulsivity [64, 65].

Histrionic personality disorder. Histrionic personality can be a risk factor for repetitive aggression in high-security forensic psychiatric setting [66]. Dissociation can be viewed as the prerequisite for a compromised and partial acting out of prohibited non-integrated elements, e.g. aggression, as a coping strategy [67].

Narcissistic personality disorder. In 2009, Warren and South highlighted the significance of considering narcissistic traits in violence risk assessment, when there is a tendency for professionals to link violence solely with ASPD [68]. Key findings from the literature in relation to NPD traits indicate that delusions of a grandiose nature, when associated with elation or anger, can present a direct pathway to serious violence [69]. This lends consideration to precipitating factors that can influence elation or anger, such as substance misuse which is known to be associated with PD, violence, and aggression [70]. Emotion dysregulation could also precipitate elation or anger, which may account for violence perpetration in the context of an inflated sense of entitlement being or feeling violated, as identified by Fisher and Hall [71]. From a Schema-focused perspective, a violated sense of entitlement could result in behavioural externalisation of aggression as a means to overcompensate for such feelings of entitlement [72]. Further insight could be taken from the tenuous relationship identified between impaired accuracy in perspective taking and trait impulsivity and recklessness [73]. Impaired perspective taking was also identified to exacerbate anger arousal [74], which may thus enhance risk of impulsive and/or reckless violence. Trait "aggressiveness" was identified to relate to NPD; however this was distinguished to refer solely to the emotional trait of aggressiveness, being anger and irritability, as opposed to physical acts of aggression [75]. Despite this, NPD comorbid with other PDs significantly enhances the risk of serious physical violence, particularly murder [68], which supports the inference that trait impulsivity, associated with ASPD and BPD, may present a significant elevating risk factor towards the perpetration of physical violence or aggression in the context of NPD traits. The trait of impulsivity has theoretical linkage to personality structure as well as aggressive or violent behaviour [76]. In fact, Elonheimo et al. discussed how they felt "violence may be attributed more to impulsiveness than actual mental disorder; it may arise out of situational factors, provocation, and an emotional surge" [77].

Perpetrators of sexual aggression had higher scores on NPD traits, which were also associated with frequent perpetration. HSNS scores were only associated with perpetration via alcohol and/or drugs. Only the maladaptive facets of NPI narcissism correlated with perpetration [78].

Avoidant personality disorder. Sex offenders with paraphilia had significantly higher rates of certain types of mental illness and avoidant personality disorder. Moreover, paraphilic offenders spent less time in prison but started offending at a younger age and reported more victims and more non-rape sexual offenses against minors than offenders without paraphilia. Sex offenders should be carefully evaluated for the presence of mental illness and sex offender management programs should have a capacity for psychiatric treatment [79].

Dependent and obsessive-compulsive personality disorders. Although obsessive-compulsive personality disorder is not commonly associated with behavioural disinhibition, the literature contains reports of occasional explosive aggressive outbursts [80, 81]. In addition, dependant personality has been related to violent behaviours, and some authors suggested that violent criminals can be divided into two categories, the under-controlled (antisocial) and the over-controlled (dependent) [82, 83].

5.4   Conclusions

The history of personality disorders is strongly intermingled with the understanding of interpersonal violence and some aspects of criminality. Most of the basic questions about the relationship between personality disorders, and especially the particular construct of psychopathy, and violence, remain open to discussion, and more research is needed. The lack of appropriate treatments for most of the more problematic personality disturbances is another major problem. Legal systems may differently deal with crimes performed by this kind of persons, and judicial decisions may be strongly influenced by the conceptualisation of these mental conditions, creating difficult ethical issues, such as indeterminate sentencing or involuntary treatments for personality disorders.

References

1. Pinel P. Traité médico-philosophique sur l'aliénation mentale. 2nd ed. Paris: Brosson; 1809.
2. Salomone G, Arnone R. Italian psychiatric nosography before Kraepelin. Giorn Ital Psicopat. 2009;15:75–88.
3. Esquirol JED. Delle malattie mentali considerate in relazione alla medicina dell'igiene e alla medicina legale. Firenze: Mariano Cecchi; 1846.
4. Fornari U. Monomania omicida. Origini ed evoluzione storica del reato d'impeto. Torino: Centro Scientifico Editore; 1997.
5. Griesinger W. Traité des Maladies Mentales, Pathologie et Thérapeutique. Paris: Adrien Delahaye, Libraire-Éditeur; Place de L'école-De-Médecine; 1865.
6. Morel B-A. Traité Thèorique et Pratique des Maladies Mentales. Paris: J.B. Baillière Éditeur, Rue de L'école-De-Médecine; 1852.
7. Danion JM, Keppi J, Singer L. A historical approach to the doctrine of degeneration and psychopathic constitution. Ann Med Psychol (Paris). 1985;143(3):271–80.

8. Magnan V. Recherches sur les Centres Nerveux, Pathologie et Physiologie Pathologique. Paris: Masson Éditeur; 1876.
9. Rush B. Medical inquiries and observations upon the diseases of the mind. Philadelphia: Grigg; 1830.
10. Stone MH. Healing the mind: a history of psychiatry from antiquity to the present. Dunmore, PA: W. W. Norton Company; 1997.
11. Prichard JC. A treatise on insanity and other disorders affecting the mind. Philadelphia, PA: E. L. Carey & A. Hart; 1837.
12. Scott P. Pioneers in criminology. XI. Henry Maudsley (1835–1918). J Crim Law Criminol Police Sci. 1956;46(6):753–69.
13. Maudsley H. The pathology of mind: a study of its distempers, deformities, and disorders. London: Macmillan; 1895.
14. Ray I. A treatise on the medical jurisprudence of insanity. In: Overholser W, editor. Series: the John Harvard library. Harvard, MA: Harvard University Press; 2014.
15. Henderson DK, Batchelor IRC. Henderson's and Gillespie's textbook of psychiatry. 9th ed. London: Oxford University Press; 1962.
16. Meyer A, Winters EE. The collected papers of Adolf Meyer. Baltimore: Johns Hopkins Press; 1950.
17. Alexander F. The neurotic character. Int J Psychoanal. 1930;11:292–311.
18. Reich W. Character analysis. New York: Orgone Institute Press; 1949.
19. Partridge GE. Current conceptions of psychopathic personalities. Am J Psychiatry. 1930;10:53–99.
20. Craft M. The natural history of psychopathic disorder. Br J Psychiatry. 1969;115(518):39–44.
21. Karpman B. On the need for separating psychopathy into two distinct clinical types: symptomatic and idiopathic. J Crim Psychopathol. 1941;3:112–37.
22. Cleckley H. The mask of sanity. St. Louis, MO: Mosby; 1941.
23. Hare RD. Manual for the revised psychopathy checklist. 1st ed. Toronto: Multi-Health Systems; 1991.
24. McCord WL, McCord J. The psychopath an essay on the criminal mind. New York, NY: Van Nostrand; 1964.
25. Robins LN. Deviant children grow up. Baltimore: William & Wilkins; 1966.
26. Gutmann P. Julius Ludwig August Koch (1841–1908): Christian, philosopher and psychiatrist. Hist Psychiatry. 2008;19(74 Pt 2):202–14.
27. Diefendorf AR. Clinical psychiatry: a textbook for students and physicians. Abstracted and adapted from the seventh German edition of Kraepelin's Lehrbuch der Psychiatrie. New York, NY: McMillan; 1923.
28. Kretschmer E. Constitution and character: research on the constitution and the doctrine of temperaments (1921). Vertex. 2015;26(122):303–17.
29. Schneider K. Le personalità psicopatiche. Roma: Giovanni Fioriti Editore; 2016.
30. Patrick CJ, Fowles DC, Krueger RF. Triarchic conceptualization of psychopathy: developmental origins of disinhibition, boldness, and meanness. Dev Psychopathol. 2009;21(3):913–38.
31. Lykken DT. A study of anxiety in the sociopathic personality. J Abnorm Soc Psych. 1957;55(1):6–10.
32. Lykken DT. The antisocial personalities. Hillsdale, NJ: Erlbaum; 1995.
33. Hare RD. The Hare Psychopathy Checklist-Revised. 2nd ed. Toronto: Multi-Health; 2003.
34. Hare RD, Neumann CS. Psychopathy as a clinical and empirical construct. Annu Rev Clin Psychol. 2008;4:217–46.
35. Cooke DJ, Michie C. Refining the construct of psychopathy: towards a hierarchical model. Psychol Assess. 2001;13(2):171–88.
36. Gretton HM, Hare RD, Catchpole RE. Psychopathy and offending from adolescence to adulthood: a 10-year follow-up. J Consult Clin Psychol. 2004;72(4):636–45.
37. Porter S, Birt AR, Boer DP. Investigation of the criminal and conditional release profiles of Canadian federal offenders as a function of psychopathy and age. Law Hum Behav. 2001;25(6):647–61.

38. Walters GD, Knight RA, Grann M, Dahle KP. Incremental validity of the Psychopathy Checklist facet scores: predicting release outcome in six samples. J Abnorm Psychol. 2008;117(2):396–405.
39. Gustavson C, Ståhlberg O, Sjödin AK, Forsman A, Nilsson T, Anckarsäter H. Age at onset of substance abuse: a crucial covariate of psychopathic traits and aggression in adult offenders. Psychiatry Res. 2007;153(2):195–8.
40. Kennealy PJ, Hicks BM, Patrick CJ. Validity of factors of the Psychopathy Checklist-Revised in female prisoners: discriminant relations with antisocial behavior, substance abuse, and personality. Assessment. 2007;14(4):323–40. Erratum in: Assessment. 2008;15(1):116–7
41. Caldwell MF, Ziemke MH, Vitacco MJ. An examination of the Sex Offender Registration and Notification Act as applied to juveniles: evaluating the ability to predict sexual recidivism. Psychol Public Pol L. 2008;14(2):89–114.
42. Cooke DJ, Michie C. An item response theory analysis of the Hare Psychopathy Checklist—Revised. Psychol Assess. 1997;9(1):3–14.
43. Harpur TJ, Hakstian AR, Hare RD. Factor structure of the Psychopathy Checklist. J Consult Clin Psychol. 1988;56(5):741–7.
44. Andershed H, Kerr M, Stattin H, Levander S. Psychopathic traits in non-referred youths: a new assessment tool. In: Blau E, Sheridan L, editors. Psychopaths: current international perspectives. Amsterdam: Elsevier; 2002.
45. American Psychiatric Association. Diagnostic and statistical manual of mental disorders. 5th ed. Washington, DC: American Psychiatric Association; 2013.
46. Wright ZE, Pahlen S, Krueger RF. Genetic and environmental influences on Diagnostic and Statistical Manual of Mental Disorders-Fifth Edition (DSM-5) maladaptive personality traits and their connections with normative personality traits. J Abnorm Psychol. 2017;126(4):416–28.
47. Krueger RF, Derringer J, Markon KE, Watson D, Skodol AE. Initial construction of a maladaptive personality trait model and inventory for DSM-5. Psychol Med. 2012;42(9):1879–90. Erratum in: Psychol Med. 2012;42(9):1891
48. Al-Dajani N, Gralnick TM, Bagby RMA. Psychometric review of the Personality Inventory for DSM-5 (PID-5): current status and future directions. J Pers Assess. 2016;98(1):62–81. Erratum in: J Pers Assess. 2018;100(4):448
49. Fossati A, Krueger RF, Markon KE, Borroni S, Maffei C. Reliability and validity of the personality inventory for DSM-5 (PID-5): predicting DSM-IV personality disorders and psychopathy in community-dwelling Italian adults. Assessment. 2013;20(6):689–708.
50. Somma A, Krueger RF, Markon KE, Fossati A. The replicability of the personality inventory for DSM-5 domain scale factor structure in U.S. and non-U.S. samples: a quantitative review of the published literature. Psychol Assess. 2019;31(7):861–77.
51. Dhillon S, Bagby RM, Kushner SC, Burchett D. The impact of underreporting and overreporting on the validity of the Personality Inventory for DSM-5 (PID-5): a simulation analog design investigation. Psychol Assess. 2017;29(4):473–8.
52. Markon KE, Quilty LC, Bagby RM, Krueger RF. The development and psychometric properties of an informant-report form of the personality inventory for DSM-5 (PID-5). Assessment. 2013;20(3):370–83.
53. Strickland CM, Drislane LE, Lucy M, Krueger RF, Patrick CJ. Characterizing psychopathy using DSM-5 personality traits. Assessment. 2013;20(3):327–38.
54. Verona E, Vitale J. Psychopathy in women: assessment, manifestations, and etiology. In: Patrick CJ, editor. Handbook of psychopathy. New York, NY: The Guilford Press; 2018.
55. Carabellese F, Felthous AR, Rossetto I, La Tegola D, Franconi F, Catanesi R. Female residents with psychopathy in a high-security Italian hospital. J Am Acad Psychiatry Law. 2018;46(2):171–8.
56. Carabellese F, Felthous AR, La Tegola D, Rossetto I, Montalbò D, Franconi F, Catanesi R. Psychopathy and female gender: phenotypic expression and comorbidity; a study comparing a sample of women hospitalized in Italy's maximum security facility with women who

were criminally sentenced and imprisoned. J Forensic Sci. 2019;64:1438–43. https://doi.org/10.1111/1556-4029.14039. Epub ahead of print

57. Harford TC, Chen CM, Kerridge BT, Grant BF. Borderline personality disorder and violence toward self and others: a National Study. J Personal Disord. 2018:1–18.
58. González RA, Igoumenou A, Kallis C, Coid JW. Borderline personality disorder and violence in the UK population: categorical and dimensional trait assessment. BMC Psychiatry. 2016;16:180.
59. Jackson MA, Sippel LM, Mota N, Whalen D, Schumacher JA. Borderline personality disorder and related constructs as risk factors for intimate partner violence perpetration. Aggress Violent Behav. 2015;24:95–106.
60. Verona E, Sprague J, Javdani S. Gender and factor-level interactions in psychopathy: implications for self-directed violence risk and borderline personality disorder symptoms. Personal Disord. 2012;3(3):247–62.
61. Allen A, Links PS. Aggression in borderline personality disorder: evidence for increased risk and clinical predictors. Curr Psychiatry Rep. 2012;14(1):62–9.
62. Sansone RA, Elliott K, Wiederman MW. Alcohol and prescription drug abuse and borderline personality disorder symptomatology among male and female perpetrators of partner violence. Prim Care Companion CNS Disord. 2014;16:6.
63. Newhill CE, Eack SM, Mulvey EP. A growth curve analysis of emotion dysregulation as a mediator for violence in individuals with and without borderline personality disorder. J Personal Disord. 2012;26(3):452–67.
64. La Grutta S, Lo Baido R, Castelli M, Marrazzo G, Schiera G, Gentile MC, Sarno L, Roccella M. Predictive signs and indicators of aggressiveness and violence: a comparison between a group of adolescents attending an external penal area, a group of prisoners and a group of patients with borderline personality disorder. Minerva Pediatr. 2006;58(2):121–9.
65. Látalová K, Prasko J. Aggression in borderline personality disorder. Psychiatry Q. 2010;81(3):239–51.
66. Langton CM, Hogue TE, Daffern M, Mannion A, Howells K. Personality traits as predictors of inpatient aggression in a high-security forensic psychiatric setting: prospective evaluation of the PCL-R and IPDE dimension ratings. Int J Offender Ther Comp Criminol. 2011;55(3):392–415.
67. Sigmund D, Barnett W, Mundt C. The hysterical personality disorder: a phenomenological approach. Psychopathology. 1998;31(6):318–30.
68. Warren JI, South SC. A symptom level examination of the relationship between Cluster B personality disorders and patterns of criminality and violence in women. Int J Law Psychiatry. 2009;32(1):10–7.
69. Ullrich S, Keers R, Coid JW. Delusions, anger, and serious violence: new findings from the MacArthur violence risk assessment study. Schizophr Bull. 2014;40(5):1174–81.
70. Pluck G, Brooker C, Blizard R, Moran P. Personality disorder in a probation cohort: demographic, substance misuse and forensic characteristics. Crim Behav Ment Health. 2015;25(5):403–15.
71. Fisher S, Hall G. 'If you show a bit of violence they learn real quick': measuring entitlement in violent offenders. Psychiatry Psychol Law. 2011;18(4):588–98.
72. Keulen-de Vos ME, Bernstein DP, Vanstipelen S, Vogel V, Lucker TP, Slaats M, Hartkoorn M, Arntz A. Schema modes in criminal and violent behaviour of forensic cluster B PD patients: a retrospective and prospective study. Leg Crim Psychol. 2016;21:56–76.
73. Seidel EM, Pfabigan DM, Keckeis K, Wucherer AM, Jahn T, Lamm C, Derntl B. Empathic competencies in violent offenders. Psychiatry Res. 2013;210(3):1168–75.
74. Day A, Mohr P, Howells K, Gerace A, Lim L. The role of empathy in anger arousal in violent offenders and university students. Int J Offender Ther Comp Criminol. 2012;56(4):599–613.
75. Fossati A, Barratt ES, Borroni S, Villa D, Grazioli F, Maffei C. Impulsivity, aggressiveness, and DSM-IV personality disorders. Psychiatry Res. 2007;149(1–3):157–67.

76. Komarovskaya I, Loper AB, Warren J. The role of impulsivity in antisocial and violent behavior and personality disorders among incarcerated women. Crim Justice Behav. 2007;34(11):1499–515.

77. Elonheimo H, Niemelä S, Parkkola K, Multimäki P, Helenius H, Nuutila AM, Sourander A. Police-registered offenses and psychiatric disorders among young males: the Finnish "From a boy to a man" birth cohort study. Soc Psychiatry Psychiatr Epidemiol. 2007;42(6):477–84.

78. Mouilso ER, Calhoun KS. Personality and perpetration: narcissism among college sexual assault perpetrators. Violence Against Women. 2016;22(10):1228–42.

79. Dunsieth NW Jr, Nelson EB, Brusman-Lovins LA, Holcomb JL, Beckman D, Welge JA, Roby D, Taylor P Jr, Soutullo CA, McElroy SL. Psychiatric and legal features of 113 men convicted of sexual offenses. J Clin Psychiatry. 2004;65(3):293–300.

80. Villemarette-Pittman NR, Stanford MS, Greve KW, Houston RJ, Mathias CW. Obsessive-compulsive personality disorder and behavioral disinhibition. J Psychol. 2004;138(1):5–22.

81. Hopwood CJ, Burt SA, Markowitz JC, Yen S, Shea MT, Sanislow CA, Grilo CM, Ansell EB, McGlashan TH, Gunderson JG, Zanarini MC, Skodol AE, Morey LC. The construct validity of rule-breaking and aggression in an adult clinical sample. J Psychiatr Res. 2009;43(8):803–8.

82. Ortiz-Tallo M, Cardenal V, Blanca MJ, Sánchez LM, Morales I. Multiaxial evaluation of violent criminals. Psychol Rep. 2007;100(3 Pt 2):1065–75.

83. Megargee EI. Undercontrolled and overcontrolled personality types in extreme antisocial aggression. Psychol Monogr. 1966;80(3):1–29.

Substance-Use Disorders and Violence

6

Fabrizio Schifano, Caroline Zangani, Stefania Chiappini,
Amira Guirguis, Stefania Bonaccorso, and John M. Corkery

6.1 Introduction

The relationship between violence and substance-use disorders (SUD) has been largely debated [1], but recent changes in drug scenarios are likely to have complicated the situation [2]. To better understand the relationship between these two constructs, focus will be here first on briefly presenting a few relevant definitions.

6.1.1 Substance-Use Disorder

SUD is a medical condition or state where the administration, consumption or other uses of at least one substance/drug causes or contributes to some form of distress or impairment that has clinical significance for an individual. Several terms (e.g. drug abuse, drug dependence, drug addiction and substance abuse) are used for referring to it [3, 4]. Different classes of substances may be involved, including alcohol, opiates/opioids, psychedelic phenethylamines, dissociatives (i.e. phencyclidine, ketamine and derivatives), hallucinogens (i.e. cannabis and synthetic cannabinoids), hypnotic/sedatives (e.g. benzodiazepines), solvents/volatile substances and gases,

F. Schifano · C. Zangani · S. Chiappini (✉) · J. M. Corkery
Psychopharmacology, Drug Misuse, and Novel Psychoactive Substances Research Unit,
School of Life and Medical Sciences, University of Hertfordshire, Hatfield, UK
e-mail: f.schifano@herts.ac.uk; j.corkery@herts.ac.uk

A. Guirguis
Swansea University Medical School, Institute of Life Sciences 2,
Swansea University, Swansea, Wales, UK
e-mail: amira.guirguis@swansea.ac.uk

S. Bonaccorso
Camden and Islington NHS Mental Health Foundation Trust, London, UK
e-mail: stefania.bonaccorso@kcl.ac.uk

© Springer Nature Switzerland AG 2020
B. Carpiniello et al. (eds.), *Violence and Mental Disorders*, Comprehensive
Approach to Psychiatry 1, https://doi.org/10.1007/978-3-030-33188-7_6

stimulants (e.g. amphetamine-type substances, cocaine, synthetic cathinones, khat) and many others [5].

6.1.2   Violence: Different Natures of Violence

The World Health Organization (WHO) describes it as "the intentional use of physical force or power, threatened or actual, against oneself, another person, or against a group or community, that either results in or has a high likelihood of resulting in injury, death, psychological harm, maldevelopment, or deprivation" [6]. The nature of the relationship between substance use and violence can be very varied, with range dimensions being included: suicide and self-abuse, child abuse, antisocial behaviour, sexual offences and physical assault/manslaughter.

6.1.2.1 Suicide and Self-Abuse

Suicide represents the 18th cause of death, with up to 800,000 deaths per year [6–9]. Risk factors for suicide include previous suicide attempts and mental health problems, but also harmful use of alcohol and drug use [10]. Notably, prevalence of risk factors for suicide has shown to be higher in drug users than in general population [11, 12]. Suicide attempts are six times more frequent in individuals with alcohol or drug abuse than in no-users [13, 14], whilst completed suicide rates are higher in both men and women with substance abuse (respectively, 2–3 times and 6.5–9 times higher) than in the general population [13, 15, 16].

Self-abuse, including acts such as self-mutilation, self-poisoning and other self-harm practices [6], has been typically associated with history of mental health problems and substance use [17, 18], with a prevalence peak in women aged 14–17 years [19]. Several studies have described a strong relationship between substance abuse [20–24].

6.1.2.2 Child Abuse

Although estimating prevalence of child abuse has several problems [6, 25, 26], their real occurrence may be more than 30 times higher than that identified by official reports [27, 28]. Indeed, a recent meta-analysis found that risk of child maltreatment increased with drug abuse and dependence severity, with the highest risk having been identified in parents with past-year dependence [29]. Moreover, children of drug abusers could get injured and be infected by HIV or by other infections [30, 31]. Conversely, adverse childhood experiences have been associated with a range of both psychopathological [27, 32] and substance-abuse disorders in later life [33].

6.1.2.3 Antisocial Behaviour

A relationship between substance-use disorder and antisocial personality disorder (ASPD) is widely recognised [34–36], with up to 14% substance users presenting comorbidity with ASPD [37]. These clients may present with high levels of poly-substance use, prevalence of sexual risky behaviour, mental and physical ill-health issues [35, 36, 38], aggression, violence and serious criminal activity [39–41].

Interestingly, a recent study found preliminary evidence of a putatively genetic association between ASPD and use of alcohol and cannabis [42].

6.1.2.4 Sexual Offences

As with other types of violence, prevalence of sexual offences [6] is hard to estimate. Several surveys, both in the USA and Europe, found an incidence of rape of about 0.1% in males and 0.3–0.5% in females [43–47]. However, cases notified to authorities can be representing generally the most violent expressions of this spectrum (i.e. rape and deaths related to sexual offences) [48–52]. Risk factors for being a sexual abuse victim include alcohol/drug use [6, 53]. Individuals under alcohol or drug effects are perceived easier to force in unwanted sexual acts without using violence [47, 54, 55]. Indeed, substance-intoxicated states could cause disinhibition and misjudgement, but also aggressiveness and violent behaviours [6, 56]. Among the others, alcohol, cannabis and cocaine have been identified as the substances more associated with sexual violence events [56–59]. At times, assaulters could deliberately intoxicate the victim with alcohol or drugs, such as gamma-hydroxybutyrate (GHB; [60]), ketamine [61], flunitrazepam or other hypnotics [62, 63].

6.1.2.5 Physical Assault/Manslaughter

It is largely accepted that substance use can be related in several ways with episodes of outward violence and aggression [56, 57, 64]. The correlation between substance use and violent behaviours might be mediated by both a direct pharmacological effect of the index drug and cognitive, social and dispositional factors (e.g. exposure to a dangerous environment or violence, childhood abuse, risk-taking personality traits) [65]. There might be a tripartite relationship between violence and drug use. The first type is a 'psychopharmacological', dopamine-related [66], violence in which the substance has a direct role in causing the harmful behaviour, either increasing aggressiveness and irritability or altering reality perception as during an induced psychotic episode [41, 67]. The second is an 'economic' violence in which heavily dependent people commit assaults or homicides in order to obtain money for drugs [67]. The last is a 'systemic' violence that involves criminal organisations, drug trafficking and street gang fights [67–70], although the proportion of drug-related homicides (DRH) remains unclear [69, 71, 72]. In a national report on deaths in England and Wales between March 2017 and March 2018, 44% of homicides were defined as 'drug related', considering all the above-mentioned possible relationships [73].

6.2   Violence, Mortality and Substance Use: Epidemiological Issues

In order to characterise and measure the nature of violence associated with substance use, different types of data sources and information are required. However, the availability of these varies over both time and place.

Health and crime data can contribute to understand both non-fatal and fatal outcomes of violence associated with alcohol and substance use.

At a general level, mortality data can give some indication of the nature and extent of violence-related fatalities in a particular region or country, especially those treated as homicide, suicide and war-related deaths. They are capable to provide evidence of changes over time, and identify 'at-risk' groups and differences between areas. Typically, such information is obtained from medical death certificates. However, for more details it is necessary to either turn to special mortality registers [74, 75] or promote national confidential inquiries that try to access a variety of sources in order to get a complete picture [76, 77].

Overall, the association between the occurrence of a violent death instance and a drug misuse intake episode may be direct or indirect. For example, a range of psychoactive substances can induce or trigger changes in mental states, including anxiety, depression, paranoia, psychosis and suicidal ideation (for a review, see [66]). Indeed, stimulants appear to be particularly and directly implicated in suicides involving violent methods such as hanging and self-injuries [78]. Other classes of drugs including alcohol, GHB and natural cannabis are also commonly involved in suicides [60]. Conversely, for its effects in reducing inhibitions, impairing judgment and increasing reaction times, alcohol is often but indirectly involved in traffic-related deaths [79] and accidental deaths for falling from heights, drowning, exposure to the elements (particularly hypothermia) and electrocution [61, 80, 81]. Similarly, distorted perceptions of reality, particularly after the use of hallucinogens and dissociatives, could indirectly cause death for falling from heights.

6.3   Dual Diagnosis and Violence

The coexistence of a mental illness and one or more substance-related disorders is indicated by the terms 'dual diagnosis' or 'co-occurring disorders' [82, 83]. Dual diagnosis may complicate the psychopathological clinical status; increase rates of risky behaviours (e.g. promiscuous sexual behaviours), psychosocial impairment (e.g. unemployment, homelessness) and criminal behaviours; and determine poor outcomes with high drop-out and hospitalisation rates [82]. In 2014, 7.9 million adult past-year substance users (39% of the total) have been reported with the co-occurrence of a mental illness in the USA [83]. In Europe, about 50% of substance users have been indicated as having both a substance use and mental health disorder [82]. Furthermore, in a sample of 374 psychiatric patients admitted over a year, almost one-third showed aggressive and violent behaviour in the month before admission; these episodes were associated with male sex, substance abuse and positive symptoms [65].

Among people with a mental disorder, occurrence of SUD has been consistently shown to be a significant risk factor for aggression and violence [84–89]. Moreover, a dual diagnosis condition has been established in 50–80% of forensic cases [41].

Most frequently reported substances abused by psychiatric clients are alcohol, cannabis, stimulants, hallucinogens, sedatives and opioids [86, 90, 91], with most vulnerable categories including homeless men and prisoners [86, 92].

The coexistence of schizophrenia and SUD has a prevalence ranging from 10% to 70% [92]. In schizophrenia, dual diagnosis, conditions violence seems more strongly related to both positive (e.g. persecutory delusions and bizarre behaviours) and negative symptoms (e.g. avolition-apathy, and social withdrawal; [93]). Conversely, self-harm/suicide has been associated with presence of command hallucinations [94–96].

A co-occurring substance abuse condition may increase the risk of violent behaviours and crimes in bipolar disorder as well [97, 98]. Risk factors for violence behaviours in this population are younger age, male gender, low education level and previous history of physical assault [97]. The presence of a bipolar spectrum diagnosis in heroin-addicted patients appeared to be associated with aggressive behaviours toward others [96].

Finally, in a sample of incarcerated women diagnosed with antisocial personality disorder, a SUD condition was highly prevalent, i.e. alcohol dependence, 56.1%; opiate dependence, 48.8%; and cocaine dependence, 61.0%, and associated with aggression and criminal behaviours [99].

6.4 Specific Substances of Abuse and Aggression

Cases of drug-related aggressiveness mostly involve a number of molecules, such as ethanol, stimulants, cannabinoids, opiates, benzodiazepines and a range of NPS [66, 100–102]. Conversely, polydrug consumption has been associated with higher number of physical and verbal aggressions compared with single drug abuse [103]. Overall, however, individuals who engage in substance use are more likely to be involved in several types of deviant behaviours [104].

6.4.1 Substances of Abuse Intake and Related Neurobiological Issues

The evidence of a relationship between violence and use of a range of recreational drugs' ingestion has been suggested to be related to their association with increased dopamine levels [66]. Dopaminergic hyperactivity in the midbrain striatum is thought to cause aberrant salience attribution [105]. Indeed, attribution of abnormally heightened salience to daily-life stimuli is considered to underlie the occurrence of persecutory delusions/psychosis and hence at times facilitate the occurrence of 'defensive aggression'/violent behaviour [106].

On the other hand, ingestion of serotoninergic compounds, including MDMA/ecstasy, has been related to several cases of aggressiveness, by inducing mania, disinhibition, akathisia or serotonin syndrome, which might unleash violence episodes [100, 107, 108]. Numerous preclinical and clinical studies have suggested that serotonin (5-hydroxytryptamine or 5-HT) plays a critical role in modulating some dimensions of personality and behaviour [108], and its increase is involved in the risk of antidepressant-related acting out episodes, including suicides [109].

Finally, modulation of 5-HT neurotransmission by gamma-aminobutyric acid (GABA) and glutamate may be of critical significance in both suppression and escalation of aggressive behaviour [110].

6.4.1.1 Alcohol

A causal link between alcohol and auto/hetero-aggressive behaviours has recently been suggested, with a statistically significant increase of aggression occurrence at an alcohol level of 0.75 g/kg or higher [111]. Alcohol may contribute to aggression by both decreasing the behavioural inhibitory activity of the frontal lobe region [100] and dysregulating higher order cognitive capacities, leading to an increase in impulsive behaviours and overreactions [111]. Considering accesses to the emergency departments related to violence, a history of chronic (mostly concurrent abuse of alcohol and cannabis) substance abuse may be identified in up to one out of three cases [56]. In a recent systematic review about outward violence within the emergency department setting, reports of patient- or visitor-perpetrated violence ranged between 1 and 172 per 10,000 presentations. Alcohol and drug exposure was associated with nearly one in every two violent patient's behaviour [112]. In the context of the emergency departments, not only alcohol intoxication but also alcohol withdrawal may be related with aggressiveness [113].

6.4.1.2 Stimulants

Cocaine and amphetamines are often implicated in impulsive and aggressive behaviours, especially if ingested together with alcohol [111]. This is possibly due to increase in self-confidence; assertiveness; impaired judgement and related paranoid ideation; disinhibition; hyperactivity; dysfunction of cognitive capacities of planning, lack of response inhibition; and emotional dysregulation [109, 111]. Chronic effects could lead to a proper 'limbic dyscontrol syndrome', which is in turn related to limbic structures' changes in both noradrenalin and serotonin levels [109]. Cocaine intake has been associated with violent behaviours, ranging from minor psychological aggressions to major physical acts, including murder and rape [114]. In a cross-sectional study including 1560 Brazilian young adults with lifetime use of crack cocaine, mortality was estimated at 20% and was typically related to drug-related murders and police confrontation [115].

Amphetamine users appeared to be significantly more agitated, violent and aggressive than patients with other toxicology-related emergency department presentations [116]. Amphetamine-type substances, including the 'ecstasy' (i.e. 3,4-methylenedeoxymethamphetamine/MDMA)-group molecules, have been associated with aggressive and violent behaviours [117]. Agitation and aggression were the main reported features in 48.2% of 2-(4-iodo-2,5-dimethoxyphenyl)-N-[(2-methoxyphenyl)methyl]ethanamine (25I-NBOMe; a psychedelic phenethylamine) toxicity cases in London nightclubs [118].

High dosage, long-term use, of stimulants is typically associated with intense psychotic symptoms, including delusions and hallucinations [119], which can drive either suicidal ideation or hetero-aggressiveness due to both high levels of DA increase and user's erroneous perception of danger [120]. Most troublesome adverse neuropsychiatric effects, including psychotic states and aggressive behaviours, occur with higher dosages and long-term use of amphetamines and methamphetamines, being associated with higher intensity drug craving and antisocial personality disorder comorbidity. Moreover, the persistent reduction in the serotonergic neurotransmission in abstinent users seems to contribute as well to increased levels of impulsivity and aggressive behaviours [119].

6.4.1.3 Cannabis

Despite the large body of related research, the strength of the association between marijuana use and aggression is still unclear [121, 122]. However, aggressiveness and chronic/heavy marijuana consumption may well be associated, due to changes in mood and behaviour during periods of both intoxication [123–125] and abstinence [122]. It is a reason of concern that daily use of marijuana during adolescence may determine the occurrence of neural connectivity impairment levels in the precuneus and fimbria of the hippocampus, together with a reduction of connectivity and inappropriate behaviour inhibition activity of the prefrontal cortex and in the subcortical regions [126, 127]. Indeed, early cannabis use has been implicated in criminal behaviour whilst being associated with both paranoid/suspicious ideation [126] and maladaptive interpersonal functioning [128].

High levels of aggressiveness have been related with delta-9-THC high-concentration cannabis, known to have potent psychotropic effects due to a strong agonist interaction with cannabinoid CB-1 receptors [128]. Overall, endocannabinoid abnormalities in specific psychopathological disorders have been reported, with preliminary evidence suggesting that the metabolising endocannabinoid enzyme fatty acid amide hydrolase genetic polymorphisms are linked to antisocial personality disorder and impulsive/antisocial psychopathic traits [129].

6.4.1.4 Opioids

Despite opioids being central nervous system depressants, they have been associated with violent behaviours. Indeed, opioid withdrawal can lead to heightened aggression levels due to increased sensitivity to pain, feelings of anxiety and agitation, and sleep disruption. Furthermore, opioids may reduce inhibition and management of acting-out behaviour, increasing the risk for violence [130]. Existing evidence suggests a strong link between opiates/opioids' drug use and involvement in crime, especially among individuals with frequent and problematic use of molecules such as heroin [131] and new synthetic opioids/fentanyls [132], but also prescribing molecules such as tramadol [133].

6.4.1.5 Benzodiazepines

Whilst being typically prescribed for the treatment of anxiety, benzodiazepines, even at therapeutic dosages, have been associated with violence, irritability and agitation (e.g. paradoxical reactions; [134]). These reactions are typically observed in poly-drug users [109], but also in the elderly [135], and in individuals with pre-existing brain damage [100]. This behavioural disinhibition may increase the risk of auto- or hetero-aggression and acting out [109, 136, 137]. Aggressive and hostile behaviours may be observed as well during the acute benzodiazepine withdrawal [136].

6.4.1.6 New Psychoactive Substances (NPS): Synthetic Cannabinoids and Synthetic Cathinones

Although sharing some properties with THC, synthetic cannabinoids exhibit full cannabinoid CB-1 receptor agonist activity, are highly lipophilic and cross the blood-brain barrier easily [138]. Effects could be unpredictable, with symptoms typically resembling cannabis intoxication, and including agitation, anxiety, irritability, hallucinations, cognitive impairment and psychosis (e.g. 'spiceophrenia'; [129, 138, 139]). In a sample of students, cannabinoid use was associated with physical outward violence, sexual risky behaviours and physical fights [140]. Among synthetic cannabinoids, most reported compounds include JWH derivatives, XRL-11, ADB-PINACA, AM-2201, MAM-2201 and 5F-PB-22 [141, 142].

Toxicity of synthetic cathinones includes significant sympathomimetic effects similar to amphetamines, related to both a dose-dependent inhibition on the reuptake of serotonin and dopamine and their affinity for serotonin 5-HT2 and dopamine D2 membrane transporters and receptors [143]. This stimulation could lead to psychotic episodes, agitation, aggression and sometimes violent and bizarre behaviours [144]. Mephedrone is one of the most reported cathinones used in the UK, and its consumption, alone or in combination with alcohol, could frequently induce these symptoms [145, 146]. In a forensic setting, the synthetic cathinone 3,4-methylenedioxypyrovalerone (MDPV) was detected in blood and urine samples of 50 individuals involved in violent crimes, including bodily harm, robberies, homicides and acts of resistance. In many cases, subjects showed highly aggressive and violent behaviour with endangerment of self and others and/or psychotic symptoms; the risk for such behaviours rose with plasma concentrations of MDPV above 30 mg/L [147]. Finally, mexedrone, a mephedrone derivative, was found in 11 of 305 patients who presented to an emergency department. All of them presented with agitation and six patients required sedation and/or physical restraint [143].

6.5   Prevention and Treatment Issues

6.5.1   Prevention

Social and ecological factors (e.g. parental neglect, authoritarian parental figures, being bullied, antisocial peer culture) represent important risk factors for the emergence of violence, especially in the youngsters [148]. Hence, early intervention on the parenting style, in terminating and preventing bullying and a healthy integration of peer, family, school and community bonds, could help to resolve some of these issues [148]. Also, violent neighbourhoods populated with gangs and drug dealers and easier access to weapons together with underemployment, high levels of transiency and overcrowding or unsafe housing constitute predisposing factors [148, 149]. Indeed, it has been shown that both neighbourhoods with positive processes (i.e. support, cohesion and involvement) and high-quality parenting (i.e. efficient monitoring, close relationship and warmth) reduce violent behaviour in children [150].

There is a clear need for drug misuse prevention and intervention efforts at the population level, highlighting social context influences and promoting greater awareness of the health risks associated with drugs, considering as well daily tobacco and marijuana use [151]. Prevention strategies should also be implemented in the emergency departments (ED), since individuals with mental disorders and substance misuse history who have been involved in serious violence episodes have visited EDs in the previous 6 months [152]. Although prior violence episodes may go under-reported [153], appropriate history taking and effective suicide risk assessment activities should be carried out [152]. Provided that the severity of the subject's ill-health condition allows for time and space for such interventions, the administration of a range of structured violence risk assessment tools may help the clinician in understanding the likelihood for violent behaviour to occur. These tools include the Dynamic Appraisal of Situational Aggression (DASA) [154], the Modified Overt Aggression Scale (MOAS) [65] and the Clinical Global Impression Scale (CGI-S) [153]. The use of such tools has facilitated the development of tailored non-pharmacological and non-coercive interventions [154, 155] as practices such as seclusion and restraint have historically been associated to increased risk levels of violence [156].

6.5.2 Drug-Related Violence and Aggressive Behaviour: Acute Treatment and Management Issues

Consumers of misusing drugs may present to EDs without providing information about the substances(s) ingested and it is likely that standard drug tests will show negative results [157]. Conversely, it is problematic to draft a universally valid treatment/management plan to cope with the behavioural and psychopathological disturbances related to the intake of the virtually few hundred [66] and up to a few thousand [158] substances currently available. Some clients may simply need reassurance, support and medical monitoring. When a medication may be needed, given the complex/unknown pharmacology of the substances arguably ingested, benzodiazepines may be the agents of choice (for a thorough review, see [157]). They may, however, need frequent re-dosing to achieve adequate sedative effect, and this may be a problem whilst in presence of alcohol. Benzodiazepines may be particularly useful for the treatment of the stimulant/synthetic cathinone-related agitation. Targeted treatment suggested includes intramuscular or intranasal midazolam, intramuscular lorazepam or intravenous diazepam to control aggression and agitation. This approach may be useful as well to stop seizures [159].

Where patients cannot be controlled with benzodiazepines alone, propofol and/ or antipsychotics may be considered, although drugs such as haloperidol, olanzapine or ziprasidone can lower seizure thresholds, and contribute to dysrhythmias. In general, the use of atypical antipsychotics has shown good efficacy in containing episode of aggression in different cohorts and different phases of illness [160, 161]. Indeed, although under-prescribed [162], clozapine presents with a specific profile against aggression, which may not be linked to its antipsychotic properties [163]. Interestingly, the psychonauts' 'ideal trip terminator' [164] olanzapine [163, 165, 166] can be considered as well. Although often used in the acute treatment of aggression [167, 168], efficacy of mood stabilisers in patients with dual diagnosis is controversial [169]. Notably, in a study focused on prevention of relapse in alcohol-dependent patients, oxcarbazepine showed efficacy in dual-diagnosis patients with high level of aggressiveness [170]. Finally, the intake of serotonergic misusing drugs (e.g. phenethylamines, hallucinogens, NBOMe compounds) may be associated with the occurrence of the serotonin syndrome, which is often associated with agitation, to be managed using both benzodiazepines and cyproheptadine [157].

Maintenance therapy should be focused on the treatment of SUD more than on violent behaviour. In fact, medications prescribed in the treatment of opioid-use disorder (e.g. buprenorphine and methadone) have been associated with reduction in prevalence of all crime (i.e. violent, nonviolent and substance related) categories in SUD individuals [171] whilst demonstrating efficacy in preventing both re-offending and re-incarceration [172, 173]. Moreover, methadone therapy has been related with a significant reduction in suicidal behaviour rates [171].

6.5.3   Longer Term Psychological Approach

Staff training, with a focus on counselling and motivational interviewing (MI), is critical, especially for patients with comorbid polysubstance-use disorder. MI was originally developed as a technique for motivating substance abusers to change [174]. MI/brief intervention techniques have been proposed as well for the treatment of aggressive behaviour in dual-diagnosis [175, 176], including adolescent [177, 178], populations albeit conflicting results have been reported [179].

6.6   Discussion and Conclusions

The rapidly evolving drug scenario phenomenon represents a challenge for medicine, and especially so for emergency physicians and mental health professionals. Indeed, drug misuse intake is typically associated with the imbalance of a range of neurotransmitter pathways/receptors, and consequently with a significant risk of psychopathological disturbances and related violence occurrence [66]. Non-adherence to prescribed medications appears linked to violent behaviours [180]; hence patients' education and counselling should be carefully considered by clinicians. The effect of the combined intake of drug, including NPS, products and whether simultaneous or sequential, could be detrimental to individuals' health [159]. In addition, the limitations of the current detection tools highlight the existing need for efficient on-site screening and detection [159].

More adequate information and understanding of how and why violent substance-related episodes, including fatalities, do occur and eventual with dissemination of timely statistics is here considered of paramount importance. Drug-related violent episodes should be recorded in sufficient detail for them to be identified, collated and analysed by a central point. This large data set may improve treatment strategies and service provision, but also inform education and prevention strategies.

Vulnerable subjects, including both children/adolescents and psychiatric patients, may be exposed to a large number of prodrug web pages, from which anecdotal levels of knowledge related to both well-known and novel psychotropics are typically provided by the 'e-psychonauts' (e.g. drug forum/blog communities' members). Hence, future approaches should consider the role of Web-based preventative strategies in targeting youngsters/vulnerable individuals at risk of approaching the drug market.

Future studies should provide better levels of misusing drugs' clinical pharmacological related knowledge, so that better tailored management/treatment strategies and guidelines can be made available. Finally, because of the complex behavioural and medical toxicity issues, raising awareness and education of healthcare professionals on drugs' health harms, interventions, harm reduction techniques and referral pathways are here deemed of particular relevance [159].

References

1. Coomber K, Mayshak R, Liknaitzky P, Curtis A, Walker A, Hyder S, Miller P. The role of illicit drug use in family and domestic violence in Australia. J Interpers Violence. 2019;11:886260519843288. https://doi.org/10.1177/0886260519843288. [Epub ahead of print].
2. Schifano F. Recent changes in drug abuse scenarios: the new/novel psychoactive substances (NPS) phenomenon. Brain Sci. 2018;8(12):E221. https://doi.org/10.3390/brainsci8120221.
3. American Psychiatric Association (APA). Diagnostic and statistical manual of mental disorders. 5th ed. Arlington, VA: American Psychiatric Publishing; 2013.
4. WHO. ICD-11 for Mortality and Morbidity Statistics (ICD-11-MMS). 2018. https://icd.who.int/browse11/l-m/en. Accessed 19 Apr 2019.
5. Papaseit E, Farré M, Schifano F, Torrens M. Emerging drugs in Europe. Curr Opin Psychiatry. 2014;27(4):243–50. https://doi.org/10.1097/YCO.0000000000000071.
6. WHO. World report on violence and health. 2002. https://www.who.int/violence_injury_prevention/violence/world_report/en/. Accessed 25 Apr 2019.
7. Nock MK, Borges G, Bromet EJ, Cha CB, Kessler RC, Lee S. Suicide and suicidal behavior. Epidemiol Rev. 2008;30(1):133–54.
8. WHO. Global health estimates 2016: estimates deaths by age, sex and cause. 2016. https://www.who.int/healthinfo/global_burden_disease/estimates/en/. Accessed 25 Apr 2019.
9. WHO. National suicide prevention strategies progress, examples and indicators. 2018. https://www.who.int/mental_health/suicide-prevention/national_strategies_2019/en/. Accessed 25 Apr 2019.
10. WHO. Preventing suicide: a global imperative. 2014. https://www.who.int/mental_health/suicide-prevention/world_report_2014/en/. Accessed 25 Apr 2019.
11. Kwon M, Yang S, Park K, Kim DJ. Factors that affect substance users suicidal behavior: a view from the Addiction Severity Index in Korea. Ann General Psychiatry. 2013;12:35.

12. Pereira-Morales AJ, Adan A, Camargo A, Forero DA. Substance use and suicide risk in a sample of young Colombian adults: an exploration of psychosocial factors. Am J Addict. 2017;26(4):388–94.
13. Dragisic T, Dickov A, Dickov V, Mijatovic V. Drug addiction as risk for suicide attempts. Mater Sociomed. 2015;27(3):188–91.
14. Maloney E, Degenhardt L, Darke S, Mattick RP, Nelson E. Suicidal behaviour and associated risk factors among opioid-dependent individuals: a case–control study. Addiction. 2007;102(12):1933–41.
15. Oyefeso A, Ghodse H, Clancy C, Corkery JM. Suicide among drug addicts in the UK. Br J Psychiatry. 1999;175:277–82.
16. Wilcox HC, Conner KR, Caine ED. Association of alcohol and drug use disorders and completed suicide: an empirical review of cohort studies. Drug Alcohol Depend. 2004;76(Suppl):S11–9.
17. McAllister M. Multiple meanings of self harm: a critical review. Int J Ment Health Nurs. 2003;12:177–85.
18. Skegg K. Self-harm. Lancet. 2010;376(9736):1471–83.
19. Whitlock J. Self-Injurious Behavior in Adolescents. PLoS Med. 2010;7(5):e1000240.
20. Hughes T, Szalacha LA, McNair R. Substance abuse and mental health disparities: comparisons across sexual identity groups in a national sample of young Australian women. Soc Sci Med. 2010;71:824–31.
21. Moller CI, Tait RJ, Byrne DG. Deliberate self-harm, substance use, and negative affect in nonclinical samples: a systematic review. Subst Abus. 2013;34(2):188–207.
22. Pattison EM, Kahan J. The deliberate self-harm syndrome. Am J Psychiatry. 1983;140:867–72.
23. Penn JV, Esposito CL, Schaeffer LE, Fritz GK, Spirito A. Suicide attempts and self- mutilative behavior in a juvenile correctional facility. J Am Acad Child Adolesc Psychiatry. 2003;42:762–9.
24. Riala K, Hakko H, Rasanen P. Nicotine dependence is associated with suicide attempts and self-mutilation among adolescent females. Compr Psychiatry. 2009;50:293–8.
25. Bross DC. World perspectives on child abuse: the fourth international resource book. Denver, CO: Kempe Children's Center, University of Colorado School of Medicine; 2000.
26. Theodore AD, Runyan DK. A medical research agenda for child maltreatment: negotiating the next steps. Pediatrics. 1999;104:168–77.
27. Hillis SD, Mercy J, Amobi A, Kress H. Global prevalence of past-year violence against children: a systematic review and minimum estimates. Pediatrics. 2016;137(3):e20154079.
28. Stoltenborgh M, van Ijzendoorn MH, Euser EM, Bakermans-Kranenburg MJ. A global perspective on child sexual abuse: meta-analysis of prevalence around the world. Child Maltreat. 2011;16(2):79–101.
29. Kepple NJ. The complex nature of parental substance use: examining past year and prior use behaviors as correlates of child maltreatment frequency. Subst Use Misuse. 2017;52(6):811–21.
30. Anda RF, Butchart A, Felitti VJ, Brown DW. Building a framework for global surveillance of the public health implications of adverse childhood experiences. Am J Prev Med. 2010;39(1):93–8.
31. Hillis SD, Anda RF, Felitti VJ, Nordenberg D, Marchbanks PA. Adverse childhood experiences and sexually transmitted diseases in men and women: a retrospective study. Pediatrics. 2000;106(1):e11.
32. Springer KW, Sheridan J, Kuo D, Carnes M. The long-term health outcomes of childhood abuse an overview and a call to action. J Gen Intern Med. 2003;18:864–70.
33. Elwyn L, Smith C. Child maltreatment and adult substance abuse: the role of memory. J Soc Work Pract Addict. 2013;13(3):269–94.
34. Goldstein RB, Compton WM, Pulay AJ, Ruan WJ, Pickering RP, Stinson FS, et al. Antisocial behavioral syndromes and DSM-IV drug use disorders in the United States: results from the National Epidemiologic Survey on Alcohol and Related Conditions. Drug Alcohol Depend. 2007;90(2–3):145–58.
35. Ladd GT, Petry NM. Antisocial personality in treatment-seeking cocaine abusers: psychosocial functioning and HIV risk. J Subst Abus Treat. 2003;24(4):323–30.

36. Luk JW, Worley MJ, Winiger E, Trim RS, Hopfer CJ, Hewitt JK, et al. Risky driving and sexual behaviors as developmental outcomes of co-occurring substance use and antisocial behavior. Drug Alcohol Depend. 2016;169:19–25.

37. Casadio P, Olivoni D, Ferrari B, Pintori C, Speranza E, Bosi M, et al. Personality disorders in addiction outpatients: prevalence and effects on psychosocial functioning. Subst Abuse. 2014;31(8):17–24.

38. Westermeyer J, Thuras P. Association of antisocial personality disorder and substance disorder morbidity in a clinical sample. Am J Drug Alcohol Abuse. 2005;31(1):93–110.

39. Brooner RK, Schmidt CW, Felch LJ, Bigelow GE. Antisocial behavior of intravenous drug abusers: implications for diagnosis of antisocial personality disorder. Am J Psychiatry. 1992;149(4):482–7.

40. Cottler LB, Price RK, Compton WM, Mager DE. Subtypes of adult antisocial behavior among drug abusers. J Nerv Ment Dis. 1995;183(3):154–61.

41. Žarkovic Palijan T, Mužinić L, Radeljak S. Psychiatric comorbidity in forensic psychiatry. Psychiatr Danub. 2009;21(3):429–36.

42. Tielbeek JJ, Vink JM, Polderman TJC, Popma A, Posthuma D, Verweij KJH. Genetic correlation of antisocial behaviour with alcohol, nicotine, and cannabis use. Drug Alcohol Depend. 2018;187:296–9.

43. Allroggen M, Rassenhofer M, Witt A, Plener PL, Brähler E, Fegert JM. The prevalence of sexual violence. Dtsch Arztebl Int. 2016;113(7):107–13.

44. Jahromi MK, Jamali S, Rahmanian Koshkaki A, Javadpour S. Prevalence and risk factors of domestic violence against women by their husbands in Iran. Glob J Health Sci. 2015;8(5):175–83.

45. U.S. Department of Justice—Full report of the prevalence, incidence, and consequences of violence against women. 2000. www.ncjrs.gov/pdffiles1/nij/183781.pdf. Accessed 5 Apr 2019.

46. WHO. Multi-country study on women's health and domestic violence against women. 2005. https://www.who.int/gender/violence/who_multicountry_study/summary_report/summary_report_English2.pdf. Accessed 5 Apr 2019.

47. World Health Organisation [WHO] (2012). Understanding and addressing violence against women. Available from https://apps.who.int/iris/bitstream/handle/10665/77434/WHO_RHR_12.37_eng.pdf;jsessionid=8E7FDC40D041025A09BF8CB75379B936?sequence=1. Accessed 8 Oct, 2019.

48. Coker AL, Smith PH, Bethea L, King MR, McKeown RE. Physical health consequences of physical and psychological intimate partner violence. Arch Fam Med. 2000;9(5):451–7.

49. Do VT, Ho HT, Nguyen TM, Do HK. Sexual violence and the risk of HIV transmission in sexual partners of male injecting drug users in Tien Du district, Bac Ninh province of Vietnam. Health Care Women Int. 2018;39(4):404–14.

50. Holmes MM, Resnick HS, Kilpatrick DG, Best CL. Rape-related pregnancy: estimates and descriptive characteristics from a national sample of women. Am J Obstet Gynecol. 1996;175(2):320–5.

51. Kaslow NJ, Thompson MP, Meadows LA, Jacobs D, Chance S, Gibb B, et al. Factors that mediate and moderate the link between partner abuse and suicidal behavior in African American women. J Consult Clin Psychol. 1998;66(3):533–40.

52. López-Castroman J, Melhem N, Birmaher B, Greenhill L, Kolko D, Stanley B, et al. Early childhood sexual abuse increases suicidal intent. World Psychiatry. 2013;12(2):149–54.

53. Sutton TE, Gordon Simons L, Tyler KA. Hooking-up and sexual victimization on campus: examining moderators of risk. J Interpers Violence. 2019:886260519842178. https://doi.org/10.1177/0886260519842178

54. Graham KR. The childhood victimization of sex offenders: an underestimated issue. Int J Offender Ther Comp Criminol. 1996;40(3):192–203.

55. Jewkes R, Sikweyiya Y, Morrell R, Dunkle K. Gender inequitable masculinity and sexual entitlement in rape perpetration South Africa: findings of a cross-sectional study. PLoS One. 2011;6(12):e29590.

56. Liakoni E, Gartwyl F, Ricklin M, Exadaktylos AK, Krähenbühl S. Psychoactive substances and violent offences: a retrospective analysis of presentations to an urban emergency department in Switzerland. PLoS One. 2018;13(3):e0195234.
57. Grisso JA, Schwarz DF, Hirschinger N, Sammel M, Brensinger C, Santanna J, et al. Violent injuries among women in an urban area. N Engl J Med. 1999;341:1899–905.
58. Parrott DJ, Lisco CG. Effects of alcohol and sexual prejudice on aggression toward sexual minorities. Psychol Viol. 2015;5:256–65.
59. Crane CA, Easton CJ. Physical health conditions and intimate partner violence perpetration among offenders with alcohol use diagnoses. J Interpers Violence. 2017 Jun;32(11):1678–91. https://doi.org/10.1177/0886260515590124.
60. Corkery JM, Loi B, Claridge H, Goodair C, Corazza O, Elliott S, et al. Gamma hydroxybutyrate (GHB), gamma butyrolactone (GBL) and 1,4 butanediol (1,4-BD, BDO): a literature review with a focus on UK fatalities related to non-medical use. Neurosci Biobehav Rev. 2015;53:52–78.
61. Schifano F, Corkery J, Oyefeso A, Tonia T, Ghodse AH. Trapped in the "K-hole": overview of deaths associated with ketamine misuse in the UK (1993–2006). J Clin Psychopharmacol. 2008;28(1):114–6.
62. Giorgetti R, Tagliabracci A, Schifano F, Zaami S, Marinelli E, Busardò FP. When "chems" meet sex: a rising phenomenon called "chemsex". Curr Neuropharmacol. 2017;15(5):762–70. https://doi.org/10.2174/1570159X15666161117151148.
63. Watts C, Zimmermann C. Violence against women: global scope and magnitude. Lancet. 2002;359(9313):1232–7.
64. Room R, Babor T, Rehm J. Alcohol and public health. Lancet. 2005;365(9458):519–30.
65. Amore M, Menchetti M, Tonti C, Scarlatti F, Lundgren E, Esposito W, et al. Predictors of violent behavior among acute psychiatric patients: clinical study. Psychiatry Clin Neurosci. 2008;62(3):247–55.
66. Schifano F, Orsolini L, Duccio Papanti G, Corkery JM. Novel psychoactive substances of interest for psychiatry. World Psychiatry. 2015;14(1):15–26. https://doi.org/10.1002/wps.20174.
67. Goldstein PJ. The drugs/violence nexus: a tripartite conceptual framework. J Drug Issues. 1985;15(4):493–506.
68. Corkery JM, Schifano F, Oyefeso A, Ghodse AH, Tonia T, Naidoo V, et al. Review of literature and information on 'khat-related' mortality: a call for recognition of the issue and further research. Annali dell'Istituto Superiore di Sanità. 2011;47(4):445–64.
69. European Monitoring Centre for Drugs and Drug Addiction (EMCDDA). Drug-related homicide in Europe: a first review of the data and literature. 2018. http://www.emcdda.europa.eu/publications/emcdda-papers/drug-related-homicide-in-europe-review-data-literature_en. Accessed 5 Apr 2019.
70. Heffernan R, Martin MJ, Romano AT. Homicides related to drug trafficking. Fed Probation. 1982;46(3):3–7.
71. Akers RL. Drugs, alcohol, and society: social structure, process, and policy. Belmont, CA: Wadsworth Publishing; 1992.
72. Hohl BC, Wiley S, Wiebe DJ, Culyba AJ, Drake R, Branas CC. Association of drug and alcohol use with adolescent firearm homicide at individual, family, and neighborhood levels. JAMA Intern Med. 2017;177(3):317–24.
73. Office for National Statistics (ONS). Homicide in England and Wales: year ending March 2018. 2018. https://www.ons.gov.uk/peoplepopulationandcommunity/crimeandjustice/articles/homicideinenglandandwales/yearendingmarch2018#drug-and-alcohol-related-homicides. Accessed 5 Apr 2019.
74. Corkery J. UK drug-related mortality—issues in definition and classification. Drugs Alcohol Today. 2008;8(2):17–25.
75. Corkery J, Claridge H, Loi B, Goodair C, Schifano F. Drug-related deaths in the UK: Annual Report 2013. Drug-related deaths reported by coroners in England, Wales, Northern Ireland, Guernsey, Jersey and the Isle of Man; Police forces in Scotland; and the Northern Ireland Statistics and Research Agency—Annual Report January–December 2012. London: International Centre for Drug Policy, St Georges University of London. 2014. https://www.sgul.ac.uk/images/docs/idcp%20pdfs/National%20programme%20on%20substance%20

abuse%20deaths/National_Programme_on_Substance_Abuse_Deaths-Annual_Report_2013_ on_Drug-related_Deaths_in_the_UK_January-December_2012_PDF.pdf. Accessed 20 Apr 2019.

76. HQIP. National Confidential Inquiry into Suicide and Homicide by People with Mental Illness. Annual Report 2017: England, Northern Ireland, Scotland and Wales. Healthcare Quality Improvement Partnership. University of Manchester. 2017. http://documents.manchester. ac.uk/display.aspx?DocID=37560. Accessed 20 Apr 2019.

77. HQIP. National Confidential Inquiry into Suicide and Safety in Mental Health – Annual Report 2018: England, Northern Ireland, Scotland, Wales. Healthcare Quality Improvement Partnership. University of Manchester. 2018. http://documents.manchester.ac.uk/display. aspx?DocID=38469. Accessed 20 Apr 2019.

78. Schifano F, Corkery J, Ghodse AH. Suspected and confirmed fatalities associated with mephedrone (4-methylmethcathinone, "meow meow") in the United Kingdom. J Clin Psychopharmacol. 2012;32(5):710–4. https://doi.org/10.1097/JCP.0b013e318266c70c.

79. Oyefeso A, Schifano F, Ghodse H, Cobain K, Dryden R, Corkery J. Fatal injuries while under the influence of psychoactive drugs: a cross-sectional exploratory study in England. BMC Public Health. 2006;6:148.

80. Chiappini S, Claridge H, Corkery JM, Goodair C, Loi B, Schifano F. Methoxetamine-related deaths in the UK: an overview. Hum Psychopharmacol Clin Exp. 2015;30(4):244–8.

81. Corkery JM, Schifano F, Ghodse AH. Mephedrone-related fatalities in the United Kingdom: contextual, clinical and practical issues. In: Gallelli L, editor. Pharmacology. Rijeka: InTech—Open Access Publisher; 2012. p. 355–80.

82. European Drug Monitoring Centre for Drugs and Drug Addiction (EMCDDA). Perspectives on drugs. Comorbidity of substance use and mental health disorders in Europe. 2016. http://www. emcdda.europa.eu/system/files/publications/2935/Comorbidity_POD2016.pdf. Accessed 4 Apr 2019.

83. Substance Abuse and Mental Health Services Administration (SAMHSA). Behavioral health trends in the United States: results from the 2014 national survey on drug use and health. 2014. https://www.samhsa.gov/data/sites/default/files/NSDUH-FRR1-2014/NSDUH-FRR1-2014. htm#idtextanchor086. Accessed 4 Apr 2019.

84. Gostin LO, Record KL. Dangerous people or dangerous weapons: access to firearms for persons with mental illness. JAMA. 2011;305(20):2108–9.

85. Latt N, Jurd S, Tennant C, Lewis J, Macken L, Joseph A, et al. Alcohol and substance use by patients with psychosis presenting to an emergency department: changing patterns. Australas Psychiatry. 2011;19:354.

86. Soyka M. Substance misuse, psychiatric disorder and violent and disturbed behaviour. Br J Psychiatry. 2000;176:345–50.

87. Swanson JW, Holzer CE III, Ganju VK, Jono RT. Violence and psychiatric disorder in the community: evidence from the Epidemiologic Catchment Area surveys. Hosp Community Psychiatry. 1990;41(7):761–70.

88. Volavka J, Swanson J. Violent behavior in mental illness: the role of substance abuse. JAMA. 2010;304(5):563–4.

89. Zhuo Y, Bradizza CM, Maisto SA. The influence of treatment attendance on subsequent aggression among severely mentally ill substance abusers. J Subst Abus Treat. 2014;47(5):353–61.

90. Mueser KT, Yarnold PR, Levinson DF, Singh H, Bellack AS, Kee K, Morrison RL, Yadalam KG. Prevalence of substance abuse in schizophrenia: demographic and clinical correlates. Schizophr Bull. 1990;16(1):31–56.

91. Stompe T, Ritter K, Schanda H. Patterns of substance abuse in offenders with schizophrenia—illness-related or criminal life-style? Front. Psychiatry. 2018;9:233. https://doi.org/10.3389/ fpsyt.2018.00233.

92. Erkiran M, Ozunalan H, Cuneyt E, Aytaclar S, Kirisci L, Tarteret R. Substance abuse amplifies the risk for violence in schizophrenia spectrum disorder. Addict Behav. 2006;31:1797–805.

93. Swanson JW, Swartz MS, Van Dorn RA, Elbogen EB, Wagner HR, Rosenheck RA, et al. A national study of violent behaviour in persons with schizophrenia. Arch Gen Psychiatry. 2006;63:490–9.

94. Haddock G, Eisner E, Davies G, Coupe N, Barrowclough N. Psychotic symptoms, self-harm and violence in individuals with schizophrenia and substance misuse problems. Schizophr Res. 2013;151(1–3):215–20.
95. Link B, Stueve A. Psychotic symptoms and the violent/illegal behavior of mental patients compared to the community. In: Monahan J, Steadman H, editors. Violence and mental disorder: development in risk assessment. Chicago: University of Chicago Press; 1994. p. 137–58.
96. Maremmani AGI, Rugani F, Bacciardi S, Rovai L, Pacini M, Dell'Osso L, et al. Does dual diagnosis affect violence and moderate/superficial self-harm in heroin addiction at treatment entry? J Addict Med. 2014;8:116–22.
97. Alnıak I, Erkıran M, Mutlu E. Substance use is a risk factor for violent behaviour in male patients with bipolar disorder. J Affect Disord. 2016;193:89–93.
98. Fazel S, Lichtenstein P, Grann M, Goodwin GM, Langström N. Bipolar disorder and violent crime new evidence from population-based longitudinal studies and systematic review. Arch Gen Psychiatry. 2010;67(9):931–8.
99. Lewis CF. Substance use and violent behavior in women with antisocial personality disorder. Behav Sci Law. 2011;29:667–76.
100. Anderson PD, Bokor G. Forensic aspects of drug-induced violence. J Pharm Pract. 2012;25(1):41–9.
101. Ferner RE. Effects of drugs on behavior. Forensic pharmacology: medicines, mayhem, and malpractice. Oxford: Oxford University Press; 1996. p. 73–8.
102. Moore TJ, Glenmullen J, Furberg CD. Prescription drugs report with associated with reports of violence towards others. PLoS One. 2010;5(12):1–5.
103. Steele JL, Peralta RL. Are polydrug users more physically and verbally aggressive? An assessment of aggression among mono- versus polydrug users in a university sample. J Interpers Violence. 2017;886260517715024. https://doi.org/10.1177/0886260517715024.
104. Osgood DW, Johnston LD, O'Malley PM, Bachman JG. The generality of deviance in late adolescence and early adulthood. Am Sociol Rev. 1996;53(1):80–92.
105. Miyata J. Toward integrated understanding of salience in psychosis. Neurobiol Dis. 2019:S0969-9961(19)30061-0. https://doi.org/10.1016/j.nbd.2019.03.002.
106. Ntounas P, Katsouli A, Efstathiou V, Pappas D, Chatzimanolis P, Touloumis C, Papageorgiou C, Douzenis A. Comparative study of aggression—dangerousness on patients with paranoid schizophrenia: focus on demographic data, PANSS, drug use and aggressiveness. Int J Law Psychiatry. 2018;60:1–11. https://doi.org/10.1016/j.ijlp.2018.06.001.
107. Rouve N, Bagheri H, Telmon N, Pathak A, Franchitto N, Schmitt L, et al. Prescribed drugs and violence: a case/noncase study in the French pharmacovigilance database. Eur J Clin Pharmacol. 2011;67(11):1189–98.
108. Wolkers CPB, Serra M, Júnior AB, Urbinati EC. Acute fluoxetine treatment increases aggressiveness in juvenile matrinxã (Brycon amazonicus). Fish Physiol Biochem. 2017;43(3):755–9.
109. Gillet C, Polard E, Mauduit N, Allain H. Acting out and psychoactive substances: alcohol, drugs, illicit substances. Encephale. 2001;27(4):351–9.
110. Miczek KA, DeBold JF, Hwa LS, Newman EL, de Almeida RMM. Alcohol and violence: neuropeptidergic modulation of monoamine systems. Ann N Y Acad Sci. 2015;1349(1):96–118.
111. Kuypers K, Verkes RJ, van der Brink W, van Amsterdam JGC, Ramaekers JC. Intoxicated aggression: do alcohol and stimulants cause dose-related aggression? A review. Eur Neuropsychopharmacol. 2018:1–34. Pii: S0924-977X(18)30147-0. https://doi.org/10.1016/j.euroneuro.2018.06.001.
112. Nikathil S, Olaussen A, Gocentas RA, Symons E, Mitra B. Workplace violence in the emergency department: a systematic review and meta-analysis. Emerg Med Australas. 2017;29(3):265–75.
113. Morgan MY. Acute alcohol toxicity and withdrawal in the emergency room and medical admissions unit. Clin Med (Lond). 2015;15(5):486–9.
114. Miller NS, Gold MS, Mahler JC. Violent behaviors associated with cocaine use: possible pharmacological mechanisms. Int J Addict. 1991;26(10):1077–88.

115. Narvaez GCM, Jansen K, Pinheiro RT, Kapczinski F, Silva RA, Pechansky F, et al. Violent and sexual behaviors and lifetime use of crack cocaine: a population-based study in Brazil. Soc Psychiatry Psychiatr Epidemiol. 2014;49(8):1249–55.

116. Bunting PJ, Fulde GWO, Forster SL. Comparison of crystalline methamphetamine ("ICE") users and other patients with toxicology-related problems presenting to a hospital emergency department. Med J Aust. 2007;187:564–6.

117. Vaughn MG, Salas-Wright CP, DeLisi M, Perron BE, Cordova D. Crime and violence among MDMA users in the United States. AIMS Public Health. 2015;2(1):64–73. https://doi.org/10.3934/publichealth.2015.1.64.

118. Wood D, Sedefov R, Cunningham A, Dargan PI. Prevalence of use and acute toxicity associated with the use of NBOMe drugs. Clin Toxicol. 2015;53:85–92.

119. Harro J. Neuropsychiatric adverse effects of amphetamine and methamphetamine. Int Rev Neurobiol. 2015;120:179–204.

120. Fulde GWO, Forster SL. The impact of amphetamine-type stimulants on emergency services. Curr Opin Psychiatry. 2015;28:275–9.

121. Ostrowsky MK. Does marijuana use lead to aggression and violent behavior? J Drug Educ. 2011;41(4):369–89.

122. Smith PH, Homish GG, Leonard KE, Collins RL. Marijuana withdrawal and aggression among a representative sample of U.S. marijuana users. Drug Alcohol Depend. 2013;132(0):63–8.

123. Allsop DJ, Norberg MM, Copeland J, Fu S, Budney AJ. The Cannabis Withdrawal Scale development: patterns and predictors of cannabis withdrawal and distress. Drug Alcohol Depend. 2011;119:123–9.

124. Budney AJ, Hughes JR. The cannabis withdrawal syndrome. Curr Opin Psychiatry. 2006;19:233.

125. Kouri EM, Pope HG Jr, Lukas SE. Changes in aggressive behavior during withdrawal from long-term marijuana use. Psychopharmacology. 1999;143:302–8.

126. Barthelemy OJ, Richardson MA, Cabral HJ, Frank DA. Prenatal, perinatal, and adolescent exposure to marijuana: relationships with aggressive behaviour. Neurotoxicol Teratol. 2016;58:60–77.

127. Volkow ND, Baler RD, Compton WM, Weiss SRB. Adverse health effects of marijuana use. N Engl J Med. 2014;370:2219–27.

128. Martinotti G, Cinosi E, Santacroce R, Papanti D, Pasquini A, Mancini V, et al. Substance-related psychopathology and aggressiveness in a nightlife holiday resort: results from a pilot study in a psychiatric inpatient unit in Ibiza. Hum Psychopharmacol Clin Exp. 2017;32:e2586.

129. Kolla NJ, Mishra A. The endocannabinoid system, aggression, and the violence of synthetic cannabinoid use, borderline personality disorder, antisocial personality disorder, and other psychiatric disorders. Front Behav Neurosci. 2018;12:41.

130. Schifano F. Substance misuse in the workplace. In: Ghodse AH, editor. Addiction at work: tackling drug use and misuse in the workplace. Aldershot: Gower Publishing Ltd; 2005. p. 53–67.

131. Hayhurst KP, Pierce M, Hickman M, Seddon T, Dunn G, Keane J, et al. Pathways through opiate use and offending: a systematic review. Int J Drug Policy. 2017;39:1–13.

132. Schifano F, Chiappini S, Corkery J, Guirguis A. Assessing the 2004–2018 fentanyl misusing issues reported to an international range of adverse reporting systems. Front Pharmacol. 2019;10:46. https://doi.org/10.3389/fphar.2019.00046.

133. El-Hadidy MA, Helaly AML. Medical and psychiatric effects of long-term dependence on high dose of tramadol. Subst Use Misuse. 2015;50(5):582–9.

134. Tae CH, Kang KJ, Min BH, Ahn JH, Kim S, Lee JH, Rhee PL, Kim JJ. Paradoxical reaction to midazolam in patients undergoing endoscopy under sedation: incidence, risk factors and the effect of flumazenil. Dig Liver Dis. 2014;46(8):710–5. https://doi.org/10.1016/j.dld.2014.04.007.

135. Reddy MSS, Achary U, Harbishettar V, Sivakumar PT, Varghese M. Paradoxical reaction to benzodiazepines in elderly—case series. Asian J Psychiatr. 2018;35:8–10. https://doi.org/10.1016/j.ajp.2018.04.037.

136. Saxon L, Borg S, Hiltunen AJ. Reduction of aggression during benzodiazepine withdrawal: effects of flumazenil. Pharmacol Biochem Behav. 2010;96(2):148–51.
137. Wallace PS, Taylor SP. Reduction of appeasement-related affect as a concomitant of diazepam-induced aggression: evidence for a link between aggression and the expression of self-conscious emotions. Aggress Behav. 2009;35:203–12.
138. Papanti D, Schifano F, Botteon G, Bertossi F, Mannix J, Vidoni D, Impagnatiello M, Pascolo-Fabrici E, Bonavigo T. "Spiceophrenia": a systematic overview of "spice"-related psychopathological issues and a case report. Hum Psychopharmacol. 2013;28(4):379–89. https://doi.org/10.1002/hup.2312.
139. Courts J, Maskill V, Gray A, Glue P. Signs and symptoms associated with synthetic cannabinoid toxicity: systematic review. Australas Psychiatry. 2016;24(6):598–601.
140. Clayton HB, Lowry R, Ashley C, Wolkin A, Grant AM. Health risk behaviors with synthetic cannabinoids versus marijuana. Pediatrics. 2017;139(4):e20162675.
141. Armenian P, Darracq M, Gevorkyan J, Clark S, Kaye B, Brandehoff NP. Intoxication from the novel synthetic cannabinoids AB-PINACA and ADB-PINACA: a case series and review of the literature. Neuropharmacology. 2018;134(Pt A):82–91.
142. Tournebize J, Gibaja V, Kahn JP. Acute effects of synthetic cannabinoids: update 2015. Subst Abus. 2017;38(3):344–66.
143. Roberts L, Ford L, Patel N, Vale JA, Bradberry SM. 11 analytically confirmed cases of mexedrone use among polydrug users. Clin Toxicol (Phila). 2017;55(3):181–6.
144. Capriola M. Synthetic cathinone abuse. Clin Pharmacol. 2013;5:109–15.
145. James D, Adams RD, Spears R, Cooper G, Lupton DJ, Thompson JP, et al. Clinical characteristics of mephedrone toxicity reported to the UK National Poisons Information Service. Emerg Med J. 2011;28:686–9.
146. Schifano F, Albanese A, Fergus S, Stair JL, Deluca P, Corazza O, Davey Z, Corkery J, Siemann H, Scherbaum N, Farré M, Torrens M, Demetrovics Z, Ghodse AH, Psychonaut Web Mapping, ReDNet Research Groups. Mephedrone (4-methylmethcathinone; 'meow meow'): chemical, pharmacological and clinical issues. Psychopharmacology. 2011;214(3):593–602. https://doi.org/10.1007/s00213-010-2070-x.
147. Diestelmann M, Zangl A, Herrle I, Koch E, Graw M, Paul LD. MDPV in forensic routine cases: psychotic and aggressive behavior in relation to plasma concentrations. Forensic Sci Int. 2018;283:72–84.
148. Gilligan J, Lee B. The psychopharmacologic treatment of violent youth. Ann N Y Acad Sci. 2004;1036(1):356–81.
149. Timmis S. Doctors should not be legally obliged to report youths at risk of knife crime. BMJ. 2019;365:l1973.
150. Miller GM, Tolan PH. The influence of parenting practices and neighborhood characteristics on the development of childhood aggression. J Community Psychol. 2019;47(1):135–46.
151. Oser CB, Harp K, Pullen E, Bunting AM, Stevens-Watkins D, Staton M. African-American women's tobacco and marijuana use: the effects of social context and substance use perceptions. Subst Use Misuse. 2019;54(6):873–84. https://doi.org/10.1080/10826084.2018.1528464.
152. Wang J, Xie H, Holland KM, Sumner SA, Balaji AB, David-Ferdon CF, et al. Self-directed violence after medical emergency department visits among youth. Am J Prev Med. 2019;56(2):205–14.
153. Fond G, Boyer L, Boucekine M, Girard V, Loubière S, Lenoir C, French Housing First Study Group, et al. Illness and drug modifiable factors associated with violent behavior in homeless people with severe mental illness: results from the French Housing First (FHF) program. Prog Neuropsychopharmacol Biol Psychiatry. 2019;90:92–6.
154. Kaunomäki J, Jokela M, Kontio R, Laiho T, Sailas E, Lindberg N. Interventions following a high violence risk assessment score: a naturalistic study on a Finnish psychiatric admission ward. BMC Health Serv Res. 2017;17(1):26.
155. Ogloff JR, Daffern M. The dynamic appraisal of situational aggression: an instrument to assess risk for imminent aggression in psychiatric inpatients. Behav Sci Law. 2006;24(6):799–813.

156. Khadivi AN, Patel RC, Atkinson AR, Levine JM. Association between seclusion and restraint and patient-related violence. Psychiatr Serv. 2004;55(11):1311–2.
157. Schifano F, Orsolini L, Papanti GD, Corkery JM. NPS: medical consequences associated with their intake. Curr Top Behav Neurosci. 2017;32:351–80. https://doi.org/10.1007/7854_2016_15.
158. Schifano F, Chiappini S, Corkery JM, Guirguis A. Abuse of prescription drugs in the context of novel psychoactive substances (NPS): a systematic review. Brain Sci. 2018 Apr 22;8(4):pii: E73. https://doi.org/10.3390/brainsci8040073.
159. Guirguis A, Corkery J, Stair J, Kirton S, Zloh M, Schifano F. Intended and unintended use of cathinone mixtures. Hum Psychopharmacol Clin Exp. 2017;32(3). https://doi.org/10.1002/hup.2598.
160. Mauri MC, Rovera C, Paletta S, De Gaspari IF, Maffini M, Altamura AC. Aggression and psychopharmacological treatments in major psychosis and personality disorders during hospitalisation. Prog Neuro-Psychopharmacol Biol Psychiatry. 2011;35(7):1631–5.
161. Swanson JW, Swartz MS, Van Dorn RA, Volavka J, Monahan J, Stroup TS, et al. Comparison of antipsychotic medication effects on reducing violence in people with schizophrenia. Br J Psychiatry. 2008;193(1):37–43.
162. Patchan K, Vyas G, Hackman AL, Mackowick M, Richardson CM, Love RC, et al. Clozapine in reducing aggression and violence in forensic populations. Psychiatry Q. 2018;89(1):157–68.
163. Volavka J. Violence in schizophrenia and bipolar disorder. Psychiatr Danub. 2013;25(1):0–33.
164. Valeriani G, Corazza O, Bersani FS, Melcore C, Metastasio A, Bersani G, Schifano F. Olanzapine as the ideal 'trip terminator'? Analysis of online reports relating to antipsychotics' use and misuse following the occurrence of novel psychoactive substance-related psychotic symptoms. Human Psychopharmacol Clin Exp. 2015;30:249–54.
165. Kasinathan J, Sharp G, Barker A. Evaluation of olanzapine pamoate depot in seriously violent males with schizophrenia in the community. Ther Adv Psychopharmacol. 2016;6(5):301–7.
166. Volavka J, Citrome L. Pathways to aggression in schizophrenia affect results of treatment. Schizophr Bull. 2011;37(5):921–9.
167. Jones RM, Arlidge J, Gillham R, Reagu S, van den Bree M, Taylor PJ. Efficacy of mood stabilisers in the treatment of impulsive or repetitive aggression: systematic review and meta-analysis. Br J Psychiatry. 2011;198(2):93–8.
168. Lindenmayer JP, Kotsaftis A. Use of sodium valproate in violent and aggressive behaviors: a critical review. J Clin Psychiatry. 2000;61(2):123–8.
169. Maremmani I, Pacini M, Lamanna F, Pani PP, Perugi G, Deltito J, et al. Mood stabilizers in the treatment of substance use disorders. CNS Spectr. 2010;15(02):95–109.
170. Martinotti G, Di Nicola M, Romanelli R, Andreoli S, Pozzi G, Moroni N, et al. High and low dosage oxcarbazepine versus naltrexone for the prevention of relapse in alcohol-dependent patients. Hum Psychopharmacol. 2007;22:149–56.
171. Molero Y, Zetterqvist J, Binswanger IA, Hellner C, Larsson H, Fazel S. Medications for alcohol and opioid use disorders and risk of suicidal behavior, accidental overdoses, and crime. Am J Psychiatry. 2018;175(10):970–8.
172. Chang Z, Lichtenstein P, Långström N, Larsson H, Fazel S. Association between prescription of major psychotropic medications and violent reoffending after prison release. JAMA. 2016;316:1798–807.
173. Hedrich D, Alves P, Farrell M, Stöver H, Møller L, Mayet S. The effectiveness of opioid maintenance treatment in prison settings: a systematic review. Addiction. 2012;107:501–17.
174. Miller WR, Rollnick S. Motivational interviewing: preparing people to change addictive behavior. New York: Guilford Press; 1991.
175. López-Castro T, Smith KZ, Nicholson RA, Armas A, Hien DA. Does a history of violent offending impact treatment response for comorbid PTSD and substance use disorders? A secondary analysis of a randomized controlled trial. J Subst Abus Treat. 2019;97:47–58.
176. McMurran M. Motivational interviewing with offenders: a systematic review. Leg Criminol Psychol. 2009;14(1):83–100.

177. Cunningham RM, Chermack ST, Zimmerman MA, Shope JT, Bingham CR, Blow FC, et al. Brief motivational interviewing intervention for peer violence and alcohol use in teens: one-year follow-up. Pediatrics. 2012;129(6):1083.
178. Zatzick D, Russo J, Lord SP, Varley C, Wang J, Berliner L, et al. Collaborative care intervention targeting violence risk behaviors, substance use, and posttraumatic stress and depressive symptoms in injured adolescents: a randomized clinical trial. JAMA Pediatr. 2014;168(6):532–9.
179. Steinauer R, Huber CG, Petitjean S, Wiesbeck GA, Dürsteler KM, Lang UE, et al. Effect of door-locking policy on inpatient treatment of substance use and dual disorders. Eur Addict Res. 2017;23(2):87–96.
180. Hedlund J, Forsman J, Sturup J, Masterman T. Psychotropic medications in Swedish homicide victims and offenders: a forensic-toxicological case-control study of adherence and recreational use. J Clin Psychiatry. 2017;78(7):e797–802.

Posttraumatic Stress Disorder, Intimate Partner Violence, and Trauma-Informed Intervention

7

Ohad Gilbar, Katherine E. Gnall, Hannah E. Cole, and Casey T. Taft

7.1 Posttraumatic Stress Disorder Diagnostic Criteria and Intimate Partner Violence

Posttraumatic stress disorder (PTSD) is a trauma-related disorder that has consistently been linked to increased risk for the perpetration of intimate partner violence (IPV) in military veterans and civilians [1]. It can be instructive to examine the features of the PTSD diagnosis as they relate to IPV. As delineated in the fifth edition of the *Diagnostic and Statistical Manual of Mental Disorders* (*DSM-5*), PTSD results from one or more exposures to "actual or threatened death, serious injury, or sexual violence" [2]. Specific examples include exposure to military combat, war, physical assault, and sexual assault; being kidnapped or taken hostage; terrorist

O. Gilbar
Boston University School of Medicine, Boston, MA, USA

VA Boston Healthcare System, Boston, MA, USA

K. E. Gnall · H. E. Cole (✉)
Boston University School of Medicine, Boston, MA, USA

VA Boston Healthcare System, Boston, MA, USA

National Center for PTSD, Behavioral Science Division, Boston, MA, USA
e-mail: Hannah.cole@va.gov

C. T. Taft (✉)
National Center for PTSD, Behavioral Science Division, Boston, MA, USA
e-mail: casey.taft@va.gov

© Springer Nature Switzerland AG 2020
B. Carpiniello et al. (eds.), *Violence and Mental Disorders*, Comprehensive
Approach to Psychiatry 1, https://doi.org/10.1007/978-3-030-33188-7_7

attacks; natural disasters; and motor vehicle accidents. The disorder involves four symptom clusters which include persistent reexperiencing of the traumatic event(s), avoidance of trauma-related stimuli and emotional numbing symptoms, negative alterations in mood or cognitions, and persistent symptoms of increased arousal or reactivity.

In the latest revision of the *DSM* [2], aggression is listed as one of the symptoms of PTSD, which is a departure from the prior version of the *DSM* that included "irritability/anger" as a hyperarousal symptom and not direct aggressive behavior. Two reasons were cited for this change: to reduce overlap between this symptom and the new Criterion D ("negative alterations in cognitions and mood that are associated with the traumatic event") symptom "persistent negative emotional state" and to reflect consistent findings that aggression is commonly correlated with PTSD. While this change may bring clinicians' attention to the significant connection between PTSD and violence, seldom part of routine assessment in PTSD clinics [3], including aggression as an actual symptom of the disorder may have negative repercussions. Specifically, its inclusion may give the misimpression that aggressive behavior just "comes with the territory" when one struggles with PTSD. We must be very careful when working with partners and caregivers of those with PTSD to explain that violence is not an inevitable consequence of PTSD and we all have a choice of whether or not to engage in violent or abusive behavior.

In 2018, the World Health Organization (WHO) published the 11th revision of the International Classification of Diseases and included two sibling trauma-based disorders [4]. The *ICD-11*, similar to *DSM-IV-TR* [5], describes three main groups of symptoms: reexperiencing, avoidance, and sense of threat [6–8]. The *ICD-11* also includes a complex PTSD diagnosis with two symptom components, PTSD and other psychological problems such as deficits in self-organization [DSO] (i.e., affective dysregulation, negative self-concept, and disturbances in relationships). In contrast, in the DSM-5, the A2 criterion, peritraumatic experiences of fear, shock, or horror, was removed from the definition of PTSD [9]. While the DSM-5 classifies PTSD as a trauma- and stressor-related disorder [2], the ICD-11 still classifies PTSD as a threat response to the traumatic experience and includes threat-related symptoms [4]. Additionally, for the *ICD-11* complex PTSD diagnosis, emotional regulation deficits are emphasized [10]. For complex PTSD, angry outbursts are considered to be a component of emotion dysregulation problems [11].

The revision of PTSD criteria for *DSM-5* and *ICD-11*'s new definition of complex PTSD raises the need for further discussion of the updated symptoms and mechanisms of PTSD and their possible impact on IPV. Particular attention should perhaps be paid to symptoms that reflect a heightened fight or flight response and classic "hyperarousal" symptoms that have been shown to be most highly associated with IPV risk among the PTSD symptom groupings [12]. Among these symptoms, cognitive biases that may reflect an overly heightened perception of threat and emotion regulation difficulties may be particularly important to consider, as discussed in the following sections.

7.2   The Role of Social Information Processing in Partner Violence

The trauma-informed social information processing model for IPV discusses how trauma can contribute to biased or faulty processing of information gathered from our social environment which can contribute to violence risk [13]. McFall's social information processing model involves three sequential stages through which elements of social information are transformed into responses or task performances [14]. In the first stage, incoming information is received, perceived, and interpreted in relation to meaning structures available to the individual. In this stage, inattention, distraction, and/or misinterpretation of social information can contribute to violence risk. The second step involves generating possible responses and evaluating response options. The enactment stage then involves carrying out the selected response and monitoring and evaluating its impact. Here, skill deficits (e.g., communication and stress management) can contribute to increased violence risk. These processes can also be influenced by several other risk factors that may be associated with trauma and PTSD, such as mood state, stress level, and substance use.

Considerable research and theory have linked deficits in social information processing to risk for IPV [15–18]. Prior research also suggests the potential importance of trauma and PTSD with respect to faulty social information processing. For example, Chemtob and his colleagues [19–21] asserted that problems with anger and aggression among veterans with PTSD may occur because they enter into a "survival mode" of functioning. They hypothesized that individuals with PTSD are more likely to perceive threats in their environment due to their prior experience of trauma and life threat, and these veterans essentially become physiologically and cognitively wired to misperceive social cues and inappropriately respond with aggression.

Our team has also obtained evidence consistent with the notion that PTSD is associated with IPV through its influence on social information processing. In a community-based sample of 161 men [22], early trauma experiences were related to the use of both physical and psychological IPV in adulthood due to their impact on both PTSD symptoms and social information-processing deficits, assessed via responses to hypothetical relationship vignettes intended to assess decoding and decision-making skills. In a subsequent study of returning military veterans [23], among 92 male Operation Enduring Freedom/Operation Iraqi Freedom veterans, we similarly found laboratory-assessed cognitive biases to mediate associations between PTSD scores and anger expression. More recently, we examined the direct and indirect effects between PTSD, cognitive biases, and IPV among both men and women in a sample of 83 civilian couples with results suggesting that for men in particular, cognitive biases mediated the association between PTSD and physical IPV and spousal injury [24].

Examining another way in which PTSD may contribute to biased social information processing, Sippel and Marshall [25], in a sample of 47 community participants, found that PTSD was related to shame-related cognitive processing, and such processing was related to the use of IPV. In other words, those with PTSD may be more likely to misperceive ambiguous partner behaviors as rejecting and this may contribute to social information-processing deficits and IPV.

7.3 Social Information-Processing Deficits and Aggressive Behavior in Children

For some, the development of deficits in social information processing begins in childhood, and similar to our trauma-informed social information processing model for adult IPV, several studies by Dodge and his colleagues demonstrate that childhood exposure to trauma and abuse contributes to deficits that pose a risk for aggressive behavior [26]. For example, Dodge, Pettit, Bates, and Valente found that children who experienced physical abuse before the age of 5 were four to five times more likely to exhibit externalizing problems [27]. Further, social information-processing deficits were shown to explain this relationship such that childhood abuse exposure predicted social information-processing deficits, and these deficits in turn predicted aggressive behavior towards others. More specifically, abused children were more likely to assume that others had hostile intentions during ambiguous scenarios, and those who displayed this attribution style were more likely to exhibit aggression. Longitudinal evidence also indicates that social information-processing deficits help explain how exposure to interparental relationship conflict during childhood contributes to later aggressiveness in romantic relationships in young adulthood [28].

Theory and research on the role of social information processing in the development of children's aggression have led to interventions that target these deficits and biases [29, 30]. Dodge et al. evaluated whether improvements in children's social information-processing abilities explained the effectiveness of the Fast Track prevention intervention [29]. This program exposed high-risk kindergarten children to a multiyear intervention aimed to enhance their social-cognitive skills via classroom teaching, parent training, tutoring and peer coaching, and small group activities. As the researchers hypothesized, the program had a positive impact on social cognition in grades one through five which led to reductions in antisocial behavior and aggression. Specifically, the intervention helped participants to make more benign attributions in response to peer provocations, to generate more competent responses to social problems, and to view aggressive response options as more detrimental.

7.4 The Role of Core Themes

Relevant for problems experienced by individuals from childhood through adulthood, the experience of trauma can have a profound effect on the way that one views the world and can underlie trauma reactions such as PTSD and/or relationship conflict [31, 32]. For example, core themes related to difficulties trusting others, low self-esteem, and conflicts related to power and control are commonly encountered in our work with individuals who have difficulties with abusive relationship behavior. It may be especially important to assist clients in gaining insight into how their negative life experiences and trauma have impacted these core beliefs, and how these beliefs in turn may contribute to their interpersonal difficulties.

Core beliefs are also important to address from a therapeutic standpoint, because "stuck points" related to these core themes can hinder therapeutic progress and can underlie social information-processing deficits. For example, someone with PTSD that resulted from a form of interpersonal violence or betrayal trauma may feel like they cannot trust anyone, or that all people are out to hurt or betray them. The individual may be more likely to view others as having negative intentions, and thus will interpret ambiguous situations in a more negative light. If the individual with PTSD develops low self-esteem from trauma, they may misperceive "threats" to their relationship or abandonment by their partner via maladaptive social information-processing processes [33]. If one's PTSD reaction included a profound sense of helplessness and uncontrollability during the event(s), they may have developed difficulties with power and control which may contribute to negative assumptions about their partner regarding dominance and power [34]. It would be critically important for the provider to assist the client in recognizing their trauma-related core themes, where they appear to be "stuck," and assist them in generating more adaptive and less biased interpretations of events and their partners.

7.5 The Role of Emotion Dysregulation

Another potentially important factor relevant for the trauma-informed social information processing model is emotion dysregulation. Emotion regulation has been defined in many ways, with Gratz and Roemer providing what has become the standard definition, which includes awareness and acceptance of emotions, impulse control, and ability to strategize and apply content-appropriate regulation of emotions [35]. An increased focus on emotion regulation in the field is reflected in the aforementioned recent changes to the *DSM-5* that emphasize uncontrollable anger in the Cluster E symptoms: "Irritable behavior and angry outbursts (with little or no provocation) typically expressed as verbal or physical aggression toward people or objects" [2]. Likewise, the WHO group working on PTSD disorders argued that a component of emotion dysregulation be part of the *ICD-11* complex PTSD diagnosis, and symptom of "temper outbursts" was suggested for the *ICD-11* CPTSD definition [11]. However, the specific "anger outbursts" symptom was not included in the final version of the disorder [4].

Emotion dysregulation has received increasing research attention in both the PTSD literature and the aggression literature, with studies showing emotion regulation related to both PTSD and impulsive aggression [36–41]. This literature extends extensive prior research on the association between PTSD and emotion deregulation [42], both under-regulation of fear and other emotions (hyperarousal symptoms) and overregulation through avoidance and dissociation [43]. Cross-sectional research [44, 45] and longitudinal studies [46] suggest that these intense negative emotions are either a symptom of PTSD or a catalyst to PTSD [47].

Literature on non-PTSD predictors for aggression has found emotion dysregulation to be a consistent correlate [48], and also to be specifically correlated with IPV [49–51]. More specifically, these findings indicate that men who report experiencing difficulties in emotion regulation are more likely to behave aggressively against an intimate partner [51], presumably in an attempt to regulate their emotional state [52]. Emotional regulation in relation to aggression also has been identified in persons who have experienced a traumatic event [53]. Recent studies that have focused on the associations between emotion dysregulation *DSM-IV/ICD-11* PTSD criteria and interpersonal aggression/IPV have been fairly consistent. One study demonstrated that difficulties with emotion regulation were associated with physical and verbal IPV perpetration among a clinical sample of 77 individuals with PTSD [54]. In a recent study of Israeli court-mandated men, there was a strong association between PTSD, emotion dysregulation symptoms, and psychological and physical IPV [55].

Some studies have attempted to examine moderators and mediators with respect to emotion regulation and its association with aggressive behavior to better understand this association. In a cross-sectional mediation model, emotion dysregulation was shown to fully account for the PTSD and impulsive aggression relationship [40]. Another study among methamphetamine users found that the higher their levels of PTSD symptoms, and the lesser their access to emotion regulation strategies, the greater their interpersonal aggression [56]. In another study of women, PTSD symptoms, emotion regulation, and escalating strategies marginally interacted to predict perpetration of IPV [57].

Further support for the mechanism of emotion dysregulation and IPV in the context of trauma was found recently in a study which examined the role of alexithymia in predicting IPV in a clinical sample of veterans [58]. Alexithymia is a deficit in the cognitive processing of emotional experience characterized by difficulty identifying and distinguishing between feelings, difficulty describing feelings, and use of an externally oriented thinking style. The results of the study demonstrated a statistically significant association between alexithymia and use of psychological IPV. Moreover, this study demonstrated that participants in trauma-informed intervention for preventing IPV based on the social information processing model showed significantly greater reductions in alexithymia over time relative to participants in an "enhanced treatment as usual" comparison condition. These findings suggest that a trauma-informed intervention may optimize outcomes, helping men who engage in IPV both to limit their use of violence and to improve deficits in emotion processing.

7.6   Potential Mediators and Moderators of the Association Between PTSD and IPV

PTSD symptomatology often statistically accounts for the commonly found relationship between trauma exposure and IPV, and PTSD predicts IPV even while adjusting for other factors, such as personality disorder features and stressors present in childhood [59, 60]. In other words, examining trauma by itself may not fully capture how it increases the risk for IPV, nor does it seem to be the primary risk factor when PTSD is also considered. Rather, the evidence suggests that the primary factor in predicting IPV in trauma-exposed samples is whether the trauma exposure precipitates symptoms of PTSD. If an individual is exposed to trauma and does not go on to develop significant PTSD symptoms, that individual's IPV risk may be similar to what we might find for someone without significant trauma exposure [61, 62]. While PTSD seems to largely account for the effects of trauma on IPV risk, much remains to be known about how and why PTSD increases such risk. Several biological, psychological, and social risk factors have been associated with IPV and PTSD and may serve as mechanisms by which PTSD is related to IPV, or they may operate together with PTSD to increase IPV risk. We will explore some of the most well-known and researched factors.

Studies have consistently shown a higher prevalence of traumatic brain (TBI) among those who engage in IPV relative to the general population and nonviolent peers. A review by Pinto and colleagues reported head injury rates of 40–61% among those who engage in IPV [63]. These high rates persisted regardless of whether the injury was determined by a medical diagnosis or reported by participants as a loss of consciousness. A recent meta-analysis by Farrer, Frost, and Hedges likewise indicated that rates of TBI among IPV perpetrators were significantly higher than comparison estimates for the general population derived from four distinct studies [64].

Head-injured men have also reported more frequent loss of temper, greater difficulty verbally communicating, and more instances of yelling and arguing with others, including their partners [65]. Neuropsychological and social deficits such as poor concentration, perseveration, cognitive rigidity, misperception of social cues, misinterpretations of nonverbal information (e.g., body language), and impaired verbal reasoning can all result from a head injury and may contribute to the risk of IPV perpetration [66].

TBI and PTSD co-occur frequently [67] and it is difficult to parse out their differential relationships with IPV, as well as their interactive effects, given that the two problems overlap in cognitive and affective symptoms [67, 68]. As such, the literature is quite mixed. For example, some studies indicate that the problematic effects of TBI may be mediated by the presence of PTSD [68], while other studies indicate that the presence of both TBI and PTSD may result in more severe symptoms than the presence of either condition in isolation [67]. Still other neuroimaging studies have raised the possibility that damage to neural circuitry following TBI may account for symptoms previously thought to be the related to PTSD [69]. The impact of comorbid PTSD and TBI on IPV risk is not yet understood as little research has directly examined the relationships between PTSD, TBI, and IPV use. A cross-sectional study explored the interaction between TBI and PTSD and its impact on IPV risk and, contrary to hypotheses, found that PTSD symptom severity increased IPV risk in the absence of a head contact event, but not in the presence of a head contact event [70]. More research is needed to delineate the precise nature of these relationships and the implications of such relationships on treatment.

Neuropsychological functioning has also been examined in populations of individuals engaging in IPV outside the context of head injuries. Use of violence has been linked to deficits in the frontal lobes, neural substrates for cognition and impulse control, as well as overactivation of the limbic structure which mediates emotions and drive-related behaviors [71]. In a study by Cohen and colleagues, individuals who used IPV scored lower on measures of executive functioning, attention, and learning and memory compared to nonviolent controls, even after controlling for verbal intellectual ability and prior head injury [72]. Studies have also demonstrated greater impulsivity and diminished inhibition among those who use

IPV compared to nonviolent controls [73, 74]. Such deficits may reduce problem-solving abilities as well as impulse and behavioral control, resulting in an increased likelihood to respond to conflict in an aggressive or violent manner [63]. As previously described, many of the symptoms associated with TBI and neuropsychological deficits overlap with symptoms of PTSD, making it difficult to determine the root of these symptoms and how these factors might interact to impact the risk of IPV. To our knowledge, no longitudinal study has examined PTSD and neuropsychological deficits (associated with and independent of TBI) in the context of IPV use so it is difficult to draw conclusions about causality, directionality, and any potential interactions of these factors.

Another commonly studied risk factor for PTSD and IPV is substance use. Research has demonstrated that men who drink heavily or use other illicit substances are at a considerably heightened risk of IPV perpetration compared to men who do not [75, 76]. PTSD and substances-use disorders (SUDs) have been consistently found to co-occur at high rates [77]. Additionally, individuals with PTSD have been shown to be 2–14 times more likely to meet criteria for a SUD than individuals without PTSD [77]. Theories such as the tension reduction hypothesis and the self-medication hypothesis posit that individuals with PTSD turn to substances in an attempt to cope with negative affect and as a means of self-soothing [78–80]. Further, the theory that substance use increases the likelihood of aggression and violent behavior through disinhibition and impaired information-processing mechanisms is supported in the literature [76, 81, 82]. A study of Vietnam veterans and their partners indicated that hyperarousal symptoms and physical aggression were positively associated, and that excessive alcohol consumption exacerbated this relationship [83]. Drug abuse dependence has also been shown to occur at a significantly higher rate in partner violent male veterans with PTSD compared to counterparts with PTSD who did not engage in violence [84].

Numerous studies have established depressive symptoms as predictors of aggression and IPV use in men and women [85–87]. Several studies have examined the specific features associated with depression that are most strongly linked to aggression and IPV including a sense of powerlessness and dysphoria [88, 89]. Notably, this sense of powerlessness echoes the disruption to the core theme of power and control discussed within the framework of PTSD, which is known to co-occur with depression at high rates [90]. There's some support for the hypothesis that in cases of comorbid PTSD and depression, dysphoric symptoms may serve as a disinhibitory influence on processes that would otherwise limit aggression [88]. Research suggests that this relationship operates particularly strongly among veterans, who experience comorbid depression and PTSD at high rates [84]. Regarding the possibility that depression can potentiate the association between PTSD and IPV, Taft et al. found a significantly higher rate of depression among a sample of partner violent male veterans with PTSD as compared to a sample of nonviolent counterparts with PTSD [84].

Perhaps the most consistent predictor of/risk factor for IPV perpetration other than PTSD is relationship conflict. In a study by Marshall and colleagues [91], conflict within a couple was strongly associated with IPV and predicted the occurrence of both men's and women's IPV use as well as the frequency of women's IPV use. Further, in a multivariate model of partner aggression [85], marital adjustment evidenced a strong and direct pathway to IPV behaviors for both men and women. Poor emotional intimacy, a facet of relationship adjustment, has been found to significantly mediate the relationship between PTSD symptoms and use of physical violence and thus represents an important piece of the link between PTSD symptomatology and IPV use [92]. Findings of a mediational effect of PTSD symptoms through relationship problems are important given consistently found associations between PTSD and indices of relationship adjustment [1].

Specific populations may be more vulnerable to risk factors associated with IPV use. For example, due to the nature of military service and culture, military service members and veterans are at an increased risk for PTSD, depression, alcohol abuse, TBI, and relationship conflict as compared to civilians [93–95]. In particular, service members and veterans who develop PTSD are at a high risk for using IPV [96, 97]. Additionally, PTSD and IPV have evidenced a stronger relationship in military samples than civilian samples [1]. A meta-analysis by Taft and colleagues [1] indicated that there may be a gender difference in the association between PTSD and IPV such that this relationship operates more strongly in men than in women. As such, men with PTSD may represent a population at increased risk of IPV use.

Individuals with PTSD who engage in partner violence have also been shown to have elevated rates of other risk factors related to IPV use, such as atrocity exposure, major depressive episode, and drug abuse dependence, as well as poorer marital adjustment [84]. Additional research is needed to understand the nature and impact of these risk factors as they relate specifically to PTSD and IPV.

It is also important to emphasize that while research has demonstrated that PTSD correlates with IPV risk, and there are a number of other factors that may mediate or moderate this relationship, evidence has not yet established a "causal" relationship. This is relevant clinically as well, since providers who work with those who engage in IPV must make it clear that we are all ultimately responsible for our own behavior. One may experience PTSD and a host of other risk factors for IPV and still refrain from engaging in abusive behavior. In fact, most of those with PTSD do not use IPV in their relationships. Ultimately, while some conditions and difficulties may pose greater challenges with respect to IPV, it is important to make clear that IPV is a learned behavior and can be unlearned regardless of the risk factors present. In other words, our behavior is not caused or predetermined by the experience of trauma or the presence of PTSD or other risk factors.

7.7 Trauma-Informed Interventions for IPV Treatment and Prevention

Psychoeducational IPV intervention programs in the United States have generally been shown to result in minimal reductions in IPV use [98–100], and there has been an increasing shift towards a more trauma-informed, therapeutic approach to IPV treatment and prevention [13]. At their conceptual core, trauma-informed interventions integrate the role of prior trauma experiences in the understanding of how IPV behaviors are learned, and intervention is geared towards increasing one's insight regarding past experiences and the development of skills to more effectively respond to social situations. This more therapeutic approach contrasts with more strict psychoeducational programs that operate primarily from a power and control framework [101]. Growing evidence suggests that a trauma-informed IPV intervention approach is effective in preventing and ending physical and psychological IPV [102, 103], and in reducing other trauma-related problems such as PTSD symptoms [104], as well as difficulties in identifying and expressing feelings [58].

Interventions for addressing IPV are delivered in individual, group, and couples' formats and range from strictly psychoeducational to more therapeutic. Although individually tailored interventions can be helpful in exploring individual factors that relate to the use of aggression [105], group process factors such as group cohesion have been shown to be an especially important facilitator of change in the use of IPV [106, 107], and some evidence suggests benefits of group intervention over individual therapy for those who use IPV [108]. Group intervention is the typical format for IPV interventions, perhaps for this reason and also because it is more feasible and cost effective to provide intervention for groups of individuals.

Unfortunately, to date, most IPV intervention evaluation research has been conducted using either nonexperimental or quasi-experimental methods, or suffers from other serious design flaws [109]. In this section, we emphasize research on interventions that have been tested via randomized controlled trials (RCTs), the gold standard in evaluating any intervention program across fields examining behavior change. It is imperative that programs are evaluated with acceptable comparison groups; simply using pre- and post-intervention reports cannot accurately account for various other factors that may influence rates of IPV (e.g., impact of court monitoring, lack of access to victim, protective orders, low follow-up response rates). This is a critically important point as a number of IPV intervention programs claim to be "empirically supported" but have not been shown to be efficacious through RCTs. As a result, many IPV intervention programs are disseminated across communities and military installations without clear evidence that they work to prevent or end IPV, which ultimately places the victims of the violence at greater risk of revictimization.

In recent years, IPV interventions have begun to shift towards more therapeutic models by incorporating cognitive-behavioral principles into their theoretical frameworks [109]. These frameworks posit that IPV is a result of distorted perceptions and maladaptive thinking patterns about the self and others, and that these can be changed through interventions focusing on cognitive reappraisal. The following is a review of evidence-based programs that show promising results in IPV treatment and prevention.

Acceptance and commitment therapy (ACT) is an intervention developed to address contextual factors relatively absent from traditional cognitive behavior-based therapies [110]. The ACT framework is a third-wave cognitive behavioral therapy approach, focusing on enhancing psychological flexibility within the context of mindfulness and acceptance strategies. ACT was adapted in a recent study of 101 treatment-seeking adults for use in preventing IPV [111]. This adapted version of ACT emphasizes bringing awareness to current distressing emotional states prior to engagement in acts of aggression, with the overall aim of choosing to respond to situations in line with one's values and goals, rather than immediately and aggressively reacting to emotional triggers. Results from this RCT demonstrated significant reductions in both psychological and physical IPV as compared to a support and discussion control group. These reductions were retained at a 6-month follow-up period, suggesting long-term effectiveness of ACT for IPV reduction.

Another study by Zarling and colleagues [112] provides additional preliminary support for ACT as an effective treatment for IPV reduction. A sample of 3474 men court-mandated to a batterer's intervention program received either a standard Duluth Model program or an ACT-based program. Results show that those who received the ACT-based program acquired significantly fewer criminal, violent, or domestic violence charges during the intervention time period, as well as 12 months post-intervention. However, this study was not a true RCT due to a lack of participant randomization to treatment conditions.

The latest shift in the field has been towards trauma-informed interventions for IPV use. These interventions were developed in response to a growing recognition of studies demonstrating high rates of trauma exposure and trauma-related symptoms (e.g., PTSD) in samples of men who engage in IPV [12, 67, 113]. Due to theoretical and clinical presentation overlap between emotion regulation difficulties and use of IPV and aggression [47, 53, 114], *dialectical behavioral therapy (DBT)* [115] has been adapted and utilized for IPV intervention [116, 117]. DBT focuses on emotion regulation skills and has been shown through RCTs to be effective in individuals with borderline personality disorder (BPD), suicidality, and self-harming behaviors [118–120]. Recent research has demonstrated that DBT may be effective in reducing anger and aggression. For instance, a randomized trial comparing a modified version of individual DBT to a case management condition in a correctional population demonstrated trending reductions in aggressive behaviors [121]. Further, a pilot RCT testing the effectiveness of a DBT-based psychoeducational workshop for males at risk for IPV suggests the possibility of preventing physical IPV through lowering individuals' risk for and desire to engage in violence [122]. However, to date, no full RCTs have demonstrated the efficacy of DBT as an IPV intervention specifically.

"Strength at Home" (SAH) is a trauma-informed group IPV intervention that is based on the social information processing model of IPV [102]. The program emphasizes a fundamental understanding that the experience of trauma may contribute to cognitive biases and deficits in one's ability to process social information, which in turn increase the risk for IPV [123]. SAH incorporates elements of cognitive-behavioral interventions for IPV and anger [124, 125] with interventions for trauma and PTSD [32, 126]. SAH is a 12-week program comprised of 2-h weekly group sessions organized into four phases: (1) psychoeducation on IPV and common reactions to trauma; (2) conflict management skills; (3) coping strategies and negative thought patterns; and (4) communication skills.

In a recent RCT of 135 male veteran or services members, individuals randomized to SAH evidenced greater reductions in both physical and psychological IPV, reported by both group members and collateral partners, compared to those in an enhanced treatment as usual (ETAU) wait-list control condition [102]. A follow-up investigation showed that those in ETAU further reduced their IPV after receiving SAH following the RCT, and physical IPV was 56% less likely for veterans receiving SAH overall [127]. Furthermore, participants with and without PTSD benefitted from SAH, showing that the intervention is broadly efficacious. An additional follow-up study found that those in the SAH condition experienced considerably greater reductions in alexithymia than those who received ETAU, suggesting that SAH may function in part by improving emotion-processing deficits [58].

Shown to be efficacious in the veteran population, SAH is currently being nationally implemented across the US Department of Veteran Affairs (VA). To date, SAH has been implemented at 46 VA sites nationwide. Year one of the program's implementation demonstrated continued efficacy in reducing IPV, PTSD symptoms, and alcohol misuse [104]. Veterans also reported high treatment satisfaction. SAH has recently been shown to be effective in reducing physical and psychological IPV in a court-mandated pilot sample of civilian men in Rhode Island [128]. However, RCTs are still needed to establish efficacy in civilian populations.

A couples group program for military couples at risk for using IPV, SAH-Couples (SAH-C), has also been developed. SAH-C is similar in structure and format to SAH, though the focus is on *prevention* of IPV rather than on violence cessation and involves groups of at-risk couples rather than groups of individuals who use violence. A randomized controlled trial of SAH-C was conducted in a sample of 69 male service members or veterans and their female partners [103]. Participants were randomized by cohort to receive either SAH-C or a supportive prevention (SP) couples group. In comparison to those in the SP condition, couples who received SAH-C engaged in less physical and psychological IPV at posttreatment as well as at 6- and 12-month posttreatment follow-ups.

Other IPV programs that describe themselves as trauma informed are widely used but a lack of RCT evidence makes them difficult to evaluate. One example is the Domestic Abuse Projects' (DAP) men's program, which operates from a cognitive-behavioral, trauma-informed perspective, and DAP's military-specific CHANGE STEP program. While DAP's men's program has shown reductions in IPV arrest recidivism in noncontrolled research, it has also demonstrated conflicting results on program completers' reductions in partner-reported experience of violence in comparison to non-completers [129].

The STOP Domestic Violence Program is an open-ended 26-week or 52-week psychoeducational treatment program used for both military members and civilians [130]. It is based on a combination of feminist, cognitive-behavioral, and self-psychological frameworks and addresses themes of power and control as well as male entitlement. The program also emphasizes consideration of men's prior experiences and involves both didactic and process activities to help men develop new skills. We are aware of only one RCT examining this program in 861 US Navy couples, which indicated no significant difference in program effectiveness relative to both rigorous monitoring and control groups [131].

In the United States, standards for IPV interventions for court-mandated individuals differ from state to state. A 2001 study of standards in 30 states found that most states (75%) have not specified orientation, method, and content [132]. By the end of the last decade, nearly every state ($N = 45$) had developed standards to regulate program practice [133]. However, despite the increase in the number of states with regulations, a review of standards shows that they are neither based on evidence, nor do they include any evaluation of the effectiveness of such interventions [133]. In addition, recently, after reviewing 400 North American social science studies which focused on the characteristics and efficacy of IPV intervention programs, a panel of researchers have recommended a model for best practices. One of the main findings of this review was that current state standards negatively impact the quality of the programs and these standards are not grounded in empirical research or scientific evidence [134]. There have been some other attempts in recent years by the World Health Organization (WHO) to establish international best practice guidelines for IPV interventions based on the results of WHO's 2001 survey [135], though to date the only WHO guidelines released are for health care for women survivors of IPV [136, 137]. Given promising results for at least some trauma-informed IPV interventions, and a growing movement towards trauma-informed care across a variety of problems and conditions, it seems clear that guidelines will need to better incorporate elements of effective trauma-informed care and allow enough flexibility for such programs to be used and evaluated.

7.8   Conclusions

Diagnostic criteria for PTSD and the research literature suggest two main mechanisms operating in the association between PTSD and IPV. The first mechanism involves social information processing deficits; the second mechanism acts by emotion dysregulation. Most previous research has been limited both by examining these mechanisms separately and by failing to examine the role of core themes underpinning relationship problems among trauma survivors. More combined models for IPV that incorporate multiple mechanisms are needed to broaden our understanding of the association between PTSD and IPV.

PTSD is a significant risk factor for the use of IPV in trauma-exposed populations. However, a number of other biological, psychological, and social risk factors have also been linked to PTSD and IPV use. These various factors have been hypothesized to moderate or mediate the relationship between PTSD and IPV use, and we are only beginning to better understand these complex relationships. Further work is needed to clarify these relationships to better capture factors that predict development and continuation of IPV.

The IPV intervention literature does not paint a particularly positive picture, though there is reason for optimism as some programs, particularly those that account for trauma experiences, show some promise. These programs require more careful study and we must evaluate whether obtained findings suggesting effectiveness generalize across cultures and populations (e.g., civilians, internationally and within same-sex relationships, women, and gender-diverse populations). Randomized controlled trials and interventions based on sound theory must remain the gold standard, and the literature is increasingly demonstrating that IPV interventions must be trauma-informed.

References

1. Taft CT, Watkins LE, Stafford J, Street AE, Monson CM. Posttraumatic stress disorder and intimate relationship problems: a meta-analysis. J Consult Clin Psychol. 2011;79(1):22.
2. American Psychiatric Association. Diagnostic and statistical manual of mental disorders (DSM-5®). Washington, DC: American Psychiatric Publishing; 2013.
3. Taft CT, Weatherill RP, Woodward HE, Pinto LA, Watkins LE, Miller MW, Dekel R. Intimate partner and general aggression perpetration among combat veterans presenting to a posttraumatic stress disorder clinic. Am J Orthopsychiatry. 2009;79(4):461–8.
4. World Health Organization. ICD-11 for mortality and morbidity statistics (ICD-11 MMS). Geneva: World Health Organization; 2018.
5. American Psychiatric Association (APA). Diagnostic and statistical manual of mental disorders (DSM-IV-TR). Washington, DC: APA; 2000.
6. Brewin CR, Cloitre M, Hyland P, Shevlin M, Maercker A, Bryant RA, Humayun A, Jones LM, Kagee A, Rousseau C, Somasundaram D. A review of current evidence regarding the ICD-11 proposals for diagnosing PTSD and complex PTSD. Clin Psychol Rev. 2017;58: 1–5.
7. Cloitre M, Shevlin M, Brewin CR, Bisson JI, Roberts NP, Maercker A, Karatzias T, Hyland P. The International Trauma Questionnaire: development of a self-report measure of ICD-11 PTSD and complex PTSD. Acta Psychiatr Scand. 2018;138(6):536–46.
8. Gilbar O, Hyland P, Cloitre M, Dekel R. ICD-11 complex PTSD among Israeli male perpetrators of intimate partner violence: construct validity and risk factors. J Anxiety Disord. 2018;54:49–56.
9. Friedman MJ, Resick PA, Bryant RA, Brewin CR. Considering PTSD for DSM-5. Depress Anxiety. 2011;28(9):750–69.
10. Maercker A, Brewin CR, Bryant RA, Cloitre M, van Ommeren M, Jones LM, Humayan A, Kagee A, Llosa AE, Rousseau C, Somasundaram DJ. Diagnosis and classification of disorders specifically associated with stress: proposals for ICD-11. World Psychiatry. 2013;12(3):198–206.
11. Cloitre M, Garvert DW, Brewin CR, Bryant RA, Maercker A. Evidence for proposed ICD-11 PTSD and complex PTSD: a latent profile analysis. Eur J Psychotraumatol. 2013;4(1):20706.
12. Taft CT, Street AE, Marshall AD, Dowdall DJ, Riggs DS. Posttraumatic stress disorder, anger, and partner abuse among Vietnam combat veterans. J Fam Psychol. 2007;21(2):270.
13. Taft CT, Murphy CM, Creech SK. Trauma-informed treatment and prevention of intimate partner violence. Washington, DC: American Psychological Association; 2016.
14. McFall RM. A review and reformulation of the concept of social skills. Behav Assess. 1982;4:1–33.
15. Eckhardt CI, Barbour KA, Davison GC. Articulated thoughts of maritally violent and nonviolent men during anger arousal. J Consult Clin Psychol. 1998;66(2):259.
16. Eckhardt C, Jamison TR. Articulated thoughts of male dating violence perpetrators during anger arousal. Cogn Ther Res. 2002;26(3):289–308.
17. Eckhardt CI, Kassinove H. Articulated cognitive distortions and cognitive deficiencies in maritally violent men. J Cogn Psychother. 1998;12(3):231.
18. Holtzworth-Munroe A. Social skill deficits in maritally violent men: interpreting the data using a social information processing model. Clin Psychol Rev. 1992;12(6):605–17.
19. Chemtob CM, Novaco RW, Hamada RS, Gross DM. Cognitive-behavioral treatment for severe anger in posttraumatic stress disorder. J Consult Clin Psychol. 1997;65(1):184.

20. Chemtob CM, Novaco RW, Hamada RS, Gross DM, Smith G. Anger regulation deficits in combat-related posttraumatic stress disorder. J Trauma Stress. 1997;10(1):17–36.
21. Novaco RW, Chemtob CM. Anger and trauma: conceptualization, assessment, and treatment. Cognitive-behavioral therapies for trauma. New York, NY: The Guilford Press; 1998.
22. Taft CT, Schumm JA, Marshall AD, Panuzio J, Holtzworth-Munroe A. Family-of-origin maltreatment, posttraumatic stress disorder symptoms, social information processing deficits, and relationship abuse perpetration. J Abnorm Psychol. 2008;117(3):637.
23. Taft CT, Weatherill RP, Scott JP, Thomas SA, Kang HK, Eckhardt CI. Social information processing in anger expression and partner violence in returning US Veterans. J Trauma Stress. 2015;28(4):314–21.
24. Gilbar O, Gnall KE, Taft CT. Gender differences in relations between social information processing, PTSD symptoms, and intimate partner violence. Poster presented at VA Research Week; 2019 May 15; Boston, MA.
25. Sippel LM, Marshall AD. Posttraumatic stress disorder symptoms, intimate partner violence perpetration, and the mediating role of shame processing bias. J Anxiety Disord. 2011;25(7):903–10.
26. Dodge KA, Coie JD, Lynam D. Aggression and antisocial behavior in youth. In: Eisenberg N, Damon W, Lerner RM, editors. Handbook of child psychology. Hoboken, NJ: John Wiley & Sons Inc.; 2006.
27. Dodge KA, Pettit GS, Bates JE, Valente E. Social information-processing patterns partially mediate the effect of early physical abuse on later conduct problems. J Abnorm Psychol. 1995;104(4):632.
28. Fite JE, Bates JE, Holtzworth-Munroe A, Dodge KA, Nay SY, Pettit GS. Social information processing mediates the intergenerational transmission of aggressiveness in romantic relationships. J Fam Psychol. 2008;22(3):367.
29. Dodge KA, Godwin J. Conduct problems prevention research group. Social-information-processing patterns mediate the impact of preventive intervention on adolescent antisocial behavior. Psychol Sci. 2013;24(4):456–65.
30. Raver CC, Jones SM, Li-Grining C, Zhai F, Bub K, Pressler E. CSRP's impact on low-income preschoolers' preacademic skills: self-regulation as a mediating mechanism. Child Dev. 2011;82(1):362–78.
31. Monson CM, Schnurr PP, Resick PA, Friedman MJ, Young-Xu Y, Stevens SP. Cognitive processing therapy for veterans with military-related posttraumatic stress disorder. J Consult Clin Psychol. 2006;74(5):898.
32. Resick PA, Schnicke MK. Cognitive processing therapy for sexual assault victims. J Consult Clin Psychol. 1992;60(5):748.
33. LaMotte AD, Meis LA, Winters JJ, Barry RA, Murphy CM. Relationship problems among men in treatment for engaging in intimate partner violence. J Fam Violence. 2018;33(1):75–82.
34. Gilbar O, Taft C, Dekel R. Intergenerational transmission of intimate partner violence: examining the roles of childhood trauma, PTSD symptoms, and dominance. J Family Psychol. Under Review.
35. Gratz KL, Roemer L. Multidimensional assessment of emotion regulation and dysregulation: development, factor structure, and initial validation of the difficulties in emotion regulation scale. J Psychopathol Behav Assess. 2004;26(1):41–54.
36. Doyle M, Dolan M. Evaluating the validity of anger regulation problems, interpersonal style, and disturbed mental state for predicting inpatient violence. Behav Sci Law. 2006;24(6):783–98.
37. Eckhardt C, Jamison TR, Watts K. Anger experience and expression among male dating violence perpetrators during anger arousal. J Interpers Violence. 2002;17(10):1102–14.
38. LaMotte AD, Gower T, Miles-McLean H, Farzan-Kashani J, Murphy CM. Trauma's influence on relationships: clients' perspectives at an intimate partner violence intervention program. J Fam Violence. 2018;1:1–8.
39. Miles SR, Tharp AT, Stanford M, Sharp C, Menefee D, Kent TA. Emotion dysregulation mediates the relationship between traumatic exposure and aggression in healthy young women. Personal Individ Differ. 2015;76:222–7.

40. Miles SR, Menefee DS, Wanner J, Teten Tharp A, Kent TA. The relationship between emotion dysregulation and impulsive aggression in veterans with posttraumatic stress disorder symptoms. J Interpers Violence. 2016;31(10):1795–816.
41. Norström T, Pape H. Alcohol, suppressed anger and violence. Addiction. 2010;105(9):1580–6.
42. McLean CP, Foa EB. Emotions and emotion regulation in posttraumatic stress disorder. Curr Opin Psychol. 2017;14:72–7.
43. Lanius RA, Vermetten E, Loewenstein RJ, Brand B, Schmahl C, Bremner JD, Spiegel D. Emotion modulation in PTSD: clinical and neurobiological evidence for a dissociative subtype. Am J Psychiatr. 2010;167(6):640–7.
44. Klemanski DH, Mennin DS, Borelli JL, Morrissey PM, Aikins DE. Emotion-related regulatory difficulties contribute to negative psychological outcomes in active-duty Iraq war soldiers with and without posttraumatic stress disorder. Depress Anxiety. 2012;29(7):621–8.
45. Tull MT, Barrett HM, McMillan ES, Roemer L. A preliminary investigation of the relationship between emotion regulation difficulties and posttraumatic stress symptoms. Behav Ther. 2007;38(3):303–13.
46. Bardeen JR, Kumpula MJ, Orcutt HK. Emotion regulation difficulties as a prospective predictor of posttraumatic stress symptoms following a mass shooting. J Anxiety Disord. 2013;27(2):188–96.
47. Miles SR, Sharp C, Tharp AT, Stanford MS, Stanley M, Thompson KE, Kent TA. Emotion dysregulation as an underlying mechanism of impulsive aggression: reviewing empirical data to inform treatments for veterans who perpetrate violence. Aggress Violent Behav. 2017;34:147–53.
48. Roberton T, Daffern M, Bucks RS. Emotion regulation and aggression. Aggress Violent Behav. 2012;17(1):72–82.
49. Bliton CF, Wolford-Clevenger C, Zapor H, Elmquist J, Brem MJ, Shorey RC, Stuart GL. Emotion dysregulation, gender, and intimate partner violence perpetration: an exploratory study in college students. J Fam Violence. 2016;31(3):371–7.
50. Dugal C, Godbout N, Bélanger C, Hébert M, Goulet M. Cumulative childhood maltreatment and subsequent psychological violence in intimate relationships: the role of emotion dysregulation. Partn Abus. 2018;9(1):18–40.
51. Tager D, Good GE, Brammer S. "Walking over 'em": an exploration of relations between emotion dysregulation, masculine norms, and intimate partner abuse in a clinical sample of men. Psychol Men Masculinity. 2010;11(3):233.
52. Jakupcak M, Lisak D, Roemer L. The role of masculine ideology and masculine gender role stress in men's perpetration of relationship violence. Psychol Men Masculinity. 2002;3(2):97.
53. Marshall AD, Robinson LR, Azar ST. Cognitive and emotional contributors to intimate partner violence perpetration following trauma. J Trauma Stress. 2011;24(5):586–90.
54. Watkins LE, Schumacher JA, Coffey SF. A preliminary investigation of the relationship between emotion dysregulation and partner violence perpetration among individuals with PTSD and alcohol dependence. J Aggress Maltreat Trauma. 2016;25(3):305–14.
55. Gilbar O, Dekel R, Hyland P, Cloitre M. The role of complex posttraumatic stress symptoms in the association between exposure to traumatic events and severity of intimate partner violence. Child Abuse & Neglect. 2019;98:104174.
56. Wahlstrom LC, Scott JP, Tuliao AP, DiLillo D, McChargue DE. Posttraumatic stress disorder symptoms, emotion dysregulation, and aggressive behavior among incarcerated methamphetamine users. J Dual Diagn. 2015;11(2):118–27.
57. Price RK, Bell KM, Lilly M. The interactive effects of PTSD, emotion regulation, and anger management strategies on female-perpetrated IPV. Violence Vict. 2014;29(6):907–26.
58. Berke DS, Macdonald A, Poole GM, Portnoy GA, McSheffrey S, Creech SK, Taft CT. Optimizing trauma-informed intervention for intimate partner violence in veterans: the role of alexithymia. Behav Res Ther. 2017;97:222–9.
59. O'Donnell C, Cook JM, Thompson R, Riley K, Neria Y. Verbal and physical aggression in World War II former prisoners of war: role of posttraumatic stress disorder and depression. J Trauma Stress. 2006;19(6):859–66.

60. Orcutt HK, King LA, King DW. Male-perpetrated violence among Vietnam veteran couples: relationships with veteran's early life characteristics, trauma history, and PTSD symptomatology. J Trauma Stress. 2003;16(4):381–90.
61. Jordan BK, Marmar CR, Fairbank JA, Schlenger WE, Kulka RA, Hough RL, Weiss DS. Problems in families of male Vietnam veterans with posttraumatic stress disorder. J Consult Clin Psychol. 1992;60(6):916.
62. Kulka RA, Schlenger WE, Fairbank JA, Hough RL, Jordan BK, Marmar CR, Weiss DS. Trauma and the Vietnam war generation: report of findings from the National Vietnam Veterans Readjustment Study. New York: Brunner/Mazel; 1990.
63. Pinto LA, Sullivan EL, Rosenbaum A, Wyngarden N, Umhau JC, Miller MW, Taft CT. Biological correlates of intimate partner violence perpetration. Aggress Violent Behav. 2010;15(5):387–98.
64. Farrer TJ, Frost RB, Hedges DW. Prevalence of traumatic brain injury in intimate partner violence offenders compared to the general population: a meta-analysis. Trauma Violence Abuse. 2012;13(2):77–82.
65. Warnken WJ, Rosenbaum A, Fletcher KE, Hoge SK, Adelman SA. Head-injured males: a population at risk for relationship aggression? Violence Vict. 1994;9(2):153.
66. Knight JA, Taft CT. Assessing neuropsychological concomitants of trauma and PTSD. In: Wilson JP, Keane TM, editors. Assessing psychological trauma and PTSD. 2nd ed. New York: The Guilford Press; 2004. p. 344–88.
67. Wall PL. Posttraumatic stress disorder and traumatic brain injury in current military populations: a critical analysis. J Am Psychiatr Nurses Assoc. 2012;18(5):278–98.
68. Hoge CW, McGurk D, Thomas JL, Cox AL, Engel CC, Castro CA. Mild traumatic brain injury in US soldiers returning from Iraq. N Engl J Med. 2008;358(5):453–63.
69. Cavalcanti-Ribeiro P, Andrade-Nascimento M, Morais-de-Jesus M, De Medeiros GM, Daltro-Oliveira R, Conceição JO, Rocha MF, Miranda-Scippa Â, Koenen KC, Quarantini LC. Post-traumatic stress disorder as a comorbidity: impact on disease outcomes. Expert Rev Neurother. 2012;12(8):1023–37.
70. Taft CT, Kachadourian LK, Suvak MK, Pinto LA, Miller MM, Knight JA, Marx BP. Examining impelling and disinhibiting factors for intimate partner violence in veterans. J Fam Psychol. 2012;26(2):285.
71. Corvo K. The role of executive function deficits in domestic violence perpetration. Partn Abus. 2014;5(3):342–55.
72. Cohen RA, Rosenbaum A, Kane RL, Warnken WJ, Benjamin S. Neuropsychological correlates of domestic violence. Violence Vict. 1999;14(4):397.
73. Westby MD, Ferraro FR. Frontal lobe deficits in domestic violence offenders. Genet Soc Gen Psychol Monogr. 1999;125(1):71.
74. Teichner G, Golden CJ, Van Hasselt VB, Peterson A. Assessment of cognitive functioning in men who batter. Int J Neurosci. 2001;111(3–4):241–53.
75. Aldarondo E, Castro-Fernandez M. Risk and protective factors for domestic violence perpetration. In: White JW, Koss MP, Kazdin AE, editors. Violence against women and children, Vol 1: mapping the terrain. Washington, DC: American Psychological Association; 2011. p. 221–42.
76. Foran HM, O'Leary KD. Alcohol and intimate partner violence: a meta-analytic review. Clin Psychol Rev. 2008;28(7):1222–34.
77. McCauley JL, Killeen T, Gros DF, Brady KT, Back SE. Posttraumatic stress disorder and co-occurring substance use disorders: advances in assessment and treatment. Clin Psychol Sci Pract. 2012;19(3):283–304.
78. Khantzian EJ. The self-medication hypothesis of substance use disorders: a reconsideration and recent applications. Harv Rev Psychiatry. 1997;4(5):231–44.
79. Epstein JN, Saunders BE, Kilpatrick DG, Resnick HS. PTSD as a mediator between childhood rape and alcohol use in adult women. Child Abuse Negl. 1998;22(3):223–34.
80. Brown PJ, Wolfe J. Substance abuse and post-traumatic stress disorder comorbidity. Drug Alcohol Depend. 1994;35(1):51–9.

81. Taft CT, O'farrell TJ, Doron-LaMarca S, Panuzio J, Suvak MK, Gagnon DR, Murphy CM. Longitudinal risk factors for intimate partner violence among men in treatment for alcohol use disorders. J Consult Clin Psychol. 2010;78(6):924.

82. Giancola PR. Executive functioning: a conceptual framework for alcohol-related aggression. Exp Clin Psychopharmacol. 2000;8(4):576.

83. Savarese VW, Suvak MK, King LA, King DW. Relationships among alcohol use, hyperarousal, and marital abuse and violence in Vietnam veterans. J Trauma Stress. 2001;14(4):717–32.

84. Taft CT, Pless AP, Stalans LJ, Koenen KC, King LA, King DW. Risk factors for partner violence among a national sample of combat veterans. J Consult Clin Psychol. 2005;73(1):151.

85. O'Leary KD, Smith Slep AM, O'Leary SG. Multivariate models of men's and women's partner aggression. J Consult Clin Psychol. 2007;75(5):752.

86. Feldbau-Kohn S, Heyman RE, O'Leary KD. Major depressive disorder and depressive symptomatology as predictors of husband to wife physical aggression. Violence Vict. 1998;13(4):347.

87. Dinwiddie SH. Psychiatric disorders among wife batterers. Compr Psychiatry. 1992;33(6):411–6.

88. Taft CT, Vogt DS, Marshall AD, Panuzio J, Niles BL. Aggression among combat veterans: relationships with combat exposure and symptoms of posttraumatic stress disorder, dysphoria, and anxiety. J Trauma Stress. 2007;20(2):135–45.

89. Caetano R, Vaeth PA, Ramisetty-Mikler S. Intimate partner violence victim and perpetrator characteristics among couples in the United States. J Fam Violence. 2008;23(6):507–18.

90. Kessler RC, Sonnega A, Bromet E, Hughes M, Nelson CB. Posttraumatic stress disorder in the National Comorbidity Survey. Arch Gen Psychiatry. 1995;52(12):1048–60.

91. Marshall AD, Jones DE, Feinberg ME. Enduring vulnerabilities, relationship attributions, and couple conflict: an integrative model of the occurrence and frequency of intimate partner violence. J Fam Psychol. 2011;25(5):709.

92. Kar HL, O'Leary KD. Emotional intimacy mediates the relationship between posttraumatic stress disorder and intimate partner violence perpetration in OEF/OIF/OND veterans. Violence Vict. 2013;28(5):790–803.

93. Tanielian T, Haycox LH, Schell TL, Marshall GN, Burnam MA, Eibner C, Karney BR, Meredith LS, Ringel JS, Vaiana ME. Invisible wounds of war. Summary and recommendations for addressing psychological and cognitive injuries. Santa Monica, CA: RAND Corp; 2008.

94. Pearson C, Zamorski M, Janz T. Mental health of the Canadian armed forces. Ottawa: Statistics Canada; 2014.

95. Goff BS, Crow JR, Reisbig AM, Hamilton S. The impact of individual trauma symptoms of deployed soldiers on relationship satisfaction. J Fam Psychol. 2007;21(3):344.

96. Klostermann K, Mignone T, Kelley ML, Musson S, Bohall G. Intimate partner violence in the military: treatment considerations. Aggress Violent Behav. 2012;17(1):53–8.

97. Rentz ED, Martin SL, Gibbs DA, Clinton-Sherrod M, Hardison J, Marshall SW. Family violence in the military: a review of the literature. Trauma Viol Abuse. 2006;7(2):93–108.

98. Arias E, Arce R, Vilariño M. Batterer intervention programmes: a meta-analytic review of effectiveness. Psychosoc Interv. 2013;22(2):153–60.

99. Babcock JC, Green CE, Robie C. Does batterers' treatment work? A meta-analytic review of domestic violence treatment. Clin Psychol Rev. 2004;23(8):1023–53.

100. Feder L, Wilson DB. A meta-analytic review of court-mandated batterer intervention programs: can courts affect abusers' behavior? J Exp Criminol. 2005;1(2):239–62.

101. Pence E, Paymar M, Ritmeester T, Shepard M. Education groups for men who batter: the Duluth model. New York: Springer Publishing Company; 1993.

102. Taft CT, Macdonald A, Creech SK, Monson CM, Murphy CM. A randomized controlled clinical trial of the strength at home men's program for partner violence in military veterans. J Clin Psychiatry. 2016;77(9):1168–75.

103. Taft CT, Creech SK, Gallagher MW, Macdonald A, Murphy CM, Monson CM. Strength at home couples program to prevent military partner violence: a randomized controlled trial. J Consult Clin Psychol. 2016;84(11):935.

104. Creech SK, Benzer JK, Ebalu T, Murphy CM, Taft CT. National implementation of a trauma-informed intervention for intimate partner violence in the Department of Veterans Affairs: first year outcomes. BMC Health Serv Res. 2018;18(1):582.

105. Murphy CM, Eckhardt CI. Treating the abusive partner: an individualized cognitive-behavioral approach. New York, NY: Guilford Press; 2005.

106. Beech A, Fordham AS. Therapeutic climate of sexual offender treatment programs. Sexual Abuse J Res Treatment. 1997;9(3):219–37.

107. Taft CT, Murphy CM, King DW, Musser PH, DeDeyn JM. Process and treatment adherence factors in group cognitive-behavioral therapy for partner violent men. J Consult Clin Psychol. 2003;71(4):812.

108. Murphy CM, Eckhardt CI, Clifford JM, Lamotte AD, Meis LA. Individual versus group cognitive-behavioral therapy for partner-violent men: a preliminary randomized trial. J Interpers Violence 2017:0886260517705666. https://doi.org/10.1177/0886260517705666

109. Eckhardt CI, Murphy CM, Whitaker DJ, Sprunger J, Dykstra R, Woodard K. The effectiveness of intervention programs for perpetrators and victims of intimate partner violence. Partn Abus. 2013;4(2):196–231.

110. Hayes SC, Strosahl KD, Wilson KG. The ACT model of psychopathology and human suffering. In: Acceptance and commitment therapy: an experiential approach to behavior change. New York: Guilford Publications; 1999. p. 49–80.

111. Zarling A, Lawrence E, Marchman J. A randomized controlled trial of acceptance and commitment therapy for aggressive behavior. J Consult Clin Psychol. 2015;83(1):199.

112. Zarling A, Bannon S, Berta M. Evaluation of acceptance and commitment therapy for domestic violence offenders. Psychol Violence. 2019;9(3):257.

113. Byrne CA, Riggs DS. The cycle of trauma: relationship aggression in male Vietnam veterans with symptoms of posttraumatic stress disorder. Violence Vict. 1996;11(3):213.

114. Shorey RC, McNulty JK, Moore TM, Stuart GL. Emotion regulation moderates the association between proximal negative affect and intimate partner violence perpetration. Prev Sci. 2015;16(6):873–80.

115. Linehan M. Skills training manual for treating borderline personality disorder. New York: Guilford Press; 1993.

116. Waltz J. Dialectical behavior therapy in the treatment of abusive behavior. J Aggress Maltreat Trauma. 2003;7(1–2):75–103.

117. Fruzzetti AE, Levensky ER. Dialectical behavior therapy for domestic violence: rationale and procedures. Cogn Behav Pract. 2000;7(4):435–47.

118. Linehan MM, Comtois KA, Murray AM, Brown MZ, Gallop RJ, Heard HL, Korslund KE, Tutek DA, Reynolds SK, Lindenboim N. Two-year randomized controlled trial and follow-up of dialectical behavior therapy vs. therapy by experts for suicidal behaviors and borderline personality disorder. Arch Gen Psychiatry. 2006;63(7):757–66.

119. Linehan MM, Korslund KE, Harned MS, Gallop RJ, Lungu A, Neacsiu AD, McDavid J, Comtois KA, Murray-Gregory AM. Dialectical behavior therapy for high suicide risk in individuals with borderline personality disorder: a randomized clinical trial and component analysis. JAMA Psychiat. 2015;72(5):475–82.

120. Verheul R, Van Den Bosch LM, Koeter MW, De Ridder MA, Stijnen T, Van Den Brink W. Dialectical behaviour therapy for women with borderline personality disorder: 12-month, randomised clinical trial in The Netherlands. Br J Psychiatry. 2003;182(2):135–40.

121. Shelton D, Sampl S, Kesten KL, Zhang W, Trestman RL. Treatment of impulsive aggression in correctional settings. Behav Sci Law. 2009;27(5):787–800.

122. Cavanaugh MM, Solomon PL, Gelles RJ. The dialectical psychoeducational workshop (DPEW) for males at risk for intimate partner violence: a pilot randomized controlled trial. J Exp Criminol. 2011;7(3):275–91.

123. Taft CT, Creech SK, Kachadourian L. Assessment and treatment of posttraumatic anger and aggression: a review. J Rehabil Res Develop. 2012;49(5):777–88.
124. Grace M, Niles BL, Quinn SM. Anger management manual for the National Center for PTSD. Behav Sci Division. Unpublished manuscript; 1999
125. Murphy CM, Scott E. Cognitive-behavioral therapy for domestically assaultive individuals: a treatment manual. Unpublished manuscript, University of Maryland, Baltimore County; 1996.
126. Monson CM, Fredman SJ. Cognitive-behavioral conjoint therapy for PTSD: harnessing the healing power of relationships. New York: Guilford Press; 2012.
127. Creech SK, Macdonald A, Benzer JK, Poole GM, Murphy CM, Taft CT. PTSD symptoms predict outcome in trauma-informed treatment of intimate partner aggression. J Consult Clin Psychol. 2017;85(10):966.
128. Taft CT, D'Avanzato C, Creech SK, Cole HE. Strength at home for civilians: a pilot study. In preparation.
129. Edleson JL, Grusznski RJ. Treating men who batter: four years of outcome data from the domestic abuse project. J Soc Serv Res. 1989 Jan 23;12(1–2):3–22.
130. Wexler DB. Stop domestic violence: innovative skills, techniques, options, and plans for better relationships: group leader's manual. New York: WW Norton & Company; 2006.
131. Dunford FW. The San Diego Navy experiment: an assessment of interventions for men who assault their wives. J Consult Clin Psychol. 2000;68(3):468.
132. Maiuro RD, Hagar TS, Lin HH, Olson N. Are current state standards for domestic violence perpetrator treatment adequately informed by research? A question of questions. J Aggress Maltreat Trauma. 2001;5(2):21–44.
133. Maiuro RD, Eberle JA. State standards for domestic violence perpetrator treatment: current status, trends, and recommendations. Violence Vict. 2008;23(2):133.
134. Babcock J, Armenti N, Cannon C, Lauve-Moon K, Buttell F, Ferreira R, Cantos A, Hamel J, Kelly D, Jordan C, Lehmann P. Domestic violence perpetrator programs: a proposal for evidence-based standards in the United States. Partn Abus. 2016;7(4):355–460.
135. Tothman E, Butchart A, Cerdá M. Intervening with perpetrators of intimate partner violence: a global perspective. Geneva: WHO; 2003.
136. Mikton CR, Butchart A, Dahlberg LL, Krug EG. Global status report on violence prevention 2014. Am J Prevent Med. 2016;50(5):652–9.
137. World Health Organization. Responding to intimate partner violence and sexual violence against women: WHO clinical and policy guidelines. Geneva: World Health Organization; 2013.

Major Neurocognitive Disorders and Violence

8

Tracy Wharton and Daniel Paulson

8.1 Introduction

Aggressive behavior by individuals suffering from Alzheimer's disease or related dementias (ADOD) is a well-documented phenomenon, with some estimates conservatively indicating that up to 40% of dementia patients present with aggressive behavior each year [1–3]. Presence of severely aggressive behaviors may increase the risk of reciprocal violence by the caregiver by as much as four times the rate [4, 5], and is the leading cause of institutionalization, although some variation of this particular outcome exists across ethnic groups [1, 6–8].

The range of behavioral syndromes related to dementia includes delusions, hallucinations, agitation (including pacing, yelling, or rejection of care), dysphoria, anxiety, disinhibition (including socially or sexually inappropriate behavior), motor disturbance (such as wandering), nighttime alertness, and aggression [9]. Prevalence rates across these syndromes vary, although nearly all individuals are anticipated to experience at least one or more during the course of the disease. Physical aggression, once it appears, often persists through advanced stages of the disease [10], although there is some evidence that mitigation of such behaviors may be possible with appropriately targeted and thoughtful intervention [11, 12].

One challenge to intervention is related to the language used to discuss the issue and cultural pressures about taking care of family or sharing relationship challenges. The terms "violence" and "aggression" are value laden and this must be considered

T. Wharton (✉)
School of Social Work, College of Health Professions & Sciences, University of Central Florida, Orlando, FL, USA
e-mail: Tracy.Wharton@ucf.edu

D. Paulson
Department of Psychology, College of Sciences, University of Central Florida, Orlando, FL, USA
e-mail: Daniel.Paulson2@ucf.edu

© Springer Nature Switzerland AG 2020
B. Carpiniello et al. (eds.), *Violence and Mental Disorders*, Comprehensive Approach to Psychiatry 1, https://doi.org/10.1007/978-3-030-33188-7_8

when working with those who provide care for those with neurocognitive disorders. While behaviors that involve physical aggression of one adult towards another may certainly rise to the level of violence, cultural pressure to empathize with those suffering from these diseases makes it a challenge to grapple with the implications of the language. For families where a primary caregiver or an elderly spouse is the victim of the violent behavior, questions of elder abuse and mandated reporting responsibilities frequently arise in countries where such laws are in place, leading many families to be reticent in raising the issue with providers. Although aggression towards a family caregiver might be considered as interpersonal violence (IPV), violence related to dementia falls into an entirely different category, devoid of the power and control issues that characterize IPV [10]. The term "violence" connotes intention, however, and even in those contexts where aggressive intent is clear, it is uncomfortable to blame someone who is suffering from such a terrible disease for actions of this type, particularly once triggering stimuli may be understood. Nonetheless, the phenomenon remains a critical issue among both professional and informal caregivers, and managing both risk and well-being remains an area of particular challenge across multiple settings.

This issue of risk to care providers has been understudied in informal care settings, although it is a well-documented phenomenon in long-term care and hospital settings in particular, but also wherever a caregiver is attempting to provide assistance with activities of daily living, such as bathing or toileting [13–15]. Aggressive behavior may put the care provider at both physical and psychological risk. The impact of such risk must be considered carefully, since it may erode the capacity to provide care or create situations where the caregiver may be at risk for physical harm, sometimes repeatedly.

8.2 Prevalence Rates and Distinguishing Dementias

According to the World Health Organization, approximately 47 million people worldwide have a type of dementia, and this number is predicted to nearly triple by 2050 [16]. Primary care or emergency care is often the first point of contact for individuals with dementia, and when behavioral disturbance is one of the presenting symptoms, referral to psychiatry for assessment and management is common. In order to have any significant impact, however, etiology of the behaviors is critical to establish, both in the context of emergency settings and in the longer term [17, 18].

Dementia is an umbrella term for a range of disorders that share a number of common characteristics, although both initial presentation and development of symptoms may be quite varied. Most diseases of this type are progressive and involve neuronal and brain function loss. Some, such as Alzheimer's, Parkinson's, or Lewy body diseases, have no current cure. Other conditions have been identified as mimicking these diseases and are potentially reversible, such as normal-pressure hydrocephalus, depression, head injury, and some vitamin deficiencies. Additionally, there are a range of conditions which present dementia-like symptoms, such as chronic traumatic encephalopathy, Creutzfeldt-Jakob disease, or Huntington's disease. Difficulty discerning etiology among these conditions can lead to challenges in identifying the appropriate treatment, so accurate diagnosis is critical [19].

Progressive dementing disorders produce neurocognitive deficits, typically affecting executive functioning (planning, inhibition, updating), memory (both formation of new memories and recollection of autobiographical memories), and verbal performance (word finding). The pattern of neurological change, discussed in more detail below, varies considerably by dementia subtype, but the pattern of neurological change associated with most dementias disproportionately affects either prefrontal structures (Alzheimer's disease, frontotemporal dementia, among others) or white matter tracts between prefrontal cortical regions and other regions (vascular dementia, among others). The initial presentation is highly varied, but referrals for assessment are typically generated in response to the identification of memory impairment by either the individual or a close affiliate (spouse, adult child, close friend). Some dementing disorders, such as Parkinson's disease and Lewy body dementia, disrupt motor performance, while motor functioning is relatively spared in other dementias. Anosognosia, the inability to appreciate one's own deficits, is a common though not universal feature of these disorders. Notably, for most types of dementia, disease progression occurs over many years; for Alzheimer's-type dementia (the most common type), the average length of time from diagnosis to end of life is 10–12 years.

The development of violence as a symptom of dementia may be a result of several different domains. There are several neurologically based drivers for such behaviors, but the majority of triggers are related to psychosocial engagement with context. For example, a healthy adult may identify a healthcare need, schedule a medical appointment, drive to that appointment, report symptoms and history to a healthcare provider, permit the provider to conduct an assessment, attend to recommendations, and return home after stopping by a pharmacy. By contrast, an individual with dementia may misapprehend the healthcare need, schedule an appointment at an inconvenient time and miscommunicate that time to others, may lack a driver's license, or endanger other motorists; may misremember the goal of the appointment or present an unreliable medical history; may experience the medical examination as an unbidden violation of personal space; or may misremember clinical guidance and incorrectly implement the prescribed treatment. Meanwhile, a caregiver's efforts to accommodate the individual may be experienced as an unwelcome violation of independence. Confronted with inexplicable violations of autonomy and personal space and bewilderment about the motivations of those attempting to assist, a person may act to gain control of the situation and anxious distress with the most basic of methods—physical aggression.

This chapter discusses two primary domains of risk for violence or aggressive behavior in neurocognitive disorders: neurocognitive risk factors for interpersonal violence and contextually based behavioral response. We present some theoretical framework for risk factors, discussion of triggers within each domain, and assessment tools, and conclude with a discussion of evidence for interventions. Given the global increase in prevalence of dementing disorders, this is a field that continues to develop, with cutting-edge research constantly under development. Consequently, this chapter attempts to provide a broad description of the field with some detail about the most well-established evidence available.

8.3   The Application of Theory

There are a number of theories that have been applied to understanding how various neuropsychiatric syndromes develop or appear in individuals whose behavior is not directly disease driven. Among the most popular is the *progressively lowered stress threshold* theory (PLST; [20]). PLST proposes that individuals with dementia have lower thresholds for stressors, and that stressors in the environment such as noise, lighting, activity, and volume of people overtax the reserves of these individuals. As a result, behavior is a response to the overtaxing of sensory input. Using a similar perspective, the *need-driven dementia-compromised behavior (NDB)* model considers not only physical and social environment, but also premorbid personality traits, cognitive and neurological factors, and physiological need [21]. The NDB posits that factors such as premorbid agreeableness or proneness to aggression may contribute to behaviors, although other research has found equivocal support for this correlation. This model also suggests that higher education and lower cognitive testing scores, and negative interactions with care providers, may be factors in the presentation of aggression, along with environmental stimulation and stressors. Consideration of the PLST and NDB theories has led to redesign of some healthcare environments, particularly acute care settings, in an effort to minimize confusion and disorientation in patients and maximize their ability to focus on interaction and tasks, engage, and heal.

Huesmann's information processing model [22], usually applied to the development of behavior in children, is also useful in considering behavioral development in dementia. This framework posits that individuals search for, evaluate, and enact responses based on cognitive and affective cues. This is a complex task that requires cognitive understanding of future states and consequences, and memory capacity to link concepts. If prosocial responses are grounded in the ability to complete this task, it is logical that individuals with impaired cognitive capacity might face challenges with this process, leading to selection of inappropriate responses, as a result of misread or misunderstood cues [23]. For example, a care provider who must administer an uncomfortable treatment or dose a distasteful medication may be perceived as someone trying to do harm by someone who no longer is able to recognize people reliably and may not understand implicit intent.

For an individual perceiving a threat to their person, fighting back is an understandable and appropriate response. Unfortunately, the mismatch between the reality of the context and the misperceived situation is a cognitive error. Once this is understood, the situation can be approached from a different strategy and the response of fighting back against an aggressor who poses a threat can be directly addressed before it occurs (see Fig. 8.1 for a graphical representation of this cycle).

More modern efforts to delineate functional neuroanatomy associated with social judgement and social behavior have generally supported Huesmann's model, and

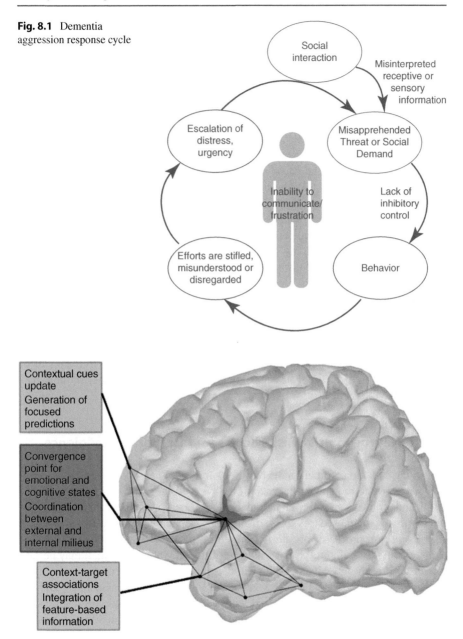

Fig. 8.1 Dementia aggression response cycle

Fig. 8.2 Social context network model (Ibañez. A & Manes, F. 2012)

have extended this framework by characterizing neuroanatomical correlates of varying concepts within this framework. Ibanez and Garcia [24] proposed the social context network model (see Fig. 8.2), which organizes social cognition around three neuroanatomical "hubs" or neural networks. Updating of external contextual cues and outcome prediction is attributed to the "frontal hub," which is comprised of the DLPFC, anterior cingulate, and orbitofrontal. Episodic and associative memory, semantic knowledge, and emotion processing are attributed to the "temporal hub" (anterior temporal cortex, amygdala, periaqueductal gray matter). It is posited that the "insular hub" is associated with emotional value and social salience.

The integration of these perspectives suggests that the expression of aggression is not typically an isolated incident, but may better be understood as one possible outcome of a cycle of social behavior (see Fig. 8.1). As suggested by the example of an individual with a medical appointment, neurocognitive disorders engender social misapprehension in myriad ways, including misapprehension of others' emotions, intentions, or some aspects of the social milieu. As in healthy adults, social distress indicates the need for a response. To understand the cognitive demands associated with script selection, we turn to Huesmann's information processing model. Individuals with cognitive impairment may struggle to select an appropriate social response. Rather than resolving social distress, an improperly selected social script may lead to other's casual disregard, misunderstanding, or active efforts to exert control. In such a situation, a neurocognitively impaired person may experience invalidation, neglect, or entrapment, leading to an escalating sense of urgency and distress. This escalating distress becomes the backdrop for further misinterpretations of others' behavior. Additional efforts to escape or control the situation advance this cycle until it ultimately resolves with an act of physical aggression; definitive efforts to manage behavior are often approached through chemical or physical restraint, behavioral strategies, or with the withdrawal of one or more parties from the interaction.

8.4   Neurocognitive Risk Factors for Interpersonal Violence

Given that dementia is an umbrella term for a family of neurodegenerative diseases, it is instructive to remember that each of these syndromes has a unique pathophysiology and produces a somewhat unique pattern of neuropathology. Though dementia is typically diagnosed as a single disorder, neuropathological studies suggest that various disease processes are fairly common [25] and generalizations about how dementia affects brain morphology may be of limited value. Instead, it may be said that in general, progressive neurological disease tends to disproportionately affect gray matter in the prefrontal cortex, temporal lobes, and/or hippocampus, and the white matter projections between and within these regions. There are several subtypes of dementia, in addition to delirium, that bear particular mention in this discussion, either because of their frequency, or because of the marked patterns of neuropsychiatric symptoms that accompany them. Specifically, Alzheimer's disease is a contributor to the vast majority of dementia presentations, and behavioral variant frontotemporal dementia (bv-FTD) is associated with very significant decrement of the prefrontal cortex and corresponding decrement in inhibitory control. Vascular dementia is also associated with executive performance deficits including inhibitory control [26]. Neuroimaging studies consistently demonstrate the extensive prefrontal cortical atrophy caused by bv-FTD, while vascular dementia is associated with accumulating disease of the periventricular and deep prefrontal white matter. In either case, planning, updating, and inhibitory control all become impaired to varying degrees [26].

Dementia and delirium are risk factors for one another [27, 28]. Delirium risk escalates as dementia progresses, and is considerably more frequently comorbid with Lewy body dementia than with Alzheimer's disease [29]. Delirium continues to be underdiagnosed and undertreated in medical settings [30]. The highly varied pathophysiology of delirium includes a diverse range of neurotransmitter [31], neurovascular, neurophysiological, behavioral, and other determinants [32]. In addition to increasing risk for morbidity and mortality [33], comorbid delirium and dementia disproportionately impact arousal levels, and cognitive performance across domains [34, 35]. By comparison to older adults with dementia, those with both dementia and delirium experienced more neuropsychiatric symptoms, including aggression across treatment environments [36], and were more likely to exhibit aggression towards medical personnel in a hospital setting [18]. While delirium symptoms frequently result in treatment with neuroleptic medications, significant empirical, pragmatic, and ethical questions surround this practice [37]. As a direct threat to orientation, delirium presents a clear barrier to successful apprehension of the social milieu and to selection of an adaptive response.

Alzheimer's, the most commonly diagnosed form of dementia, is associated with atrophy of the hippocampus and frontotemporal association areas. This produces the range of deficits associated with Alzheimer's disease, including memory impairment, verbal deficits, and executive decline, among others. To relate this pattern of changes to the previously mentioned theoretical frameworks, the temporal hub described by Ibañez and Garcia is associated with episodic and associative memory, semantic knowledge, and emotion processing. This information is employed to construct context in novel social information. Huesmann's model suggests that individuals with symptoms characterized by Ibañez and Garcia as temporal hub deficits may employ incomplete or inaccurate social information in the selection of a social script. A script selected under such limitations is likely to be incompatible with whatever social pressures may exist. The impaired person may then inaccurately assess others' reactions to the social script, thus perpetuating escalation of behaviors until the cycle resolves.

In the discussion of aggressive behaviors in dementia, bv-FTD bears particular mention, as this diagnosis is a well-known risk factor for aberrant behavior. This disorder is characterized neurologically by aggressive thinning of the prefrontal cortex, and behaviorally by gross disinhibition. This is characterized by frequent inappropriate comments and actions, often of an aggressive or sexual nature. By contrast to those with Alzheimer's disease and healthy controls, individuals with behavior-variant frontotemporal dementia demonstrated deficits in recognition of positive, negative, and self-conscious emotions [38], with particular deficits in recognition of anger and disgust [39]. A study contrasting patients with bv-FTD to healthy older adults demonstrated disease-associated impairment in identifying both static and dynamic body expressions [40]. Furthermore, evidence exists for a moral processing deficit among those with bv-FTD. Ibañez and Garcia's [24] model posits that the frontal hub is aimed to update social cues and to "predict the meaning of actions by integrating relevant contextual information" (p. 9). From the perspective of Huesmann's model, this specific deficit relates to impaired assessment of how a selected behavioral script may impact one's social environment. In other words, aggressive behavior may be thus conceptualized as the disinhibited expression of poorly selected social scripts, unchecked and unregulated by empathy and other emotional information. It is important to note, however, that expression of these behaviors may be outwardly difficult or impossible to distinguish from those of a patient with delirium or Alzheimer's disease.

8.5   Contextually Based Aggression in Neurocognitive Disorders

While there are certainly biological reasons for disrupting behavior, not all behavior is the result of physiological triggers. In fact, the overwhelming majority of aggressive or verbally assaultive behavior is communicative in nature or related to environmental or contextual stimuli. Addressing issues of aggression in the case of dementia is particularly complex, due to social expectations, taboos, and norms. No one wants to blame someone with a disease for things that they cannot control, and yet behaviors in this domain may generate high levels of risk for those providing care. Recognizing the risk that may be posed to those who are providing care or support is equally as critical as discovering what may be triggering behaviors in the first place.

8.6   Triggers

The theories delineated above can help to construct understanding of what may prompt disruptive behaviors. Operationally, evidence suggests that there are both internal and external triggers for aggression in the context of neurocognitive disorders [41].

As with other mental health disorders, comorbid conditions may be contributing factors [8, 13, 20]. Depression or anxiety, in particular, may lead to misread cues or overstimulation related to physical environment, consistent with the theories described above. Similarly, misunderstandings related to encounters with other people, such as inability to recognize others, may lead to fear or behavior perceived as either protective or defensive. Unfamiliar surroundings or changes to routine may create confusion and prompt disruptive behavior when the individual is unable to effectively process stimuli in the environment. Similarly, perceptions of restraint or inability to move about may trigger frustration or anger, particularly for individuals who may have once been quite independent [13].

While most seriously aggressive behavior is traceable to contextual stimuli or inability to communicate, unmet needs may also trigger violent behavior. In particular, pain, infection, or other physical discomfort can lead to aggression when the person is unable to express what is happening. Management of routine activities such as dressing, wound care, toileting, or bathing may be triggers for violent behavior if pain is present, since there is a high amount of movement and physical contact involved [13]. Additionally, medications such as benzodiazepines or polypharmacy problems may create disorientation, sleep disruption, or physical discomfort. Patients may respond to these conditions with aggressive or lashing out behavior, as they try to make sense of the situation and attempt to seek assistance to fix it [42, 43].

Among other things, dementia may erode feelings of security and attachment. An individual may not understand, for example, that a caregiver is trying to provide helpful care if the medication being dosed is painful to administer, or if they are being physically touched by someone who is unfamiliar in that moment. Bathing is one of the most common situations in which individuals become violent, particularly in long-term care settings. Often, this behavior can be mitigated by addressing environmental factors, such as providing more privacy, same gendered assistance, body covering, or room temperature. For the person with dementia, being approached by a stranger who attempts to remove clothing, leaves open a door where bypassing people can view the room, or approaches too abruptly and startles the person, an aggressive or violent response is a logical outcome from a person who believes that he/she is defending himself/herself. One can imagine the natural reaction of an older woman from a conservative religious background, for example, who is faced with a strange man who attempts to remove her clothing.

8.7   Assessment

Determining the etiology of behavior involves some detective work. Vision and hearing screening are an appropriate and easy place to start. Research has shown that changes in sensory input are highly correlated to violent behavior [13]. A full medical workup should occur regularly, particularly as language capacity is lost. Common issues such as dehydration, tooth pain, constipation, injury or infection, or GI discomfort, coupled with a limited communicative capacity, may be present [44]. Imagine the frustration and anger that you might experience if you were in constant or acute pain, but were expected to continue to function as usual, unable to tell anyone. Once physical causes are ruled out, patterns of stimuli and response must be investigated (see Table 8.1).

Person-centered care, often applied in medical settings, is a perfect approach for assessing etiology of violent behavior. Working with patients with neurocognitive impairment, it is critical to remember that perceptive reasoning, sensory input, and expressive capacity may all be altered. This can at times be compared to the "word salad" that is produced by individuals with schizophrenia, and may require a liberal application of intuition and metaphorical interpretation, along with direct observation to untangle. Related to this, the information processing theory explains that

Table 8.1 Practice guidelines for addressing aggressive behaviors in dementia

1. Assessment for presence of delirium.
2. Physical examination and appropriate testing to rule out pain, infection, or other somatic causes (such as gut discomfort, hearing or visual changes, dental or mouth problems, and nutrition).
3. Consider polypharmacy and nutritional interactions and adequacy.
4. Ensure that appropriate etiology of dementia has been diagnosed.
5. Explore potential triggers in the environment.
6. Establish whether a pattern exists for triggering behavior. Document occurrences and antecedents.
7. Apply non-pharmacological strategies in modifying or disrupting either the behaviors or the triggering antecedents.
8. Utilize non-pharmacological strategies to divert escalating behavior or redirect energy towards alternative activities.
9. Engage pharmacological management if non-pharmacological strategies are unsuccessful after repeat sincere attempts or utilize concurrently to treat comorbid conditions such as depression or pain: start low, go slow.
10. Address future planning and emergency management plans with caregivers, and refer caregivers for support for strain and burden.

cues may be misinterpreted, so consideration of potential misunderstanding and responsive reaction by the patient must be constantly considered.

8.7.1 Systematic Frameworks for Assessment

There are a number of frameworks that may be applied in order to systematically assess the underlying causes of aggressive behavior. These may be applied, in fact, to any behaviors that manifest in the presence of neurocognitive deficit. Gitlin, Kales, and Lyketsos recommend a six-step assessment that begins by screening for symptoms using a standardized tool, such as the Neuropsychiatric Inventory. Once symptoms are identified, they should be described in consultation with a key informant (such as the caregiver or another family member). Questions in this phase include the following: Is the behavior sudden or recent onset? How much distress is being caused? Is there a safety concern? Step 3 is to identify potential modifiable triggers. Step 4 is to develop a treatment plan that incorporates family goals and focuses on the most distressing or dangerous symptoms first, using generalized approaches such as activities, environmental modification, and structured routines. Steps 5 and 6 of their approach involve following up with the family to evaluate effectiveness of attempted approaches, whether they were implemented appropriately and reliably, and finally to reassess for new behavioral symptoms in an ongoing manner [45].

One of the most well-known assessment frameworks was developed from behavioral therapy and adapted for use in the context of dementia: the A-B-C model. This approach involves consideration of antecedent (A), detailed documentation of the behavior (B), and identification of the consequence, or reaction to the behavior (C). While this may seem rather straightforward, extensive coaching is often required to enable caregivers to think this through with enough detail, particularly when they may be exposed to high-risk behaviors (such as violence) or suffering with high levels of stress [45–47]. Through observation and documentation, patterns in the A-B-C sequence can be identified, and a targeted plan can be created. The principal focus of A-B-C assessment in this context should be the antecedent. Patterns will often emerge that clarify triggers for behavior, which can then be creatively problem-solved. For example, a patient may regularly assault his wife as she returns from getting the mail (B). Upon further investigation, it might be discovered that she retrieves the mail late in the afternoon, after her husband is beginning to experience the strain normally identified as "sundown syndrome" (A). One theory might be that the violent behavior towards his wife could be related to inability to recognize her reliably at that time of the day, leading to what the patient perceives as a defense against an invader to their home, even if in reality this is a cognitive error (C). Recognition of this pattern of B and A could assist in identifying potential interpretations of C, and lead to potential interventions to mitigate or derail the presenting consequence.

The DICE approach (describe, investigate, create, and evaluate) builds on this A-B-C sequence [9]. The DICE process begins by asking for contextualization and characterization of the behavior, in detail (describe). Following creation of the description of the behavior, the investigate stage calls for examining possible underlying causes of behavior, including medical, interpersonal, and environmental factors. At either of these stages, safety risk may prompt psychotropic drug use, in order to address eminent harm or risk. Short-term medication interventions may be recommended to manage risk and allow for a more thorough investigation of behavior and associated patterns [9]. Once underlying causes or triggers for the behavior have been identified, the create stage calls for collaboration with the caregiver and any other treatment team members to create and implement a plan, followed by evaluation (the final stage of DICE) for effectiveness and symptom persistence and ongoing monitoring for changes or new emergent behaviors. The consistent throughline for these assessment models lies in thorough and persistent questioning that identifies details, context, and patterns which may be preceding and triggering the behavior.

8.8   Intervention

The instinct when attempting to change behavior is either to medicate the disruption or to manage reward or consequences. Management of consequences, however, may be ineffective for individuals with dementia, since they are unlikely to be able to recall such things reliably. To be effective in this goal, the context or stimuli that are triggering the pattern must be addressed [48]. Research on best practices tells us that multiple non-pharmacological strategies may be needed in order to successfully redirect behavior. Similarly, while aggression often drives caregivers to seek help from the doctor, pharmacological interventions are usually off-label for behavioral aggression in dementia, and rarely effective, while increasing offset risks such as

QT prolongation, increased fall risk, and increased risk for delirium [13, 20, 49–51]. Consistent evidence indicates that while atypical antipsychotics or medications such as divalproex, quetiapine, trazadone, olanzapine, or lorazepam may be used for treatment of psychosis, sleep disruption, or disturbing psychiatric symptoms (such as hallucinations, depression, or psychotic features of dementia) with some success, such interventions may generate intolerable side effects or only minimal improvement, and should be guided by the axioms to "first do no harm" and "start low, go slow" [52]. For this reason, except in cases of psychosis, severe risk, or need for emergency intervention, medication should be considered as a short-term approach or as a second- or third-line approach, and non-pharmacological approaches should be continued in parallel, guided by a tailored treatment plan that considers a multifaceted view of patient need and situation, as well as professional knowledge and experience [11, 51, 53].

Importantly, a combination of pharmacological and behavioral approaches may be best applied to treat comorbid conditions, such as depression or pain, which alleviate contextual factors that may lead to agitation or aggression by the individual [51]. Full medical evaluation for potential causes of the behavior is important, with a focus on assessment of nutrition, gut-related discomfort, eyesight and hearing, sores or infection, or undiagnosed pain, as well as elimination of delirium as a potential cause. Validated measures, such as the Neuropsychiatric Inventory (NPI; [54]) or the BEHAVE-AD, Ryden Aggression Scale, or similar measures, can be useful in delineating a baseline against which to measure improvement and identify risk [55, 56].

Among the most well-established approaches for disrupting behavior patterns, distraction and environmental modification are the most frequently recommended. Reasoning with someone who has become aggressive will not work, but distracting with an alternate activity (e.g., "Would you like toast for breakfast?" or "Look! Your favorite TV show is on!") may have traction. Making environments safe is an ongoing process, with immediate and longer term approaches. Dangerous objects and weapons should be removed immediately. Over the longer term, reducing clutter, simplifying storage or organization of items around the home, and labeling of items may assist in reducing frustration due to overstimulation or misinterpretation of placement of items in the environment [44, 52]. It is important to remember that as dementia progresses, individuals are not able to adapt to changes in the environment, so the environment must be changed to adapt to them.

There are a range of interventions with unclear evidence, but little risk of harm. These include music therapy, animal or pet therapy, horticulture, Snoezelen rooms, light therapy, and exercise. While research is promising for these approaches, rigorous investigation continues to be lacking [44]. These approaches seem to engage positive affect and pleasurable activities, however, so as long as there is no risk of harm (including to an animal which might be present), these are inexpensive and easy approaches to try which may have gain for quality of life. Critically, there is evidence that training the care provider, whether a professional/formal caregiver or an informal/family caregiver, to shift perception from viewing the behavior as an obstacle to overcome and viewing it instead as an understandable human response to a stimuli reduces prevalence of dangerous behaviors [43, 57].

8.8.1   Evidence-Based Practices for Intervention

There are a number of structured interventions that have demonstrated efficacy for addressing disruptive behaviors and lowering caregiver burden, although few of these have specifically named violent behavior reduction as an outcome. Nonetheless, for families attempting to maintain in community settings, accessing training may prove advantageous. There are, in fact, over 200 programs that have identified statistically significant outcomes related to management of caregiver burden and behavioral disruption, although shockingly few have been translated for community implementation in noncontrolled environments [58]. These interventions cover a range of approaches, from psychoeducation to skill development and mindfulness-based approaches. Despite positive indications of efficacy, they tend to be resource intensive, involving multi-week or months-long commitment of providers to work with families.

The most common and well-documented interventions are *The Savvy Caregiver* groups or (newly developed) online intervention [59], the *Resources for Advancing Alzheimer's Caregiver Health (REACH)*-derived interventions [47, 60–62], and the *NYU Caregiving intervention* [63]. Some newer interventions have produced very promising evidence, such as the *WeCare Advisor* [64] and the *Worker Interactive Networking Caregiver program* [65]. Each of these has strengths and weaknesses and should be considered in light of available resources.

Fewer non-pharmacological interventions have been targeted for those with non-Alzheimer's-type dementia. One promising intervention, called Life Enhancing Activities for Family Caregivers (LEAF), is aimed at families living with frontotemporal dementia (FTD; [66]). Using mindfulness, altruistic activities, and attainable goals, this program improved positive affect and engagement between the care recipient and caregiver, which seemed to lead to improved behavior management overall.

Interventions such as these may provide skill-based training and psychoeducation to caregivers, and assist in ensuring safe environmental modifications where appropriate. However, limited availability and requirements for resources and funding in order to be sustainable make them less ubiquitous across healthcare settings. Although they are excellent options for intervention, when available, more basic approaches may be more appropriate for broad contexts, such as assessing using the DICE model; always assessing for delirium, medical need, and/or polypharmacy issues; training caregivers to use distraction and redirection methods; and constant modification of the environment to adapt to the changing needs of the individual as the disease progresses, in order to lower the risk of overstimulation.

One important factor to include in interventions related to mitigation of aggression or violence is the impact on the caregiver. Often termed "the invisible patient" [67], little emphasis is usually paid to the sometimes substantial strain on the individual responsible for providing care for the patient. When violence is present in the home environment, for whatever reason, the added risk compounded with burden associated with daily tasks may lead to poor long-term health outcomes, repeat injury, neglect, responsive aggression (e.g., hitting back), or institutionalization of the care recipient. Inclusion of strategies to recognize and mitigate the extraordinary burden of this type of behavior on caregivers is critical to preserving the ability to continue providing care under difficult circumstances that may last for years.

8.9   Conclusions and Clinical Implications

While some disorders, such as bv-FTD, may produce impulsive behavior that may be manageable with psychopharmacological options, other disorders, such as Alzheimer's disease, generally produce behavior that is communicative in nature and not likely to be impacted by drug therapies. Current best practice guidelines for care (see Table 8.1) require ruling out delirium and other somatic reasons for behavior, such as pain, infection, or other medical considerations (such as B12 deficiency, thyroid issues, or diabetes-related complications), considering potential polypharmacy or nutritional interactions, and then considering environmental and non-pharmacological interventions as a first line of intervention prior to initiating medication regimens for behavioral management [12, 17, 68]. Triggers for aggressive behavior, in particular, may be related to one of several domains: neurobiological causes, acute medical conditions, premorbid psychiatric disorder, environmental triggers, or unmet needs [9, 44, 64].

Applying comprehensive medical screening for physical or comorbid triggers for behavior and utilizing validated measures to establish baselines for behavior should be the standard approach. This should be followed by utilization of systematic investigation of potential stimuli and triggers, by using ABCs, the DICE method, or a similar approach. Effective management of severely aggressive or violent behavior in an individual with dementia usually incorporates a range of non-pharmacological approaches to modification of environment and stimuli, caregiver education and training, and careful and closely monitored medical and pharmacological care. For the majority of cases, pharmacological intervention is an approach that is targeted solely on symptoms, while non-pharmacological, person-centered approaches can lead to discovery of causes and triggers and bring about a more reliable change.

Additionally, it is critical that families experiencing this type of syndrome plan for the future. While remaining at home may continue to be a goal, plans should be made for providing care to the individual with dementia should the care provider get hurt or sick and need to be in hospital, even temporarily. Such unplanned disruptions can throw a family into legal, financial, and emotional crisis. Consider, for example, what would happen should the caregiving spouse have an acute illness that requires hospitalization; if that person is responsible for feeding, grooming, medication dosing, and other activities of daily life for a spouse, sudden absence in the home could be disastrous or fatal for the care recipient. For care providers who are repeatedly exposed to violence, injury becomes increasingly likely. Yet, despite such ongoing experiences, it is necessary to continue to provide care and to make critical decisions for the person inflicting the violence. Although compassion may be high and understanding and patience may run deep, the risk is quite real for the physical safety of the person providing care and replacing that compassionate care can be extremely complicated.

For families where repeat incidents of violence have occurred, it is critical that the family have care plans in place and healthcare decision-making/proxy documents legally executed that involve backup options for all individuals who live in the home. Providers should include an assessment of the well-being of the caregiver in their meetings with the patient, and engage allied health professionals in identifying and extending support to those who bear the heaviest burden of caregiving in contexts where aggression or violence may present itself.

8.9.1   Final Thought

While presentation of violent or aggressive behavior by an individual with neurocognitive disorder may present one of the more challenging diagnostic pictures, such symptoms are not untreatable. By using a patient-centered approach that engages patience, intuition, logic, and compassion alongside critical clinical observation, appropriate diagnostics, and skilled interpretation, psychiatrists can untangle the complex underlying factors leading to the behavior. Thorough and patient assessment and cautious intervention approaches that engage multidisciplinary team members in supporting non-pharmacological interventions and resource supports for families can improve the quality of life and lower the risk for both the patient and their caregiver.

References

1. Sun F, Durkin DW, Hilgeman MM, Harris G, Gaugler JE, Wardian J, et al. Predicting desire for institutional placement among racially diverse dementia family caregivers: the role of quality of care. Gerontologist. 2012;53(3):418–29.
2. Ornstein K, Gaugler JE, Devanand DP, Scarmeas N, Zhu C, Stern Y. The differential impact of unique behavioral and psychological symptoms for the dementia caregiver: how and why do patients' individual symptom clusters impact caregiver depressive symptoms? Am J Geriatr Psychiatry. 2013;21:1–10. 09/27. 2012;epub.
3. Kunik M, Snow A, Davila J, Steele A, Balasubramanyam V, Doody R, et al. Causes of aggressive behavior in patients with dementia. J Clin Psychiatry. 2010;71(9):1145–52.
4. Paveza G, Cohen D, Eisdorfer C, Freels S, Semla T, Ashford J, et al. Severe family violence and Alzheimer's disease: prevalence and risk factors. Gerontologist. 1992;32(4):493–7.
5. VandeWeerd C, Paveza GJ, Walsh M, Corvin J. Physical mistreatment in persons with Alzheimer's disease. J Aging Res. 2013;2013:1–10.
6. Brodaty H, Low L. Aggression in the elderly. J Clin Psychiatry. 2003;64(S4):36–43.
7. Orengo C, Khan J, Kunik M, Snow AL, Morgan R, Steele A, et al. Aggression in individuals newly diagnosed with dementia. Am J Alzheimer's Dis Other Dementias. 2008;23(3):227–32.
8. O'Leary D, Jyringi D, Sedler M. Childhood conduct problems, stages of Alzheimer's disease, and physical aggression against caregivers. Int J Geriatr Psychiatry. 2005;20:401–5.
9. Kales H, Gitlin L, Lyketsos C. Assessment and management of behavioral and psychological symptoms of dementia. BMJ. 2015;350(7):h369.

10. Wharton T, Ford B. What is known about dementia care recipient violence and aggression against caregivers? J Gerontol Soc Work. 2014;57:460–77.
11. Kolanowski A, Boltz M, Galik E, Gitlin LN, Kales HC, Resnick B, et al. Determinants of behavioral and psychological symptoms of dementia: a scoping review of the evidence. Nurs Outlook. 2017;65(5):515–29.
12. Kales H, Gitlin L, Lyketsos C. Management of neuropsychiatric symptoms of dementia in clinical settings: recommendations from a multidisciplinary expert panel. J Am Geriatr Soc. 2014;62(4):762–9.
13. Enmarker I, Olsen R, Hellzen O. Management of person with dementia with aggressive and violent behaviour: a systematic literature review. Int J Older People Nurs. 2011;6(2):153–62.
14. Galinsky T, Feng H, Streit J, Brightwell W, Pierson K, Parsons K, et al. Risk factors associated with patient assaults of home healthcare workers. Rehabil Nurs. 2010;35(5):206–15.
15. Sloan PD, Hoeffer B, Mitchell S, McKenszie DA, Barrick AL, Rader J. Effect of person centered care showering and the towel bath on bathing associated aggression, agitation, and discomfort in nursing home residents with dementia: a randomized, controlled trial. J Am Geriatr Soc. 2004;52:1975–804.
16. WHO. Global action plan on the public health response to dementia 2017–2025. Geneva, Switzerland; 2017.
17. Bawa R, Thirtala T, Lippmann S. A checklist of approaches for alleviating behavioral problems in dementia. Curr Psychiatr. 2016;15(1):33–4.
18. Wharton T, Paulson D, Macri L, Dubin L. Delirium and mental health history as predictors of aggression in individuals with dementia in inpatient settings. Aging Ment Health. 2018;22(1):121–8.
19. NIA Alzheimer's and Related Education and Referral (ADEAR) Center. Types of Dementia [Internet]; 2019. Available from: www.nia.nih.gov/health/types-dementia.
20. Desai A, Grossberg G. Recognition and management of behavioral disturbances in dementia. Prim Care Companion J Clin Psychiatry. 2001;3(3):93–109.
21. Whall AL, Colling KB, Kolanowski A, Kim H, Son Hong G-R, DeCicco B, et al. Factors associated with aggressive behavior among nursing home residents with dementia. Gerontologist. 2008;48(6):721–31.
22. Huesmann L. An information processing model for the development of aggression. Aggress Behav. 1988;14:13–24.
23. Wharton T, Paulson D, Burcher K, Lesch H. Delirium and antipsychotic medications at hospital intake: screening to decrease likelihood of aggression in inpatient settings among unknown patients with dementia. Am J Alzheimer's Dis Other Dementias. 2018;34(2):118–23.
24. Ibanez A, Manes F. Contextual social cognition and the behavioral variant of frontotemporal dementia. Neurology. 2012;78:1354–62.
25. Korczyn A. Mixed dementia—the most common cause of dementia. Ann N Y Acad Sci. 2002;977(1):129–34.
26. Kramer JH, Mungas D, Weiner MW, Chui HC. Executive dysfunction in subcortical ischaemic vascular disease. J Neurol Neurosurg Psychiatry. 2002;72:217–20.
27. Davis DHJ, Muniz-Terrera G, Keage HAD, Stephan BCM, Fleming J, Ince PG, et al. Association of delirium with cognitive decline in late life. JAMA Psychiat. 2017;74(3):244.
28. Gross AL, Jones R, Habtemariam D, Fong T, Tommet D, Quach L, et al. Delirium and long-term cognitive trajectory among persons with dementia. Arch Intern Med. 2012;172(17):1.
29. Fitzgerald J, Perera G, Chang-Tave A, Price A, Rajkumar A, Bhattarai M, et al. The incidence of recorded delirium episodes before and after dementia diagnosis: differences between dementia with Lewy bodies and Alzheimer's disease. J Am Med Dir Assoc. 2019;20:604–9.
30. Ritter S, Cardoso AF, Lins M, Zoccoli T, Freitas M, Camargos EF. Underdiagnosis of delirium in the elderly in acute care hospital settings: lessons not learned. Psychogeriatrics. 2018;18(4):268–75.
31. Mulkey MA, Hardin SR, Olson DM, Munro CL. Pathophysiology review: seven neurotransmitters associated with delirium. Clin Nurse Spec. 2018;32(4):195–211.

32. Oldham M, Flaherty J, Maldonado J. Refining delirium: a transtheoretical model of delirium disorder with preliminary neurophysiologic subtypes. Am J Geriatr Psychiatry. 2018;26(9):913–24.
33. Pitkala KH, Laurila JV, Strandberg TE, Tilvis RS. Prognostic significance of delirium in frail older people. Dement Geriatr Cogn Disord. 2005;19(2–3):158–63.
34. Boettger S, Passik S, Breitbart W. Delirium superimposed on dementia versus delirium in the absence of dementia: phenomenological differences. Palliat Support Care. 2009;7(4):495–500.
35. Meagher DJ, Leonard M, Donnelly S, Conroy M, Saunders J, Trzepacz PT. A comparison of neuropsychiatric and cognitive profiles in delirium, dementia, comorbid delirium-dementia and cognitively intact controls. J Neurol Neurosurg Psychiatry. 2010;81(8):876–81.
36. Edlund A, Lundström M, Sandberg O, Bucht G, Brännström B, Gustafson Y. Symptom profile of delirium in older people with and without dementia. J Geriatr Psychiatry Neurol. 2007;20(3):166–71.
37. Hui D, Valentine A, Bruera E. Neuroleptics for delirium: more research is needed. JAMA Intern Med. 2017;177(7):1052–3.
38. Goodkind MS, Sturm VE, Ascher EA, Shdo SM, Miller BL, Rankin KP, et al. Emotion recognition in frontotemporal dementia and Alzheimer's disease: a new film-based assessment. Emotion. 2015;15(4):416–27.
39. Bora E, Velakoulis D, Walterfang M. Meta-analysis of facial emotion recognition in behavioral variant frontotemporal dementia: comparison with Alzheimer disease and healthy controls. J Geriatr Psychiatry Neurol. 2016;29(4):205–11.
40. Van den Stock J, De Winter FL, de Gelder B, Rangarajan JR, Cypers G, Maes F, et al. Impaired recognition of body expressions in the behavioral variant of frontotemporal dementia. Neuropsychologia. 2015;75:496–504.
41. Kunik M, Snow AL, Davila J, McNeese T, Steele A, Balasubramanyam V, et al. Consequences of aggressive behavior in patients with dementia. J Neuropsychiatry Clin Neurosci. 2010;22(1):40–7.
42. Desai A, Schwartz L, Grossberg G. Behavioral disturbance in dementia. Curr Psychiatry Rep. 2012;14(4):298–309.
43. Chrzescijanski D, Moyle W, Creedy D. Reducing dementia-related aggression through a staff education intervention. Dementia. 2007;6(2):271–86.
44. Desai A, Wharton T, Struble L, Blazek M. Person-centered primary care strategies for assessment and intervention for aggressive behaviors in dementia. J Gerontol Nurs. 2017;43(2):9–17.
45. Gitlin LN, Kales HC, Lyketsos CG. Nonpharmacologic management of behavioral symptoms in dementia. JAMA. 2012;308(19):2020–9.
46. Teri L, Logsdon R, Uomoto J, McCurry S. Behavioral treatment of depression in dementia patients: a controlled clinical trial. J Gerontol Ser B Psychol Sci Soc Sci. 1997;52:159–66.
47. Burgio LD, Collins IB, Schmid B, Wharton T, McCallum D, Decoster J. Translating the REACH caregiver intervention for use by area agency on aging personnel: the REACH OUT program. Gerontologist. 2009;49(1):103–16.
48. Bidewell JW, Chang E. Managing dementia agitation in residential aged care. Dementia. 2011;10(3):299–315.
49. Maust D, Kales H, McCammon R, Blow FC, Leggett A, Langa KM. Distress associated with dementia-related psychosis and agitation in relation to healthcare utilization and costs. Am J Geriatr Psychiatry. 2017;25(10):1074–82.
50. Maust DT, Kim HM, Seyfried LS, Chiang C, Kavanagh J, Schneider LS, et al. Antipsychotics, other psychotropics, and the risk of death in patients with dementia. JAMA Psychiat. 2015;8:6–12.
51. Tible OP, Riese F, Savaskan E, von Gunten A. Best practice in the management of behavioural and psychological symptoms of dementia. Ther Adv Neurol Disord England. 2017;10(8):297–309.
52. Rayner A, O'Brien J, Schoenbachler B. Behavior disorders of dementia: recognition and treatment. Am Fam Physician. 2006;73(4):647–52.

53. Gitlin L, Kales H, Lyketsos C. Nonpharmacologic management of behavioral symptoms in dementia. JAMA. 2012;306(19):2020–9.
54. Cummings J, Mega M, Gray K, Rosenbergthompson S, Carusi D, Gornbein J. The neuropsychiatric inventory: comprehensive assessment of psychopathology in dementia. Neurology. 1994;44(12):2308–14.
55. Zeisel J, Silverstein NM, Hyde J, Levkoff S, Lawton MP, Holmes W. Environmental correlates to behavioral health outcomes in Alzheimer's special care units. Gerontologist. 2003;43(5):697–711.
56. Ryden M. Aggressive behavior in persons with dementia living in the community. Alzheimer's Disord Assoc Disord Int J. 1988;2(4):342–55.
57. Janzen S, Zecevic A, Kloseck M, Orange J. Managing agitation using nonpharmacological interventions for seniors with dementia. Am J Alzheimer's Dis Other Dementias. 2013;28(5):524–32.
58. Gitlin L, Marx K, Stanley I, Hodgson N. Translating evidence-based dementia caregiving interventions into practice: state-of-the-science and next steps. Gerontologist. 2015;55(2):210–26.
59. Hepburn KW, Lewis M, Sherman CW, Tornatore J. The savvy caregiver program: developing. Gerontologist. 2003;43(6):908–15.
60. Schulz R, Martire LM, Klinger JN. Evidence-based caregiver interventions in geriatric psychiatry. Psychiatr Clin North Am. 2005;28(4):1007.
61. Wisniewski S, Belle S, Coon D, Marcus S, Ory M, Burgio L, et al. The Resources for Enhancing Alzheimer's Caregiver Health (REACH): project design and baseline characteristics. Psychol Aging. 2003;18(3):375–84.
62. Nichols LO, Martindale-Adams J, Burns R, Zuber J, Graney MJ. REACH VA: moving from translation to system implementation. Gerontologist. 2016;56(1):135–44.
63. Gaugler JE, Reese M, Mittelman MS. Effects of the NYU caregiver intervention-adult child on residential care placement. Gerontologist. 2013;53:985–97.
64. Werner NE, Stanislawski B, Marx KA, Watkins DC, Kobayashi M, Kales H, et al. Getting what they need when they need it. Appl Clin Inform. 2017;8(1):191–205.
65. Mahoney D, Mutschler P, Tarlow B, Liss E. Real world implementation lessons and outcomes from the Worker Interactive Networking (WIN) project: workplace-based online caregiver support and remote monitoring of elders at home. Telemed e-Health. 2008;14(3):224–34.
66. Dowling GA, Merrilees J, Mastick J, Chang VY, Hubbard E, Moskowitz JT. Life enhancing activities for family caregivers of people with frontotemporal dementia. Alzheimer Dis Assoc Disord. 2013;28:175–81.
67. Adelman RD, Tmanova LL, Delgado D, Dion S, Lachs MS. Caregiver burden. JAMA. 2014;311(10):1052–9.
68. Ngo J, Holroyd-Leduc JM. Systematic review of recent dementia practice guidelines. Age Ageing. 2015;44(1):25–33.

Part III

The Contexts of Violence

Studying Patients with Severe Mental Disorders Who Act Violently: Italian and European Projects

9

Giovanni de Girolamo, Giorgio Bianconi,
Maria Elena Boero, Giuseppe Carrà, Massimo Clerici,
Maria Teresa Ferla, Gian Marco Giobbio,
Giovanni Battista Tura, Antonio Vita, and Clarissa Ferrari

G. de Girolamo (✉)
Unit of Epidemiological and Evaluation Psychiatry, IRCCS Istituto Centro San Giovanni di Dio Fatebenefratelli, Brescia, Italy
e-mail: gdegirolamo@fatebenefratelli.eu

G. Bianconi
Department of Mental Health, ASST Ovest Milanese, Milan, Italy
e-mail: giorgio.bianconi@asst-ovestmi.it

M. E. Boero
Clin. Psychol., Rehabilitation Hospital Beata Vergine Della Consolata, Torino, Italy
e-mail: mboero@fatebenefratelli.eu

G. Carrà
Department of Medicine and Surgery, University of Milano Bicocca, Monza, Italy
e-mail: giuseppe.carra@unimi.it

M. Clerici
Department of Medicine and Surgery, University of Milano Bicocca, Monza, Italy

Department of Mental Health, ASST of Monza, Monza, Italy
e-mail: massimo.clerici@unimib.it

M. T. Ferla
Department of Mental Health, ASST-Rhodense G. Salvini of Garbagnate, Milan, Italy
e-mail: mtferla@asst-rhodense.it

G. M. Giobbio
Villa Sant'Ambrogio Hospital, Sacro Cuore di Gesù Center, Fatebenefratelli, Milan, Italy
e-mail: gmgiobbio@fatebenefratelli.eu

G. B. Tura
IRCCS Istituto Centro San Giovanni di Dio Fatebenefratelli, Brescia, Italy
e-mail: gbtura@fatebenefratelli.eu

© Springer Nature Switzerland AG 2020
B. Carpiniello et al. (eds.), *Violence and Mental Disorders*, Comprehensive Approach to Psychiatry 1, https://doi.org/10.1007/978-3-030-33188-7_9

A. Vita
Department of Clinical and Experimental Sciences, University of Brescia, Brescia, Italy
e-mail: antonio.vita@unibs.it

C. Ferrari
Unit of Statistics, IRCCS Istituto Centro San Giovanni di Dio Fatebenefratelli, Brescia, Italy
e-mail: cferrari@fatebenefratelli.eu

9.1   Introduction

The risk of violence posed by patients with severe mental disorders has long been a hot topic for many reasons: in particular, since the start of deinstitutionalization some critics expressed the fear that the release of many inmates from mental hospitals would have increased the risk of violence by people with severe mental disorders (SMDs), although current data do not give support to this hypothesis [1–4]. However, it is certainly true that violence committed by people suffering from SMDs tends to gain disproportionate media coverage, creating an exaggerated sense of personal risk [5], and this underlines the need for proper management of patients at risk of violent behavior and for a careful planning and management of services which care for these patients.

Italy has been at the forefront of deinstitutionalization processes: after legislative changes in 1978, Italian psychiatry underwent a thorough overhaul, with the gradual closure of all mental hospitals, completed around the year 2000 [6]. Today a nationwide network of 163 departments of mental health deliver outpatient and inpatient care, but also run semi-residential and residential facilities (RFs). Hospital care is delivered through small psychiatric units (with no more than 15 beds): for more details, one of the authors of this chapter has extensively published quantitative data about the Italian psychiatric reform [7, 8].

More recently a radical change has also occurred in the area of forensic care: recent laws (n. 9/2012 and 81/2014) set the deadline of 31 March 2015 for the gradual discharge of all patients from the six forensic mental hospitals (FMHs), which hosted on average 1300 inmates, and their relocation to special high-security units, with no more than 20 beds each [9, 10]. In addition, many patients at lower risk of reoffending are currently cared for by ordinary departments of mental health (DMHs). This change involves increasing legal responsibility of both individual psychiatrists and DMHs and also requires a substantial organizational change for mental health services compared to the past.

Given this radical change and given the marked paucity of Italian studies in this area, we set up a specific project, the "VIOlence Risk and MEntal Disorder" (VIORMED) study, with three main aims: (a) to assess the sociodemographic, clinical, and treatment-related characteristics of patients in different treatment settings (e.g., living in RFs or living in the community and in outpatient treatment) with a lifetime history of interpersonal violence (named thereafter "cases"), and compare them with matched controls with no history of violence; (b) to monitor fortnightly any episode of aggressive and violent behavior with the Modified Overt Aggression Scale (MOAS) over a 1-year follow-up in these patients; and (c) to find predictors of aggressive and violent behavior. We also wanted to assess the association of violent behavior with personality disorders and with substance-use disorders (SUD), and the relationship between self-harm behavior (SHb) and aggression against other people.

We hypothesized that people with a history of violence would display more aggressive and violent behavior during the 1-year follow-up, but that the risk of violence would be significantly affected by the treatment setting: cases living in RFs, where treatment is granted and substance abuse prevented, would be less likely to show aggressive and violent behavior as compared to cases living in the community. We also hypothesized that patients with a recent history of SUD would be more likely to behave violently, and that a history of SHB would also increase the risk for violent behavior.

The objective of this chapter is to provide an overview of the main results of the overall VIORMED project: for more details about the many data gathered in this project we refer to specific publications [11–15]. Finally we will briefly sketch the ongoing European project EU-VIORMED, which will provide important information about the state of forensic care in Europe and will compare for the first time forensic patients in treatment in five different countries and systems of forensic care.

9.2 Materials and Methods

9.2.1 Study Design

The VIORMED study, a prospective cohort study, involved patients living in RFs (VIORMED-1) and in outpatient treatment in Northern Italy (VIORMED-2). In the residential sample, all patients with a history of severe interpersonal violence (cases), living in 22 RFs in four sites (Brescia, Cernusco, Pavia, and Turin) in the index period May–September 2013, were recruited by treating clinicians. Outpatient recruitment was carried out at four DMHs in Lombardy (Northern Italy): recruitment started in the second half of 2015 and study participants were then consecutively recruited during 6 months. Inclusion criteria were a primary psychiatric diagnosis and age between 18 and 65 years. Exclusion criteria included a diagnosis of mental retardation, dementia, or sensory deficits.

Cases were recruited first. The selection of these patients was based solely on a comprehensive and detailed documentation (as reported in clinical records) about a history of violent behavior(s). Violent patients had to meet any of the following criteria: (1) to have been admitted at least once to a FMH for any violent acts against people and then discharged and/or (2) to have a documented lifetime history of violent acts against people in the last 10 years (as reported in the official clinical records), which caused physical harm to the victim, or having committed armed robbery, pyromania, or sexual violence; these behaviors led to legal prosecution or to arrest. The control group included patients who did not meet any of these conditions during their lifetime.

All participants provided written informed consent before entering the study. Before signing consent, the treating clinician with the local research assistant provided the potential participant with detailed information about the observational nature of the study, of the study aims and methods. The participant information sheets and consent/assent forms made explicit the voluntary nature of subjects' involvement and the possibility to withdraw from the study at any time. All patients were assessed with several standardized instruments within 14 days of recruitment. Ethical approval was granted by the ethical committee of the coordinating center (IRCCS Saint John of God, Fatebenefratelli; n° 64/2014) and by ethical committees of all other recruiting centers (for more details see [12, 14].

9.2.2   Measures and Assessments

A specific patient schedule was developed to collect information on selected sociodemographic characteristics, clinical and treatment-related factors, and history of violence (to be completed for cases only). The Structured Clinical Interview for DSM-IV Axis I (SCID-I) and Axis II (SCID-II) [16, 17] were administered to confirm clinical diagnoses. Symptom severity and psychosocial functioning were assessed using the Brief Psychiatric Rating Scale-Expanded (BPRS-E) [18], and the Specific Levels of Functioning scale (SLOF) [19].

Aggressiveness, impulsiveness, and hostility were evaluated through a set of self-reported measures, notably (a) the Brown-Goodwin Lifetime History of Aggression (BGLHA) [20], an 11-item questionnaire assessing lifetime aggressive behavior across two stages of life (adolescence and adulthood) by directly asking how many times the aggressive behavior occurred for each item; (b) the Buss-Durkee Hostility Inventory (BDHI) [21], a 75-item questionnaire containing eight subscales (e.g., direct and indirect aggression, irritability, negativism, resentment, suspiciousness, verbal aggression, and guilt) and producing an index of inhibition of aggression (a higher score indicating more hostility); and (c) the Barratt Impulsiveness Scale (BIS-11) [22], a 30-item 4-point Likert scale questionnaire that investigates personality and behavioral impulsiveness, with scores ranging from 30 to 120 (a higher score indicating more impulsiveness). The State-Trait Anger Expression Inventory 2 (STAXI-2) [23], which includes 57 items grouped into six scales (state and trait anger, anger directed inside and outside, control and expression of anger) plus an anger expression index and an overall measure of total anger expression (a higher score indicates more anger) evaluated on a 4-point Likert scale, was employed to provide specific measures of anger.

9.2.3   Monitoring of Aggressive and Violent Behavior

Aggressive and violent behavior exhibited by patients during the 1-year follow-up was rated every 15 days with the Modified Overt Aggression Scale (MOAS) [24], for a total of 24 MOAS evaluations for each patient. All MOAS evaluators (treating clinicians and other mental health staff, and family relatives) were very familiar with the patients and had daily, or very frequent, contact with them. The MOAS includes four aggression subdomains: verbal, against objects, against self, and physical-interpersonal. A score from 0 to 4 is assigned: 0 indicating no aggressive behavior and higher scores showing increasing severity. The score in each category is multiplied by a factor assigned to that category, which is 1 for verbal aggression, 2 for aggression against objects, 3 for aggression against self, and 4 for aggression against other people. The total weighted score for each evaluation ranges from 0 (no aggression) to 40 (maximum grade of aggression); since there were 24 ratings during a 1-year period, the individual MOAS total score for that time period ranged from 0 to 960. We will subsequently refer to the weighted MOAS total score (our primary outcome) simply as the MOAS score, and the MOAS score is the main dependent variable in our project.

9.2.4 Statistical Analyses

Categorical data were analyzed in inter-group comparisons with Chi-squared, or Fisher's exact test, when appropriate ($n < 5$ in any cell in binary comparison). The Cramer values were reported as an association index. Student t-test was used to compare quantitative variables. Nonparametric tests were used for comparing non-Gaussian variables. The monitoring of violent behavior was performed by analyzing the MOAS total score and MOAS subscales along all the 24 time points during follow-up. Considering the non-Gaussian (skewed and zero-inflated) distribution of MOAS score, generalized estimating equation (GEE) models with Tweedie distribution and log-link function were adopted to analyze MOAS repeated measures. Similarly, the relation between the total scores of MOAS subscales (mean across the 24 time points) was investigated by generalized linear models with Tweedie distributions. The model goodness of fit was evaluated by Akaike information index (AIC: the lower the index value, the better the model fit). Finally, the analyses of predictive factors for violence were performed by adopting generalized linear models (GLMs) with Tweedie distribution and log-link function (MOAS score (total and subscales) used as the dependent variable and all other measurements as independent ones). The model goodness of fit was evaluated by Akaike information criterion (AIC: lower value indicates a better model). All tests were two-tailed, with statistically significant level set at alpha = 0.05. All data were coded and analyzed using the Statistical Package for Social Science (SPSS, version 21) for Windows (Chicago, Illinois 60,606, USA), and R: A language and environment for statistical computing, (R Core Team, 2015), R Foundation for Statistical Computing, Vienna, Austria.

9.3 Results

In the residential sample a total of 139 inpatients with a primary diagnosis of mental disorders met the study entry criteria: 82 had a lifetime history of severe aggression against people (cases) and 57 were controls. Another 10 patients (6.7%) were contacted but refused to participate in the study (7 with a history of violence). The mean age of the violent patients was 44.9 years (SD = 11.4) compared to 46.7 (SD = 9.5) for the controls (Table 9.1). More patients in the violent group (38.3%) were

Table 9.1 Sociodemographic characteristics of violent patients and controls at baseline

	Outpatients (N = 247)				Residential patients (N = 139)			
	Violent group N (%)	Controls N (%)	Test*	p-value	Violent group N (%)	Controls N (%)	Test*	p-value
Gender								
Male	103 (81.7)	90 (74.4)	1.96	0.161	74 90.2)	47 (82.5)	0.114	0.179
Female	23 (18.3)	31 (25.6)			8 (9.8)	10 (17.5)		
Nationality								
Italian	121 (96.0)	119 (98.3)	1.20	0.240	76 (92.7)	56 (98.2)	0.122	0.150
Others	5 (4.0)	2 (1.7)			6 (7.3)	1 (1.8)		
Age								
18–35	20 (15.9)	25 (20.8)	2.80	0.247	11 (13.4)	5 (8.8)	0.09	0.558
36–50	70 (55.6)	54 (45.0)			38 (46.3)	31 (54.4)		
51+	36 (28.6)	41 (34.2)			33 (40.2)	21(36.8)		
Marital status								
Married or cohabiting	51 (40.5)	47 (38.8)	0.07	0.793	5 (6.1)	3 (5.3)	0.201	0.232
Single	75 (59.5)	74 (61.2)			77 (93.9)	54 (94.7)		
Education								
Low level	82 (65.1)	63 (52.1)	4.31	0.038	67 (81.7)	45 (79.0)	0.165	0.584
Medium-high level	44 (34.9)	58 (47.9)			15 (18.3)	12 (21.0)		
Occupation								
Employed	52 (41.6)	60 (50.4)	1.91	0.167	31 (38.3)	11 (19.6)	0.445	0.020
Unemployed	73 (58.4)	59 (49.6)			50 (61.7)	45 (80.4)		

Economic independence								
Yes	54 (44.3)	55 (47.0)	0.18	0.670	13 (15.9)	15 (26.3)	0.128	0.130
No	68 (55.7)	62 (53.0)			69 (84.1)	42 (73.7)		
Social support in the last year								
Present	86 (72.3)	94 (83.2)	3.97	0.046	48 (62.3)	31 (55.0)	0.120	0.572
Not present	33 (27.7)	19 (16.8)			29 (37.7)	26 (45.0)		
Time spent doing nothing								
Less than 3 h per day	46 (37.4)	66 (55.5)	7.94	0.005	22 (26.8)	24 (42.1)	0.161	0.165
More than 3 h per day	77 (62.6)	53 (44.5)			60 (73.2)	33 (57.9)		

employed as compared to controls (19.6%; $\chi^2 = 0.445$, $p = 0.020$). As expected, 51.2% of the violent patients were admitted to the RF from a prison or a FMH, compared to none in the control group ($\chi^2 = 0.618$, $p = 0.001$). The most common primary diagnosis was schizophrenia, with a lifetime history of alcohol abuse. There was also a relevant proportion of patients meeting the criteria for personality disorders and the difference between the two groups was statistically significant: 79.3% in the violent group versus 63.2% in the control one ($\chi^2 = 4.39$, $p = 0.036$). No significant difference (Mann–Whitney $p = 0.221$) between groups was detected in terms of length of stay in RF: 840 days (median = 314) for violent patients, and 897 days (median = 484) for the control group. Concerning the BGLHA, there was a statistically significant difference between the two groups, indicating a more severe history of lifetime aggressive behavior in violent patients during adolescence and adulthood.

In the outpatient sample, among the 274 patients who were asked to join the study, 27 (9.8%) refused; therefore, the outpatient sample included 247 subjects with a primary diagnosis of SMDs: 126 of them had a lifetime history of violence (i.e., cases) and 121 had no such history (i.e., controls). The two groups did not differ in age, gender, nationality, marital status, or occupation. Compared to the controls, the cases had a lower educational level ($\chi^2 = 4.3$, $p = 0.038$), spent more time doing nothing (more than 3 h per day; $\chi^2 = 7.9$, $p = 0.005$), and had received less social support during the past year ($\chi^2 = 4.0$, $p = 0.046$). Regarding a lifetime history of violence, the proportion of participants who had witnessed or were involved in at least one episode of domestic violence was higher among cases ($\chi^2 = 20.2$, $p < 0.001$). The most frequent primary diagnoses included schizophrenia spectrum disorders (up to 41.3%) and personality disorders (up to 28.1%). The mean duration of illness was 17.7 years (SD = 10.5) for the violent group and 16.0 years (SD = 10.0) for the control group ($F = 1.8$, $p = 0.186$). Cases had a higher number of past compulsory admissions to psychiatric hospital wards ($\chi^2 = 19.8$, $p < 0.001$) and were less able to collaborate with treating clinicians during the previous year ($\chi^2 = 5.1$, $p = 0.023$). Cases obtained higher scores on the BGLHA (mean score: 40.4, SD = 12.4, for cases vs. 33.6, SD = 9.7, for controls; $p < 0.001$) (Table 9.2).

9.3.1 History of Violence in the Outpatient Sample

In the outpatient sample we assessed in details the history of violence: outpatient cases committed a large number of violent offenses, including physical aggression (87.2%), stalking (3.2%), sexual violence (2.4%), armed robbery (1.6%), murder (1.6%), attempted murder (0.8%), and other violent acts (3.2%). In more than one-fourth of cases, violent behavior was committed in the presence of psychotic symptoms, and in 20.5% of the instances the offenders were under the influence of alcohol. The history of violence was more frequently due to an episode of impulsive violence (92.4%). Victims of violence were more frequently the patients' parents or partners (respectively, 28.0% and 24.6%), followed by clinical staff (6.8%), patients' friends (6.8%), other relatives (6.8%), other patients (2.5%), or others (24.6%). The large majority of patients (88.8%) recognized their acts as violent, while the remaining 11.2% denied the violent nature of the offenses. Almost

Table 9.2 Baseline clinical characteristics of patients with a history of violence and controls

	Outpatients (N = 247)				Residential patients (N = 139)			
	Violent group N (%)	Controls N (%)	Test*	p-value	Violent group N (%)	Controls N (%)	Test*	p-value
Primary diagnosis by the treating clinician								
Schizophrenia	52 (41.3)	52 (43.0)	34.20	0.331	50 (61.0)	37 (64.9)	0.223	0.228
Personality disorder	47 (37.3)	34 (28.1)			16 (19.5)	10 (17.6)		
Other	27 (21.4)	35 (29.0)			16 (19.5)	10 (17.5)		
Illness duration (years) (mean, SD)	17.7 (±10.5)	16.0 (±9.9)	1.76	0.186	20.1 (±10.5)	23.3 (±10.2)	−1.70	0.092
Age of first contact with DMHs (years)	28.6 (±10.4)	29.8 (±11.5)	0.72	0.396	28.7 (±11.4)	25.7 (±7.8)	1.504	0.135
Lifetime compulsory admissions								
None	66 (54.1)	88 (72.7)	19.81	<0.001	9 (12.0)	17 (37.0)	0.503	0.001
1–3	40 (32.8)	33 (27.3)			60 (80.0)	39 (63.0)		
≥4	16 (13.1)	0 (0.0)			6 (8.0)	0 (0)		
BPRS *total score (range 24–168)*	41.0 (±11.7)	36.8 (±8.9)	−2.43	0.015	50.2 (±24.2)	57.0 (±19.1)	6.8	0.103
SLOF								
Physical functioning (range 5–25)	24.1 (±1.4)	24.2 (±1.34)	0.83	0.406	24.2 (1.4)	23.7 (1.3)	0.47	0.476
Self-care (range 7–35)	33.2 (±3.1)	33.4 (±3.1)	0.44	0.663	30.1 (2.8)	28.0 (2.7)	1.89	0.363
Interpersonal relationships (range 5–25)	23.9 (±5.9)	24.9 (±5.6)	1.46	0.143	17.5 (1.8)	16.5 (1.8)	0.9	0.731
Social acceptability/adjust (range 7–35)	23.7 (±4.0)	26.9 (±2.7)	6.81	<0.001	27.6 (4.2)	28.2 (3.2)	0.62	0.403
Activities (range 11–55)	48.5 (±7.4)	49.8 (±6.0)	1.03	0.303	41.8 (6.8)	40.7 (6.9)	1.13	0.543
Work skills (range 6–30)	21.5 (±6.6)	23.2 (±6.1)	1.91	0.056	19.2 (5.4)	16.9 (5.1)	1.29	0.066
BGLHA *total score (range 22–88)*	40.4 (±12.4)	33.6 (±9.7)	−3.91	<0.001	40.5 (±13.5)	34.9 (±12.0)	2.5	0.014
BIS-11 *total score (range 30–120)*	64.8 (±11.6)	62.1 (±10.4)	−1.62	0.105	66.1 (±12.2)	67.2 (±13.1)	−0.51	0.611
BDHI *total score (range 0–75)*	35.6 (±14.6)	34.6 (±12.6)	0.19	0.665	36.9 (±12.3)	32.5 (±11.4)	2.09	0.039
STAXI-2 *anger expression index (range 0–96)*	46.4 (±16.8)	39.9 (±15.1)	−2.84	0.005	39.1 (±13.4)	37.6 (±14.4)	0.6	0.526

*Standardized value of V Cramer

one-fourth (23.4%) of the violent patients were arrested for the violent offenses; 72.8% of patients already had a diagnosis of SMD at the time of their violent offense, and 67.5% were under care at the local DMH.

9.3.2 Psychopathology

In the residential sample, at baseline, there were no differences in the mean BPRS total score between cases and controls: a statistically significant difference was found only for the withdrawal subscale (mean score: 11.0, SD = 5.0, for the controls versus 8.4, SD = 4.3, for cases; $p = 0.001$), which includes "emotional withdrawal," "motor retardation," and "blunted affect," with higher scores pointing to a higher level of symptomatology.

Among outpatients cases showed statistically significant higher scores in the BPRS-E total score compared to controls (mean score: 41.0, SD = 11.7, for cases vs. 36.9, SD = 8.9, for controls; $p = 0.015$) and in the BPRS-E activation subdomain (mean score: 11.7, SD = 4.8, for cases vs. 9.6, SD = 3.1, for controls; $p < 0.001$).

9.3.3 Psychosocial Functioning

Among residents, there were no statistically significant group differences regarding the SLOF, although subjects with a history of violence reported higher scores on almost all SLOF domains, pointing to a higher level of psychosocial functioning. Among outpatients, although cases had lower scores on all SLOF domains, a statistically significant difference was found only for the social acceptability subscale (mean score: 23.7, SD = 4.0, for the violent group vs. 27.0, SD = 2.7, for controls; $p < 0.001$).

9.3.4 Impulsiveness and Anger

In both samples we did not find any differences in BDHI and BIS-11 scores between cases and controls. With the STAXI-2, among outpatients a statistically significant difference was found only on two STAXI-2 subscales and for the Anger Expression Index: (1) anger control-out (mean score: 27.9, SD = 13.6, for the violent group vs. 33.0, SD = 15.4, for the control group; $p = 0.006$); (2) anger control-in (mean score: 31.2, SD = 15.5, for the violent group vs. 35.1, SD = 16.6, for the control group; $p = 0.040$); and (3) Anger Expression Index (mean score: 46.5, SD = 16.8, for the violent group vs. 39.9, SD = 15.2, for the control group; $p = 0.005$).

9.3.5 Aggressive and Violent Behavior During the 1-Year Follow-Up

Among residential patients, with regard to the monitoring of MOAS total scores during the 1-year follow-up, there were no statistically significant differences between the mean total scores in the two groups (mean = 11.6, SD = 18.3, for violent group and mean = 7.56, SD = 16.7, for controls). The most common aggressive behavior displayed by residential patients was verbal aggression: 54% of patients were verbally aggressive at least once during the 1-year follow-up, compared with 25.9% of patients scoring ≥1 for aggression against objects, and 19.4% for interpersonal violence.

Among outpatients, cases compared to controls displayed statistically higher scores on the MOAS total score (mean = 25.7, SD = 36.3, for the violent group and mean = 8.4, SD = 17.4, for controls; $U = -4.7$, $p < 0.001$). The MOAS subratings were also higher for the violent group when compared to controls. This was true for MOAS verbal aggression (mean = 10.2, SD = 12.1, vs. mean = 4.8, SD = 8.5; $U = -4.1$, $p < 0.001$), MOAS aggression against objects (mean = 4.7, SD = 8.4, vs. mean = 1.7, SD = 5.6; $U = -3.9$, $p < 0.001$), MOAS physical aggression (mean = 7.4, SD = 17.0, vs. mean = 1.0, SD = 5.0; $U = -5.1$, $p < 0.001$), and MOAS self-aggression (mean = 3.3, SD = 10.8, vs. mean = 0.8, SD = 3.9; $U = -1.8$, $p = 0.067$).

While in previous publications we have separately shown figures with MOAS data in the two samples, here we wish to assess the overall sample, including both residential subjects and outpatients. This would allow (and to our knowledge it is the first time that this comparison is made so far) to establish whether staying in a RF, for patients with a history of violence, is associated with a lower risk of violent behavior: the results of this analysis are shown in Fig. 9.1.

Compared to both controls and residential cases, outpatient cases displayed statistically higher scores on the MOAS total score when compared to both controls and residential cases (mean = 25.7, SD = 36.3, for outpatient cases, mean = 11.4, SD = 18.0, for residential cases and mean = 8.1, SD = 17.1, for all controls; $K = 32.7$, $p < 0.001$). Our initial hypothesis (e.g., stay in a RF where treatment is granted, SUD is prevented, and there is a close overall supervision of patients that may be associated with a lower risk violence as compared to being treated in the community) is confirmed.

9.3.6 Predictors of Aggressive and Violent Behavior

We tried to identify predictors of new episodes of violence during follow-up in both samples: in the residential sample we defined as "new violent" a patient with a total MOAS score (sum across the 24 time points) >3. Residential patients with a total weighted MOAS score >3 during the 1-year follow-up were 46% ($N = 64$): none of the sociodemographic and clinical characteristics stood out as a significant predictor of new violent behavior.

In the outpatient sample univariate GLMs (without considering the group distinction between cases and controls) were performed to analyze factors associated with higher MOAS scores. The best predictor of new aggressive and violent behavior(s) was the BDHI suspicion score ($p = 0.030$, AIC = 1156.1, $\beta = 1.14$), followed by the BGLHA total score ($p = 0.002$, AIC = 1208.9, $\beta = 1.05$). Among outpatients a higher MOAS total score was predicted by lower levels of social

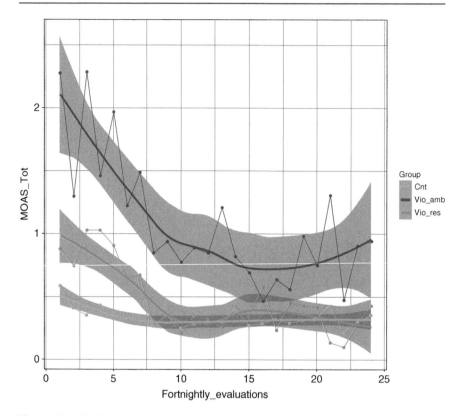

Fig. 9.1 Longitudinal evaluation of MOAS total score during the 1-year follow-up in three different clinical groups (Cnt = all controls, Vio-amb = outpatient cases, Vio_res = residential cases). Trend estimated through smoothing spline functions with corresponding 95% confidence bands (from Barlati et al., 2019)

acceptability, as assessed with the SLOF social acceptability score, among both cases and controls ($p < 0.001$, AIC = 1521.0).

With regard to the relationship between the three MOAS subscales, in both samples we found that verbal aggression was a significant predictor of aggression against objects ($p < 0.001$) and of interpersonal violence ($p < 0.001$), while aggression against objects was a significant predictor ($p < 0.001$) of interpersonal violence. This result has important clinical implications: as in the case of suicidal behavior, a continuum in aggressive and violent behavior seems to exist: a patient may start becoming verbally aggressive; this may in turn lead to aggression against objects and finally the second step may predict a final escalation to interpersonal violence. Health staff dealing with patients with SMDs should stay alert whenever a patient starts behaving aggressively; they should pinpoint the need for immediate interventions to prevent escalation and should not minimize signs of minor aggression (such as verbal aggression), especially among people with a history of violence.

9.3.7 Personality Disorders and Violence

People with personality disorders and schizophrenia are more likely to commit violent acts than healthy individuals. In our sample we did want to investigate the association between clinically significant maladaptive personality traits, PDs, schizophrenia, and risk of aggressive behavior. All recruited subjects underwent a baseline assessment also including, besides the assessment tools listed above, the Millon Clinical Multiaxial Inventory-III (MCMI-III) [25, 26]. In both samples, the most significant predictor of aggressive and violent behaviors over time was endorsing a primary diagnosis of personality disorders, and subjects meeting diagnostic criteria for personality disorders exhibited higher MOAS scores than subjects with schizophrenia. In the outpatient sample cases scored significantly higher than controls on the MCMI-III Antisocial, Sadistic, Borderline, and Paranoid personality scales (Candini et al. 2016).

These findings support the importance of routinely assessing maladaptive personality traits and features in patients with a history of violence. Identifying the most crucial risk factors for violent recidivism would contribute to both effectively preventing and reducing the risk of re-offending in this population.

9.3.8 Substance-Use Disorders and Violent Behavior

In all the samples (both residential and outpatient) we also investigated the clinical characteristics of patients with mental disorders who reported current episodes of substance use (CSU) at the time of assessment compared with patients who had only a lifetime history of substance use (LSU) and patients who had no reported episodes of substance use (NSU) over the life span (Cavalera et al., under review). We assessed the differences among these three groups in hostility, impulsivity, and aggressive behavior among 244 outpatients and 134 residential patients. Patients with CSU were more likely to be younger and of male gender than patients with LSU or NSU and showed significantly higher scores for aggressive and violent behavior (as assessed with the MOAS during the 1-year FU) compared with patients with NSU or only previous LSU. Patients with CSU also showed significantly higher scores for irritability, negativism, hostility, and verbal assault compared with NSU patients, while patients with LSU showed significantly higher scores for lifetime history of aggressive behaviors compared with patients with NSU. Whereas patients with schizophrenia showed a prevalence of NSU, patients with personality disorders showed higher rates of past or current substance use.

These findings suggest that patients with comorbid SMDs and CSU should be referred for specific interventions to reduce aggressive behavior and ensure patient well-being and community safety. In this perspective a close collaboration between mental health and addiction services appears of paramount relevance and should be at the forefront of any reorganization of mental health services.

9.3.9   Self-Harm and Aggression Against Other People

We also evaluated the differences between patients with SMDs with and without a history of self-harm behavior (SHb) and/or violent behavior against other people (Vb) in relation to a variety of dependent variables, in particular violent behavior during a 1-year FU as assessed with the MOAS, and tried to identify predictors of SHb and Vb during the FU (Scocco et al., under review); because of organizational problems this analysis was restricted to outpatients. To do this we divided the overall outpatient sample into four groups: patients with lifetime Vb (V), patients with both Vb and SHb (V-SH), patients with only SHb (SH), and patients with no history of SHb and Vb (control group, CONT). Overall 246 patients were included in this specific analysis. Outpatients with a lifetime history of Vb and SHb showed more severe psychopathological symptoms compared to those with only a history of SHb or Vb or no such history. V and V-SH patient groups reached higher scores in all MOAS subscales: a history of violence against others and self-harm, or only a history of violence partially predicted future aggressive behavior at 1-year FU. Ninety percent of controls and 82% of SH did not show any aggressive behavior during the FU period, whereas 40% of Vb and SH patients aggressively behaved at least once. Of these, 13% showed both externally directed aggression and SHb. Age among the SH group and BPRS-E affect-anxiety subscale among the V group significantly predicted aggression against people.

In summary, among people with SMDs a history of SHb or Vb is associated with different medium-term outcomes, and this represents another important point for mental health practitioners in planning care for people with SMDs.

9.4   Discussion

As mentioned in the introduction and in other chapters of this book, the recent Italian law (81/2014) which enacted a significant reorganization of the forensic system has prompted a deeper investigation into the risk of aggressive and violent behavior among patients in treatment at DMHs. To our knowledge, this is the first Italian study, and one of very few international ones, to use a large set of standardized multidimensional evaluation tools and to prospectively examine the frequency and severity of aggressive and violent behavior in outpatients with SMDs. Our study demonstrates that outpatients with SMDs who have a history of serious violence are more likely to show higher levels of aggressive and violent behavior (in terms of frequency and severity) as compared to patients who do not have such a history, and this raises important clinical problems in terms of prevention and management. On the contrary, among patients with a history of violence who are hosted in residential settings, with 24-h cover, the difference in the frequency of aggressive and violent behavior between patients with and without a history of violence becomes negligible. Living in a controlled environment, with compliance granted and no possibility of substance-use disorders, may have a preventive effect on aggressive and violent behavior, while life in the community, where treatment compliance is not warranted and there is a greater risk of SUD, has a potential detrimental effect on the risk of recurrence. To our knowledge, this is the first time ever that a study with the same prospective design has compared patients with a history of violence treated in different settings, and has shown a marked difference in behavioral patterns associated with different regimes of care (with higher or lower protection).

9.4.1 What Predicts Violence?

We identified several predictive and protective factors for community violence. Social acceptability was a predictor of nonaggressive behavior, indicating that better social acceptability is associated with lower MOAS scores among both cases and controls. With specific regard to physically aggressive behavior, higher levels of anger expression did predict aggressive behavior, while hostility was predictive only among controls. Other predictors of aggressive and violent behavior that we found in our study (i.e., lifetime substance-use disorders, early age at the first contact with DMHs, longer illness duration) are in line with findings from previous studies (REF).

9.4.2 How to Manage Violent Patients in the Community

This study provides useful indications for planners and clinicians who have the relevant task of planning and managing services which currently have also to care for mentally ill offenders in Italy. While patients with a history of interpersonal violence can be effectively managed in RFs, where treatment and clinical supervision are granted, our study shows that outpatients living in the community still pose a higher risk of reiteration of aggressive and violent behavior as compared to patients with no history of violence. It will be necessary to develop appropriate training programs for mental health staff entrusted with the care of patients with a history of violence, and the most effective pharmacological and non-pharmacological strategies of intervention need to be disseminated. An active collaboration between mental health services and addiction services (which is of paramount relevance given the importance of SUD as a primary risk factor for aggressive and violent behavior), which is often missing, is urgently required and new strategies of collaborative work involving different treatment agencies have to be developed. It will be necessary to set up appropriate monitoring systems to well understand the main unmet needs of this difficult-to-treat clinical population and identify the clinical skills which mental health workers have to learn to well manage these patients.

9.4.3 Findings of Other Prospective Studies to Assess the Risk of Violence in Outpatient Samples

Table 9.3 shows the findings of the main 20 cohort studies (concurrent or retrospective), done in Western countries, in which the authors have performed a monitoring of aggressive and violent behaviors over different periods of time. Some of these studies have involved large sample sizes (up to a maximum of 1435 patients studied in the framework of the CATIE project); in eight studies the monitoring has been done with the MOAS (or the OAS); in both studies the assessed time span was very long (up to 10 years), but the assessments of aggressive and violent behaviors were done at very long time intervals (every 2 years in one case, at 1, 2, 5, and 10 years in the other study). In only one study [35] there was a comparison sample of community citizens randomly sampled in the areas where the majority of study subjects were living.

Overall these studies show that a sizeable proportion of patients with SMDs behave aggressively or violently, and that the risk of violence is related to a variety of unmodifiable (e.g., age, sex, previous history of violence) and modifiable (treatment compliance, illness severity, SUD, etc.) factors: services should focus on the latter variables to prevent antisocial behaviors and consequently improve patients' integration, cooperation, and outcomes.

It is worth to note that no study as the VIORMED has ever performed such a close monitoring of aggressive and violent behavior, with 24 ratings every 2 weeks over the course of 1 year.

9.4.4   The European Study of Forensic Psychiatry (EU-VIORMED)

While the VIORMED study has provided valuable data about the risk of violent behavior among patients with SMDs in treatment in ordinary mental health services, it has not studied offenders currently treated in forensic settings. From this perspective available information seems to show that treatment programs and care pathways for mentally disordered offenders vary substantially across Europe. This is partially due to differences in legal frameworks, policies, and clinical resources in the different European countries. One consequence of these differences is that research to help understand the nature of the association between violence and severe mental illness has been inconsistent.

The 3-year EU-VIORMED project (Grant Number PP-2-3-2016, November 2017–October 2020) (de Girolamo et al., in press) aims to assess pathways for forensic psychiatric care in different European countries and their legal and ethical underpinnings, to identify risk factors for violence and self-harm in people with schizophrenia spectrum disorders, to evaluate tools which can predict the risk of violence and self-harm, to assess effective treatments for people with schizophrenia in forensic services, and to examine patients' capacity to consent to treatment in forensic settings. The EU-VIORMED will expand and develop knowledge on the process of violence risk assessment and will elucidate what works in terms of treatment and practice, to help us to deliver more timely, effective, and evidence-based care for offenders. The hope is that it will help the harmonization of forensic psychiatric treatment pathways across the EU, with the ultimate objective to improve the overall quality of forensic psychiatric care in its member states.

Table 9.3 List of prospective studies assessing aggressive and violent behavior in outpatient samples

Author (country)	Sample (N) Male (%)	Diagnoses	Study design (FU, assessment tool, frequency of monitoring)	Main findings
Amore et al. [27] (Italy)	186 (M 68.3%, age 40.6 ± 14.5)	SSD 52.1%; PDs 28.5%; MDD 14.6%; SA 43.0%. All patients discharged from a GHPW	1-year FU. OAS at inclusion (in hospital), 1 month and 1 year after discharge	23.6% showed aggression at 1-month FU and 22.2% at 1-year FU contacts. Overall, 8.3% of these pts resulted to be persistently aggressive in both of the FU assessments. Risk factors for physical violence in the short time period were social problems and a longer time from the first psychiatric contact. Living in residential facilities and physical aggressiveness during hospitalization were correlated to violence in the long-time period.
Appelbaum et al. [28] (USA)	1136 (M 58.7%, age 25–40: 75.3%, 18–24: 24.7%)	MDD 40.3%, SCZ or SchAff. 17.2%, BDs 13.3%, other mental disorders 3.5%, SUD 23.9%, PDs only 1.8%.	1-year FU. MACVI every 10 weeks (five assessments)	The proportions of patients who committed acts of violence across the 5 FU evaluations were 13.5%, 10.3%, 6.9%, 7.6%, and 6.3%, respectively, with a 1-year aggregate violence rate of 27.5%. Delusional symptoms did not increase the overall risk of violence in pts with mental illness in the year after discharge from hospitalization.
Bobes et al. [29] (Spain)	895 (M 66.9%, age 38.7 ± 11.5)	SCZ 100%	MOAS for the week prior to the study visit	Prevalence of recent violent behavior (defined as a score ≥3 in any of the MOAS subscores) 5.1%, where 47.0% reached the violent threshold. Most episodes were verbal (44%), followed by violence towards objects (29%), violence towards others (19%), and self-directed violence (8%). Variables associated with recent violent behavior included a history of violence, relapses in the previous year, and low treatment satisfaction.

(continued)

Table 9.3 (continued)

Author (country)	Sample (N) Male (%)	Diagnoses	Study design (FU, assessment tool, frequency of monitoring)	Main findings
Brucato et al. [30] (USA)	200 (M 72%, age 20.1 ± 3.8)	Psychosis-risk cohort. 30% of the participants developed psychosis during the FU.	2-year FU. MACVI for the past 6 months and at any FU contact	28% of pts reported violent ideation at baseline, 6% reported violent behavior within 6 months pre-baseline, and 4% committed acts of violence during the FU period. Both violent ideation and violent behavior at baseline, as well as a diagnosis of psychosis, predicted violent behavior during FU, independent of clinical and demographic variables.
Colasanti et al. [31] (Italy)	269 (M 63.2%, age 44.1 ± 13.6)	Psychotic disorders 68.0%, mood disorders 28.2%, others 4.0%	MOAS for the week prior to hospital admission	Aggressive and violent behaviors were highly prevalent, respectively, in 45% and 33% of the cases. Violence before admission was independently associated with drug abuse, involuntary admission status, and severe psychopathology. A diagnosis of a psychotic disorder did not increase the risk of aggression or violence, compared to the other psychiatric diagnoses. Personality disorders were significantly more associated to aggressive behaviors than psychotic disorders.
Dean et al. [32] (UK)	495 (M 57.9%, age 30.7 ± 10.8)	SCZ 72.5%, mania 13.5%, depressive psychosis 13.9%	Psychiatric and personal history schedule administered to the patients + review of clinical records	Almost 40% (N = 194) of the samples were aggressive at first contact with services; approximately half of these were physically violent (N = 103). Younger age, African-Caribbean ethnicity, and a history of previous violent offending were independently associated with aggression. Aggressive behavior was associated with a diagnosis of mania and individual manic symptoms were also associated with aggression both for the whole sample and for those with schizophrenia. Factors differentiating violent from nonviolent aggressive patients included male gender, lower social class, and past violent offending.

Ekinci and Ekinci [33] (Turkey)	133 (M 66.2%, age 36.4 ± 10)	SCZ 100%	MOAS for the week prior to the study visit	35.3% pts classified as violent (OAS >7), 64.7% as nonviolent. Nonviolent with more depressive symptoms, lower scores on positive symptoms, better clinical insight, more self-reflectivity.
Keane et al. [34] (Ireland)	132 (M 53%, age 33.3 ± 11.7)	SSD 74.5%, mood disorders 23.5%	MOAS for the week prior to the study visit	36% and 29% of the samples were rated as aggressive and violent, respectively. Aggression was independently associated with involuntary and inpatient treatment status in the week prior to presentation. Violence was associated with involuntary and inpatient status in the week prior to presentation.
Langeveld et al. [35] (Norway, Denmark)	178 (M 55.5%, 28.3 ± 9.2)	First-episode psychosi	10-year FU. Patient interviews at inclusion, 3 months, 1, 2, 5 and 10-years	During the FU, 20% of pts had been apprehended or incarcerated. At 10-year FU, 15% of pts had exposed others to threats or violence in the year before assessment. SUD at baseline and 5-year FU, younger age, and a longer duration of psychotic symptoms predicted violence.
Mauri et al. [36] (Italy)	400 (M 52.7%, age 49.7 ± 14.7)	SCZ 23.3%, PDs 13.5%, BD 17.0%, other diagnoses of the remaining sample.	MOAS for the week prior to the study visit	21.5% of pts with MOAS >0, 11.5% MOAS 0–10, 9% MOAS 11–20, and 1% MOAS >20. Violence related to unemployment, compulsory admission, suicide attempts, and PDs.
Pinna et al. [37] (Italy)	678 (M 45.4%, age 49.6 ± 15.3)	ADs 30.7%, SSDs 25.0%, BD 18.3%, MDD 17.2%, PDs 2.9%, MR 2.6%	Retrospective evaluation of clinical records	27.6% of the sample had committed at least one act of violence during the lifetime, 10.5% over the previous year. 56.7% of those who committed violence acts had acted violently twice or more during the lifetime. Risk of violent behavior: males, younger age, low education, unemployment, living with parents, early age at onset and at first psychiatric treatment, longer DOI, previous hospital admissions and violent events, schizophrenia and other PDs, MR, and comorbidity between two or more psychiatric disorders.

(continued)

Table 9.3 (continued)

Author (country)	Sample (N) Male (%)	Diagnoses	Study design (FU, assessment tool, frequency of monitoring)	Main findings
Steadman et al. [38] (USA)	951 (57.6%, age 18–24 23.7%, 25–40 76.3%)	SCZ 20.4%, MDD 23.7%, BD 37.2%, PDs 37.0%, SUD 56.4%	1-year FU. Interviews every 10 weeks (5 assessments) with the patient and informants	The proportion of patients with at least 1 act of violence during the 1-year FU was 4.5% using agency records alone; 23.7% adding patient self-reported acts that had not been in agency records; and 27.5% adding collateral informant–reported acts that had not been in either agency records or patient self-reports. In a community sample used for comparison (N = 519) 4.6% reported violence and 15.1% aggressive acts only. There was no significant difference at 2 out of 5 FUs between the prevalence of violence by pts without SUD and the prevalence of violence by others living in the same neighborhoods who were also without SUD. SUD significantly raised the rate of violence in both groups, and a higher portion of pts than of others in their neighborhoods reported SUD. Violence in both patient and comparison groups was most frequently targeted at family members and friends, and most often took place at home.

Swanson et al. [39] (USA)	1410 (M 74.3%, age 40.5)	SCZ 100%	MACVI for the past 6 months	The 6-month prevalence of any violence was 19.1%, with 3.6% of participants reporting serious violent behavior. Distinct, but overlapping, sets of risk factors were associated with minor and serious violence. "Positive" psychotic symptoms, such as persecutory ideation, increased the risk of minor and serious violence, while "negative" psychotic symptoms, such as social withdrawal, lowered the risk of serious violence. Minor violence was associated with co-occurring substance abuse and interpersonal and social factors. Serious violence was associated with psychotic and depressive symptoms, childhood conduct problems, and victimization.
Swanson et al. [40] (USA)	802 (M 65.1%, age 41.9 ± 9.9)	SCZ 44.8%, SCZAff 19.5%, BD 16.9%, MDD 11.3%, other 7.0%. Comorbid with SUD 45.4%	Specific assessment instrument	The 1-year prevalence of serious violent behavior was 13.6%. Variables associated with violent behavior included past violent victimization, violence in the surrounding environment, SA, homelessness, PTSD, poor subjective mental health status, earlier age at onset of psychiatric illness, and psychiatric hospital admission. Physical abuse occurring before age 16 significantly increased the risk of violence.
Swanson et al. [41] (USA)	1011 (M range 32.4–64.5%, age range 41.3–46.7)	SCZ 41.5–49.5%. Comorbid with SA 13.9%–35.5%	MCVI for the previous 6 months	18–21% of pts reported having committed violent acts in the past 6 months; 3–9% reported having used or made threats with a lethal weapon, committed sexual assault, or caused injury. Variables associated with violent behavior included younger age, male gender, poorer clinical functioning, more years in treatment, more frequent hospitalizations, and negative attitudes towards medication adherence.

(continued)

Table 9.3 (continued)

Author (country)	Sample (N) Male (%)	Diagnoses	Study design (FU, assessment tool, frequency of monitoring)	Main findings
Tyrer et al. [42] (UK)	70 (M 100%, age 44.5 ± 10.5)	SCZ, SCZaff, BD (83%), PDs (17%)	8.6-month FU. MOAS and QOVS based on patient notes	Mean MOAS monthly score: 1.91 ± 4.39. No of incidents of severe violence: 3.
Tosato et al. [43] (Italy)	80 (M 51%, age 42.1 ± 12.2)	SCZ (100%)	OAS for the previous 6 years from multiple sources	% of males with no recorded episodes of aggression 58.1%; 11.6% had only one recorded episode, and 30.3% had more than one episode. The corresponding percentages for females were 51.4%, 13.5%, and 35.1%.
Winsper et al. [44, 45] (UK)	670 (M 69%, age 21.3 ± 4.9)	FEP	1-year FU, assessment at inclusion, 6- and 12-month AOSQ	13.7% (8.6% at 6 months; 8.5% at 12 months) of the total sample were violent at 6 or 12 months. Past drug use (OR, 1.15; 95% CI, 1.00–1.32), longer DUP (OR, 1.66; 95% CI, 1.06–2.58), positive symptoms (OR, 1.15; 95% CI, 1.09–1.21), and younger age at illness onset (OR, 0.91; 95% CI, 0.87–0.96) were all significantly associated with violent behavior.
Zanarini et al. [46] (USA)	290 (M 22.9%, age 27.0 ± 6.3)	BPD	10-year FU study ABQ-R FUV 5 times (every 2 years)	BPD pts reported higher rates of verbal, emotional, and physical aggression towards others, but the rates of these forms of aggression towards others declined over time. The strongest predictors of adult aggression towards others were the severity of adult experiences of adversity and a concurrent SA disorder.

ªStandardized value of V Cramer

9.5   Conclusions

Our data show that outpatients with a history of violence are more aggressive than patients with no lifetime violent behavior, as well as residential patients with a history of violence. Indeed, more intensive care, as found in RFs, where treatment is granted and prevention of SUD is avoided, is associated with a substantial decrease in the frequency and severity of aggressive and violent behavior even among people with a history of violence.

Violence by the mentally ill has a profound detrimental effect on public opinion, is associated with stigma and discrimination, and places a great burden on family members, who are generally the victims of such a violence. Risk assessment plays a key role in the prevention and/or decrease of violent behavior [REF]. Better prediction also means better prevention by developing more appropriate treatments tailored to the psychopathological dimensions associated with violence (e.g., impulsivity, hostility). If community psychiatry can prevent the violence associated with mental disorders, the full integration of patients and their families will be much easier: therefore the management of mentally ill offenders in the community is one of the great challenges imposed on community psychiatry.

Acknowledgements The VIORMED-2 (Violence Risk and Mental Disorder 2) project was funded by the Health Authority of Regione Lombardia, Italy, grant CUP E42I14000280002 for "Disturbi mentali gravi e rischio di violenza: uno studio prospettico in Lombardia" with Decreto D.G. Salute N.6848, date16.7.2014.

The VIORMED-2 Group also includes Valentina Candini, PhD.; Cesare Cavalera, PhD.; Giovanni Conte, M.D.; Giulia Gamba, M.D.; Laura Iozzino, PhD.; Assunta Martinazzoli, M.D.; Giuliana Mina, M.D.; Alessandra Ornaghi, M.D.; Alberto Stefana, PhD.; and Bruno Travasso, M.D. The authors wish to thank the many clinicians, mental health staff, and family relatives who provided invaluable help for the realization of the project; the authors wish to particularly thank the patients who gave their time and their collaboration to the realization of the project.

Declaration of interest: All authors have no competing interests to disclose.

References

1. Large M, Smith G, Nielssen O. The relationship between the rate of homicide by those with schizophrenia and the overall homicide rate: a systematic review and meta-analysis. Schizophr Res. 2009;112:123–9.
2. Large M, Smith G, Swinson N, Shaw J, Nielssen O. Homicide due to mental disorder in England and Wales over 50 years. Br J Psychiatry. 2008;193:130–3.
3. Nielssen O, Large M. Penrose updated: deinstitutionalization of the mentally ill is not the reason for the increase in violent crime. Nord J Psychiatry. 2009;63:267. https://doi.org/10.1080/08039480902825258.
4. Nielssen O, Large M. Rates of homicide during the first episode of psychosis and after treatment: a systematic review and meta-analysis. Schizophr Bull. 2010;36:702–12.
5. Arboleda-Flórez J. Mental illness and violence. Curr Opin Psychiatry. 2009;22:475–6.
6. de Girolamo G, Cozza M. The Italian psychiatric reform: a 20-year perspective. Int J Law Psychiatry. 2000;23:197–214.
7. de Girolamo G, Bassi M, Neri G, Ruggeri M, Santone G, Picardi A. The current state of mental health care in Italy: problems, perspectives and lessons to learn. Eur Arch Psychiatry Clin Neurosci. 2007;257:83–91.

8. Picardi A, Lega I, Candini V, Dagani J, Iozzino L, de Girolamo G. Monitoring and evaluating the Italian mental health system: the "Progetto Residenze" study and beyond. J Nerv Ment Dis. 2014;202:451–9.

9. Di Lorito C, Castelletti L, Lega I, Gualco B, Scarpa F, Völlm B. The closing of forensic psychiatric hospitals in Italy: determinants, current status and future perspectives. A scoping review. Int J Law Psychiatry. 2017;55:54–63.

10. Ferracuti S, Pucci D, Trobia F, Alessi MC, Rapinesi C, Kotzalidis GD, Del Casale A. Evolution of forensic psychiatry in Italy over the past 40 years (1978–2018). Int J Law Psychiatry. 2019;62:45–9.

11. Bulgari V, Iozzino L, Ferrari C, Picchioni M, Candini V, De Francesco A, Maggi P, Segalini B, de Girolamo G, VIORMED-1 Group. Clinical and neuropsychological features of violence in schizophrenia: a prospective cohort study. Schizophr Res. 2017;181:124–30.

12. de Girolamo G, Buizza C, Sisti D, Ferrari C, Bulgari V, Iozzino L, Boero ME, Cristiano G, De Francesco A, Giobbio GM, Maggi P, Rossi G, Segalini B, Candini V, VIORMED-1 Group. Monitoring and predicting the risk of violence in residential facilities. No difference between patients with history or with no history of violence. J Psychiatr Res. 2016;80:5–13.

13. Candini V, Ghisi M, Bottesi G, Ferrari C, Bulgari V, Iozzino L, Boero ME, De Francesco A, Maggi P, Segalini B, Zuccalli V, Giobbio GM, Rossi G, de Girolamo G. Personality, schizophrenia, and violence: a longitudinal study. J Pers Disord. 2017;31:1–17.

14. Barlati S, Stefana A, Bartoli F, Bianconi G, Bulgari V, Candini V, Carrà G, Cavalera C, Clerici M, Cricelli M, Ferla MT, Ferrari C, Iozzino L, Macis A, Vita A, de Girolamo G, VIORMED-2 Group. Violence risk and mental disorders (VIORMED-2): a prospective multicenter study in Italy. PLoS One. 2019;14(4):e0214924. https://doi.org/10.1371/journal.pone.0214924. eCollection 2019. PubMed PMID: 30990814; PubMed Central PMCID: PMC6467378

15. Bottesi G, Candini V, Ghisi M, Bava M, Bianconi G, Bulgari V, Carrà G, Cavalera C, Conte G, Cricelli M, Ferla MT, Iozzino L, Macis A, Stefana A, de Girolamo G, VIORMED-2 Group. Personality, schizophrenia, and violence: a longitudinal study: the second wave of the VIORMED Project. J Pers Disord. 2019;14:1–19.

16. First MB, Gibbon M, Spitzer RL, Williams JBW, Benjamin S. Structured clinical interview for DSM-IV axis II personality disorders (SCID-II). Washington, D.C.: American Psychiatric Press, Inc.; 1997.

17. First MB, Spitzer RL, Gibbon M, Williams JBW. Structured clinical interview for DSM-IV-TR axis I disorders, research version, patient edition (SCID-I/P). Biometrics Research. New York State Psychiatric Institute: New York, NY; 2002.

18. Dazzi F, Shafer A, Lauriola M. Meta-analysis of the Brief Psychiatric Rating Scale-Expanded (BPRS-E) structure and arguments for a new version. J Psychiatr Res. 2016;81:140–51.

19. Montemagni C, Rocca P, Mucci A, Galderisi S, Maj M. Italian version of the "Specific Level of Functioning". J Psychopathol. 2015;21:287–96.

20. Brown GL, Goodwin FK, Ballenger JC, Goyer PF, Major LF. Aggression in humans correlates with cerebrospinal fluid amine metabolites. Psychiatry Res. 1979;1:131–9.

21. Buss AH, Durkee A. An inventory for assessing different kinds of hostility. J Consult Psychol. 1957;21:343–9.

22. Barratt ES. Factor analysis of some psychometric measures of impulsiveness and anxiety. Psychol Rep. 1965;16:547–54.

23. Spielberger CD, Johnson EH, Russell SF, Crane RJ, Jacobs GA, Worden TJ. The experience and expression of anger: construction and validation of an anger expression scale. In: Chesney MA, Rosenman RH, editors. Anger and hostility in cardiovascular and behavioral disorders. New York: Hemisphere/McGraw-Hill; 1985. p. 5–30.

24. Margari F, Matarazzo R, Cassacchia M, Roncone R, Dieci M, Safran S, et al. Italian validation of MOAS and NOSIE: a useful package for psychiatric assessment and monitoring of aggressive behaviours. Int J Methods Psychiatr Res. 2005;14:109–18.

25. Millon T, Davis RD. The MCMI-III: present and future directions. J Pers Assess. 1997;68:69–85.

26. Millon T, Davis RD, Millon C. Millon Clinical Multiaxial Inventory-III (MCMI-III) manual. 2nd ed. Minneapolis, MN: National Computer Systems; 1997.

27. Amore M, Tonti C, Esposito W, Baratta S, Berardi D, Menchetti M. Course and predictors of physical aggressive behaviour after discharge from a psychiatric inpatient unit: 1 year FU. Community Ment Health J. 2012;49:451–6.
28. Appelbaum PS, Robbins PC, Monahan J. Violence and delusions: data from the MacArthur Violence Risk Assessment Study. Am J Psychiatry. 2000;157:566–72.
29. Bobes J, Fillat O, Violence AC. Violence among schizophrenia outpatients compliant with medication: prevalence and associated factors. Acta Psychiatr Scand. 2009;119:218–25.
30. Brucato G, Appelbaum PS, Lieberman JA, Wall MM, Feng T, Masucci MD, et al. A longitudinal study of violent behavior in a psychosis-risk cohort. Neuropsychopharmacology. 2018;43:264–71.
31. Colasanti A, Natoli A, Moliterno D, Rossattini M, De Gaspari IF, Mauri MC. Psychiatric diagnosis and aggression before acute hospitalisation. Eur Psychiatry. 2008;23:441–8.
32. Dean K, Walsh E, Morgan C, Demjaha A, Dazzan P, Morgan K, Lloyd T, Fearon P, Jones PB, Murray RM. Aggressive behaviour at first contact with services: findings from the AESOP First Episode Psychosis Study. Psychol Med. 2007;37:547–57.
33. Ekinci O, Ekinci A. Association between insight, cognitive insight, positive symptoms and violence in patients with schizophrenia. Nord J Psychiatry. 2013;67:116–23.
34. Keane S, Szigeti A, Fanning F, Clarke M. Are patterns of violence and aggression at presentation in patients with first-episode psychosis temporally stable? A comparison of 2 cohorts. Early Interv Psychiatry. 2018;13:888–94. https://doi.org/10.1111/eip.12694. [Epub ahead of print].
35. Langeveld J, Bjørkly S, Auestad B, Barder H, Evensen J, ten Velden Hegelstad W, et al. Treatment and violent behavior in persons with first episode psychosis during a 10-year prospective FU study. Schizophr Res. 2014;156:272–6.
36. Mauri MC, Cirnigliaro G, Di Pace C, Paletta S, Reggiori A, Altamura CA, Dell'Osso B. Aggressiveness and violence in psychiatric patients: a clinical or social paradigm? CNS Spectr. 2019;4:1–10. https://doi.org/10.1017/S1092852918001438. [Epub ahead of print].
37. Pinna F, Tusconi M, Dessì C, Pittaluga G, Fiorillo A, Carpiniello B. Violence and mental disorders. A retrospective study of people in charge of a community mental health center. Int J Law Psychiatry. 2016;47:122–8.
38. Steadman HJ, Mulvey EP, Monahan J, Robbins PC, Appelbaum PS, Grisso T, Roth LH, Silver E. Violence by people discharged from acute psychiatric inpatient facilities and by others in the same neighborhoods. Arch Gen Psychiatry. 1998;55:393–401.
39. Swanson JW, Swartz MS, Van Dorn RA, Elbogen EB, Wagner HR, Rosenheck RA, Stroup TS, McEvoy JP, Lieberman JA. A national study of violent behavior in persons with schizophrenia. Arch Gen Psychiatry. 2006;63:490–9.
40. Swanson JW, Swartz MS, Essock SM, Osher FC, Wagner HR, Goodman LA, et al. The social–environmental context of violent behavior in persons treated for severe mental illness. Am J Public Health. 2002;92:1523–31.
41. Swanson JW, Van Dorn RA, Monahan J, Swartz MS. Violence and leveraged community treatment for persons with mental disorders. Am J Psychiatry. 2006;163:1404–11.
42. Tyrer P, Cooper S, Herbert E, Duggan C, Crawford M, Joyce E, Rutter D, Seivewright H, O'Sullivan S, Rao B, Cicchetti D, Maden T. The quantification of violence scale: a simple method of recording significant violence. Int J Soc Psychiatry. 2007;53:485–97.
43. Tosato S, Bonetto C, Di Forti M, Collier D, Cristofalo D, Bertani M, Zanoni M, Marrella G, Lazzarotto L, Lasalvia A, De Gir, De Gironcoli M, Tansella M, Dazzan P, Murray R, Ruggeri M. Effect of COMT genotype on aggressive behaviour in a community cohort of schizophrenic patients. Neurosci Lett. 2011;495:17–21.
44. Winsper C, Ganapathy R, Marwaha S, Large M, Birchwood M, Singh SP. A systematic review and meta-regression analysis of aggression during the first episode of psychosis. Acta Psychiatr Scand. 2013;128:413–21.
45. Winsper C, Singh SP, Marwaha S, Amos T, Lester H, Everard L, et al. Pathways to violent behavior during first-episode psychosis. JAMA Psychiat. 2013;70:1287.
46. Zanarini MC, Temes CM, Ivey AM, Cohn DM, Conkey LC, Frankenburg FR, et al. The 10-year course of adult aggression toward others in patients with borderline personality disorder and axis II comparison subjects. Psychiatry Res. 2017;252:134–8.

Prevalence and Risk Factors of Violence by Psychiatric Acute Inpatients: Systematic Review and Meta-Analysis—A 2019 Update

10

Ester di Giacomo, Laura Iozzino, Clarissa Ferrari, Cosmo Strozza, Matthew Large, Olav Nielssen, and Giovanni de Girolamo

10.1 Introduction

Physical violence, defined as an act intended to cause physical harm, in psychiatric settings is a concern of patients and their families, mental health professionals, and hospital administrators. Violence in this setting is likely to be associated with the loss of inhibition and increased perception of threat associated with some forms of mental illness, the attitudes and background of the violence person, and the increased potential for conflict associated with being a psychiatric inpatient. In acute

E. di Giacomo
School of Medicine and Surgery, University of Milan-Bicocca, Monza, Italy

Department of Mental Health and Addiction, ASST Monza, Monza, Italy

L. Iozzino · G. de Girolamo (✉)
Unit of Epidemiological and Evaluation Psychiatry, IRCCS Centro San Giovanni di Dio Fatebenefratelli, Brescia, Italy
e-mail: liozzino@fatebenefratelli.eu; gdegirolamo@fatebenefratelli.eu

C. Ferrari
Unit of Statistics, IRCCS Centro San Giovanni di Dio Fatebenefratelli, Brescia, Italy
e-mail: cferrari@fatebenefratelli.eu

C. Strozza
Department of Statistical Science, 'La Sapienza' University, Rome, Italy

Interdisciplinary Centre on Population Dynamics (CPOP), Southern Denmark University, Odense, Denmark

M. Large
Prince of Wales Hospital Sydney, Sydney, Australia

University of New South Wales, Sydney, Australia

O. Nielssen
Faculty of Medicine and Health Science, Macquarie University, Sydney, Australia

© Springer Nature Switzerland AG 2020
B. Carpiniello et al. (eds.), *Violence and Mental Disorders*, Comprehensive Approach to Psychiatry 1, https://doi.org/10.1007/978-3-030-33188-7_10

psychiatric wards violence can be perpetrated against other patients, staff members, and even visitors to the ward [1]. Inpatient violence can result in serious injuries to both patients and staff, and is harmful to the care of all patients because of the reduced perception of safety within the ward.

The psychological effects of being exposed to violence by other patients include anger, shock, fear, depression, anxiety, and sleep disturbance. Staff members may experience the same psychological reaction, even if they were not directly assaulted. The perceived threat of violence may result in greater use of coercive measures such as seclusion, restraint, and enforced medication, which patients often describe as traumatic [1] and can, in turn, trigger aggressive responses from patients, instead of engagement and cooperation with treatment [2, 3]. Physical violence against staff is thought to contribute to low morale, high rates of sick leave, and high staff turnover [4], which in turn has an adverse effect, as low staffing levels and use of temporary staff are associated with more adverse incidents [5], higher service costs, and lower standards of care [6]. Surveys show that between 75% and 100% of nursing staff on acute psychiatric units have been assaulted by patients at some stage in their careers [7, 8].

Awareness of the extent of violence in psychiatric wards, and the factors influencing the likelihood of violence, are central to efforts to reduce the prevalence and prevent episodes of violence. However, individual studies report large variation in the rates of acts of violence committed by psychiatric inpatients during their stay in acute psychiatric wards. The differences might be due to real different rates of violence, but might also be due to differences in the definition of acts of violence, differences in the period of observation, methods of data collection, and variation in the underreporting of violence by mental healthcare workers.

10.2   Previous Knowledge

The initial attempts to understand inpatient violence were based on the analysis of the sociodemographic and clinical characteristics associated with inpatient aggression and violence in individual patients. A history of previous aggressive incidents, longer hospitalization, involuntary admission, impulsiveness, hostility, and being of the same gender as the victim were the most important factors associated with acts of inpatient violence [9, 10]. A recent meta-analysis of the patient-level risk factors for either aggression or violence in a diverse range of inpatient settings by Dack and colleagues [11] found aggression to be associated with young age, male sex, involuntary admission, not being married, a diagnosis of schizophrenia, a greater number of previous admissions, a history of violence, a history of self-destructive behavior, and a history of substance use. Hence the factors associated with inpatient violence appear to be similar to those associated with violence among outpatients and in the wider community. However, the factors influencing the *proportion* of inpatients who will commit an act of violence are not as well understood.

An earlier meta-analysis of 35 eligible studies with a total of 23,972 patients found that as many as 1 in 5 patients committed an act of physical violence while in adult psychiatric units [12]. Studies with higher proportions of male patients, involuntary patients, patients with schizophrenia, and patients with alcohol-use disorder reported higher rates of inpatient violence. This update was prompted by the publication of a number of further studies, potentially reflecting improvements in ward design and procedures for managing difficult patients.

10.3   Knowledge Update

10.3.1 Study Selection and Data Extraction

We performed further searches of the same databases as the previous study (PubMed, Scopus, and Cumulative Index to Nursing and Allied Health Literature (CINAHL)) by extending the publication dates to include the period January 2015 to April 2019 using the same search terms ("violence" OR "aggression" OR "aggressive behavior" OR "assault") AND ("mental disorders" OR "psychosis" OR "acute psychiatric inpatients") AND ("hospital" OR "hospitalization" OR "acute psychiatric wards") in either the title or thes abstract. We included studies that reported the proportion of adult patients admitted to acute psychiatric wards in high-income countries (http://www.worldbank.org/) who had committed at least one act of violence while in hospital. Studies that reported only rates of verbal hostility and self-harm behavior were excluded, as were studies that did not make a distinction between different types of aggressive behavior. We also excluded studies conducted in forensic hospitals or wards, studies conducted in wards admitting only adolescents (up to 18 years of age) or psychogeriatric patients (older than 65), studies performed in outpatient settings, studies of psychiatric patients admitted to nonpsychiatric wards, studies conducted in long-stay wards that did not accept acute admissions, and studies from any type of nonhospital residential facility for psychiatric patients.

We identified 293 additional publications in the 4 years since the last searches were performed, of which 7 [13–19] met the inclusion criteria for this research update (see Fig. 10.1).

The effect size data collected was based on the number of admissions and the number of violent patients. Potential moderators of the proportion of violent patients collected included year of publication, country in which the study was conducted, study setting (single vs. multicenter), average number of ward beds, average length of stay, sample size, mean age of patients, proportions of males, involuntary admissions, psychiatric diagnoses, diagnosis of alcohol- and drug-use disorder, and proportion of patients with a history of previous violence. The methods used to record violence were also examined (Staff Observation Aggression Scale, SOAS; the Staff Observation Aggression Scale-Revised, SOAS-R; the Overt Aggression Scale, OAS; the Modified Overt Aggression Scale, MOAS; or others). These scales have a range of definitions of violence: for example, in the SOAS, an aggressive patient is defined as having an incident of physical aggression against others reported by a staff member, whereas the MOAS scale includes verbal aggression, physical violence against objects and violence against self, as well as physical violence against

Fig. 10.1 PRISMA 2009
flow diagram: article years
2015–2019

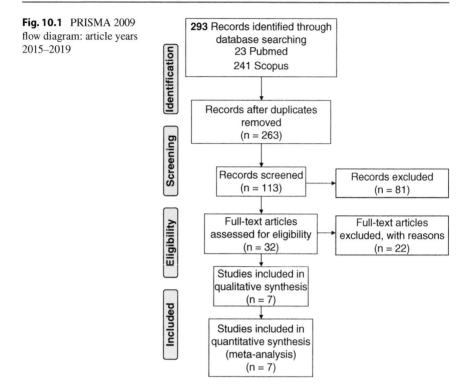

others. However, in each of the included studies that used the MOAS we were able to extract the number of patients who committed an act of physical violence against another person. Satisfactory intercoder agreement was established for the screening (95.6%, range: 85–100%; $k = 35$) and data extraction (97%, range: 85–100%; $k = 35$), respectively.

10.3.2 Assessment of Study Quality

Study quality was again assessed using a four-point "strength of reporting" scale, derived from the Strengthening the Reporting of Observational Studies in Epidemiology (STROBE) statement checklist [20]. A score of 1 was accorded if each of the following methodological features was present: (1) recruitment by consecutive patients; (2) data collected prospectively; (3) presence of detailed definitions of outcomes, exposures, predictors, potential confounders, and effect modifiers; and (4) detailed description of the methods of violence assessment and the use of structured or semi-structured measurement. The included studies were divided between those with a strength of reporting score of less than 3 and those with a score of 3 or more in order to assess the association between study quality and reported proportion of violent patients.

10.3.3 Data Analysis

Random-effects meta-analysis was used to calculate a pooled estimate of the proportion of inpatients who committed an act of violence and 95% confidence intervals (CI). A random-effects model was chosen as a conservative approach because we assumed that that would be significant between study heterogeneity in patient populations and methods of measurement of violence. The Q-statistic and I^2 index (% of total variability due to heterogeneity) were used to assess heterogeneity among studies. A significant Q value and high (larger than 50) I^2 index indicate lack of homogeneity of findings among studies [21].

Several characteristics were identified to analyze their effect on violence prevalence. Categorical characteristics were treated as moderators and were compared across subgroups formed by country (with categories: Europe, the UK-Ireland, the USA-Canada, Australia), year of publication (1995–2006 vs. 2007–2019), violence measurement tool (SOAS/OAS/MOAS vs. other tools), study setting, and study quality (less than 3, or greater than or equal to 3). Continuous characteristics including number of beds in the ward, sample's mean age, average length of stay in days, proportion of the study sample of males, total number of admissions, total number of involuntary admissions, patients with bipolar disorder, patients with schizophrenia, patients with diagnosis of personality disorder, patients with alcohol-use disorder, and patients with lifetime history of violence were examined as covariates using random-effects (restricted maximum likelihood estimation) meta-regression. Finally, multivariable meta-regression analyses were carried out to test the independence of the individual moderator variables that were significantly associated between study heterogeneity at alpha = 0.050.

Publication bias was evaluated by rank correlation test (Begg's test) [22] and Duval and Tweedie's "trim and fill" method [23] that allows for the calculation of an adjusted effect size and confidence interval [24].

All statistical analyses were performed using R: A language and environment for statistical computing, version 3.03 (R Core Team, 2013; R foundation for Statistical Computing), and its R-metafor package. The level of statistical significance was set at $p < 0.05$.

10.4   Results

Including data from our previous meta-analysis, 42 papers satisfied inclusion criteria, with a total sample of 29,303 patients. The sample had a mean age of 37.8, 51% were males, and most (61%) had a diagnosis of schizophrenia (61%).

Nineteen studies were from Europe (1 from Germany, 1 from Greece, 7 from Italy, 2 from the Netherlands, 5 from Norway, 1 from Sweden, and 2 from Switzerland), 9 from the UK and Ireland, 1 from Israel, 7 from the USA and Canada, and 7 from Australia. Most of the studies (37 out of 42) were given a high-quality score (≥ 3).

Thirty-three studies [15, 18, 19, 25–60] used a standardized tool to rate violent incidents, of which 23 studies used either SOAS, SOAS-R, OAS, or MOAS (see Table 10.1 for principal information and Table 10.2 for additional data).

10.4.1 Meta-analysis and Meta-regression

The pooled prevalence of inpatients who committed at least one act of violence while admitted to an acute psychiatric ward was 18% (CI 15–21%) (see Fig. 10.2). Heterogeneity between study was significant ($I^2 = 98.7\%$, $Q = 1735.3$, $p < 0.0001$). All the subgroups had a significant between-study heterogeneity ($p < 0.0001$). Heterogeneity was higher than 90% in all the subgroups we analyzed and higher than 95% in all the subgroups except for studies conducted in the UK-Ireland (see Table 10.3).

The proportion of violent patients was not influenced by the year in which the study was conducted or the study's quality, but varied depending on the country where the study was led, with a lower estimate in Europe (13%, CI 10–17%) or overestimate in the UK-Ireland (20%, CI 16–25%) and higher in the USA-Canada (25%, CI 16–35%). Single-center studies (14%, CI 11–17%) had a lower proportion of violent patients when compared to multicenter studies (21%, CI 16–26%), and studies assessing violence through MOAS-SOAS-OAS (16%, CI 12–20%) had a lower rate than studies conducted using other tools (20%, CI 16–25%) (see Table 10.3).

The univariate meta-regression models revealed that the proportion of male patients explained almost 18% of between-study heterogeneity ($p = 0.003$). A similar percentage of heterogeneity was explained by the ward size, represented by the number of beds in the wards studied (almost 17%). Other characteristics of the primary researches that explained between-study heterogeneity were the proportion of involuntary admissions (13%) and the proportion of patients diagnosed with alcohol-use disorder (36%).

A multivariable regression model was performed. It included ward size instead of the proportion of alcohol abusers (included in the previous meta-analysis) and was able to explain a high percentage of study heterogeneity (about 74%).

10.4.2 Publication Bias

Begg's rank correlation test and the "trim and fill" procedure showed substantially no publication bias. Begg's test resulted significant only in the univariate model for ward size moderator (due to the study by Ash et al. in 2003 that was subsequently excluded from the multivariable model analysis) (see Table 10.4).

Table 10.1 Summary information of the studies included in meta-analysis

Author, Year	Country	Multiple (M) or single (S) study	Average number of beds	Sample (N)	Number of violent patients	Male gender (N)	Average length of stay (days)	Admissions (N)	Involuntary admissions (N)	Mean age
Aberhalden et al., 2006	Switzerland	M	4	519	37	315	22.4	519	319	37.8
Aberhalden et al., 2008	Switzerland	M		2364	314	1262	19	2364	1040	39.5
Amore et al., 2008	Italy	S	20	303	75	182		374		41.6
Ash et al., 2003	Australia	S	20	119	26	83		143	51	35
Barlow et al., 2000	Australia	M	16	1269	174	662	13.8	2536		37
Beauford et al., 1997	USA	S		328	38	170	16	328	285	41.9
Biancosino et al., 2009	Italy	M		1324	37	677		1324	178	
Bjorkdahl et al., 2006	Sweden	S	10	73	11	37	13.6	73		39.6
Boggild et al., 2004	USA	S	36	105	44			259		40.5
Bowers et al., 2003	UK	M		238	38	140		238	100	40
Carr et al., 2008	Australia	M	21	3877	551	2210	14.6	5546	2640	37.1
Cohen et al., 2008	Ireland	S	18	99	18	50		99		40

(continued)

Table 10.1 (continued)

Author, Year	Country	Multiple (M) or single (S) study	Average number of beds	Sample (N)	Number of violent patients	Male gender (N)	Average length of stay (days)	Admissions (N)	Involuntary admissions (N)	Mean age
Cookson et al., 2012	Australia	M	25	79	35	43	19.6	310	212	40.8
Daffern et al., 2010	Australia	S	50	122	10		15	395	63	39.5
Dumais et al., 2012	Canada	S		77	16	47		77		36.4
Eaton et al., 2000	UK	S	20	52	17	46		79		32
Ehmann et al., 2001	Canada	S	20	78	20	53		78		34.5
Grassi et al., 2001	Italy	S	15	1534	116	798	12.8	2461	674	39.5
Hartvig et al., 2011	Norway	M	41	1017	92	536	15	1469	389	42.7
Ketelsen et al., 2007	Germany	M	17	2210	171	1226	28.2	2246	323	46.9
Krakowsi et al., 2004	USA	M		1487	222	1026		1487		36.1
Lam et al., 2000	USA	S		390	76	205		390	344	41.8
Mauri et al., 2011	Italy	S	15	244	82	179	12.2	244	74	41.9
Mellesdal et al., 2003	Norway	S	12	934	98	476	11.6	1507	1053	41.1
Nijman et al., 1997	Netherlands	S	20	123	31			123		

Study	Country									
Nijman et al., 2002	Netherlands	S	20	89	23	54		98	38	36
Oulis et al., 1996	Greece	M		136	8	72		136		
Owen et al., 2005	Australia	M		855	174			855	427	
Raja et al., 1997	Italy	S	12	313	22	143		360	36	41.8
Raja et al., 2005	Italy	S	12	2395	70	1067		2395	604	41.9
Ross et al., 2011	UK	M		522	110	279		522		41
Saverimuttu et al., 2000	UK	S	5	170	57	136		170		
Soliman et al., 2001	UK	M	15	329	49	239	36.4	474	50	39.6
Troisi et al., 2003	Italy	S		80	20	80		80	24	34.1
Valeer et al., 2011	Norway	M	4	118	13	66	5.6	118	57	36.3
Podubinski et al., 2016	Australia	M	56	200	19	132	14.59	746		38.32
Eriksen et al., 2017	Norway	M	38	362	59	158	20	558	160	41
Cullen et al., 2018	UK	M		1980	204	825		1980		
Lockertsen et al., 2018	Norway	M	38	512	81	229	12.3	684	138	40.8

(continued)

Table 10.1 (continued)

Author, Year	Country	Multiple (M) or single (S) study	Average number of beds	Sample (N)	Number of violent patients	Male gender (N)	Average length of stay (days)	Admissions (N)	Involuntary admissions (N)	Mean age
Shafi et al., 2017	UK	M		442	107	244	40.8	442	191	43.7
Sanghani et al., 2017	USA	S	208	806	356	431	37.1	806	361	40.3
Renwick et al., 2016	UK	M		522	106	279		522		41.1

Table 10.2 Additional information of the studies included in meta-analysis

Author, year	Diagnosis of schizophrenia (N)	Diagnosis of bipolar disorder (N)	Diagnosis of personality disorder (N)	Previous history of violence (N)	Lifetime history of alcohol or/and drug abuse (N)	Measurements	Quality score (range 0–4)
Aberhalden et al., 2006	196				120	SOAS-R, BVC	4
Aberhalden et al., 2008	734				574	SOAS-R, BVC	4
Amore et al., 2008	151	26	85	105	117	OAS	4
Ash et al., 2003	56		49		57	Not specified	3
Barlow et al., 2000	271	91	38			AIF	4
Beauford et al., 1997	75	71				OAS	3
Biancosino et al., 2009	472	206	168		117	Retrospective chart records	4
Bjorkdahl et al., 2006	15	14	9			SOAS-R	3
Boggild et al., 2004	0			30	76	Nursing chart record	3
Bowers et al., 2003	169					PCC	3
Carr et al., 2008	1473	543	733	318	1729	AIF, OAS	4
Cohen et al., 2008	26	23	9		8	SOAS-R	3

(continued)

Table 10.2 (continued)

Author, year	Diagnosis of schizophrenia (N)	Diagnosis of bipolar disorder (N)	Diagnosis of personality disorder (N)	Previous history of violence (N)	Lifetime history of alcohol or/and drug abuse (N)	Measurements	Quality score (range 0–4)
Cookson et al., 2012						OAS	3
Cullen et al., 2018	1136	395	76			Not specified	2
Daffern et al., 2010						OAS	3
Dumais et al., 2012	40	26	5			DASA	3
Eaton et al., 2000	33			40	39	Clinical record and hospital incident forms	1
Ehmann et al., 2001	53	9		35	28	MOAS	4
Eriksen et al., 2017	104	47	28			SOAS-R	4
Grassi et al., 2001	632	136	216		31	SOAS	4
Hartvig et al., 2011	208	122	92			REFA	3
Ketelsen et al., 2007	512	236	102		924	SOAS	4
Krakowsi et al., 2004						MOAS	3
Lam et al., 2000	87	87		53	102	Retrospective records	2

Study						Instrument	
Lockertsen et al., 2018	126	56	49			SOAS-R	4
Mauri et al., 2011	130	17	51	147		MOAS	4
Mellesdal et al., 2003	290	523	141	157		REFA	4
Nijman et al., 1997						SOAS	3
Nijman et al., 2002	50					SOAS-R	3
Oulis et al., 1996	88	11				MOAS	4
Owen et al., 2005						Violence and Aggression Checklist	4
Podubinski et al., 2016	111	17	14			OAS	2
Raja et al., 1997	110	82	32	34		Nursing chart record	4
Raja et al., 2005	295	386	55	437		Modified version of the Morrison's scale	4
Renwick et al., 2016	219		54	202	296	Patient Conflict Checklist-PCC	3
Ross et al., 2011	215					PCC	3
Sanghani et al., 2017	169	84	74			New York Incident Management and Reporting System (NIMRS)	3

(continued)

Table 10.2 (continued)

Author, year	Diagnosis of schizophrenia (N)	Diagnosis of bipolar disorder (N)	Diagnosis of personality disorder (N)	Previous history of violence (N)	Lifetime history of alcohol or/and drug abuse (N)	Measurements	Quality score (range 0–4)
Saverimuttu et al., 2000	73	34	18		21	Violent incident forms	2
Shafi et al., 2017	228	54	57	164		Not specified	3
Soliman et al., 2001	110	53	44	52	122	SOAS	3
Troisi et al., 2003	53	20	3		4	MOAS	4
Valeer et al., 2011	54				33	SOAS-R	4

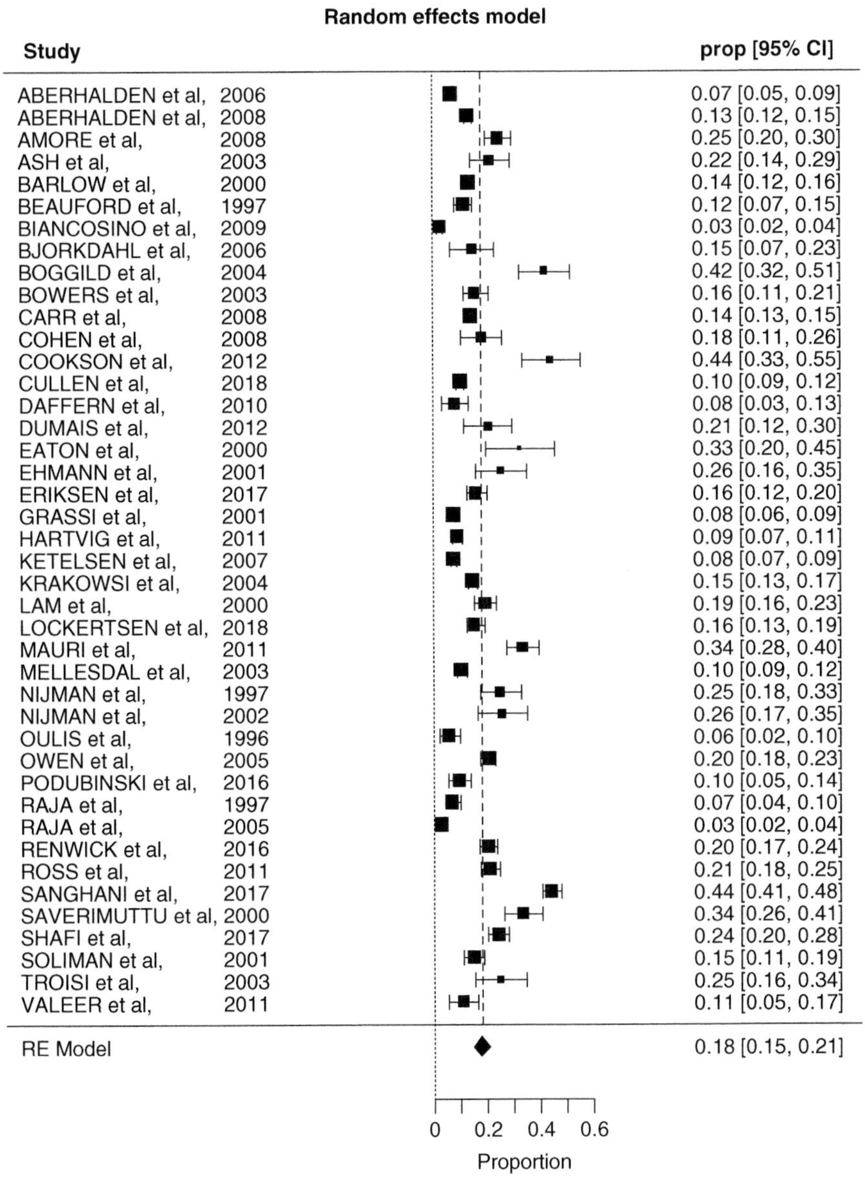

Random effects model

Study		prop [95% CI]
ABERHALDEN et al,	2006	0.07 [0.05, 0.09]
ABERHALDEN et al,	2008	0.13 [0.12, 0.15]
AMORE et al,	2008	0.25 [0.20, 0.30]
ASH et al,	2003	0.22 [0.14, 0.29]
BARLOW et al,	2000	0.14 [0.12, 0.16]
BEAUFORD et al,	1997	0.12 [0.07, 0.15]
BIANCOSINO et al,	2009	0.03 [0.02, 0.04]
BJORKDAHL et al,	2006	0.15 [0.07, 0.23]
BOGGILD et al,	2004	0.42 [0.32, 0.51]
BOWERS et al,	2003	0.16 [0.11, 0.21]
CARR et al,	2008	0.14 [0.13, 0.15]
COHEN et al,	2008	0.18 [0.11, 0.26]
COOKSON et al,	2012	0.44 [0.33, 0.55]
CULLEN et al,	2018	0.10 [0.09, 0.12]
DAFFERN et al,	2010	0.08 [0.03, 0.13]
DUMAIS et al,	2012	0.21 [0.12, 0.30]
EATON et al,	2000	0.33 [0.20, 0.45]
EHMANN et al,	2001	0.26 [0.16, 0.35]
ERIKSEN et al,	2017	0.16 [0.12, 0.20]
GRASSI et al,	2001	0.08 [0.06, 0.09]
HARTVIG et al,	2011	0.09 [0.07, 0.11]
KETELSEN et al,	2007	0.08 [0.07, 0.09]
KRAKOWSI et al,	2004	0.15 [0.13, 0.17]
LAM et al,	2000	0.19 [0.16, 0.23]
LOCKERTSEN et al,	2018	0.16 [0.13, 0.19]
MAURI et al,	2011	0.34 [0.28, 0.40]
MELLESDAL et al,	2003	0.10 [0.09, 0.12]
NIJMAN et al,	1997	0.25 [0.18, 0.33]
NIJMAN et al,	2002	0.26 [0.17, 0.35]
OULIS et al,	1996	0.06 [0.02, 0.10]
OWEN et al,	2005	0.20 [0.18, 0.23]
PODUBINSKI et al,	2016	0.10 [0.05, 0.14]
RAJA et al,	1997	0.07 [0.04, 0.10]
RAJA et al,	2005	0.03 [0.02, 0.04]
RENWICK et al,	2016	0.20 [0.17, 0.24]
ROSS et al,	2011	0.21 [0.18, 0.25]
SANGHANI et al,	2017	0.44 [0.41, 0.48]
SAVERIMUTTU et al,	2000	0.34 [0.26, 0.41]
SHAFI et al,	2017	0.24 [0.20, 0.28]
SOLIMAN et al,	2001	0.15 [0.11, 0.19]
TROISI et al,	2003	0.25 [0.16, 0.34]
VALEER et al,	2011	0.11 [0.05, 0.17]
RE Model		0.18 [0.15, 0.21]

0   0.2   0.4   0.6

Proportion

Fig. 10.2 Forest plot

Table 10.3 Subgroup analysis for prevalence of violence

Study subgroups	No. of studies	Prevalence of violence		Heterogeneity	Group heterogeneity			Publication bias Begg's test	
		Estimate	CI 95%	I² (%)	Q	df (Q)	p-value	Tau	p-value
Total	42	18	[15–21]	98.7%	1735.3	41	<0.0001	0.2	0.10
Country group									
Europe	19	13	[10–17]	98.8%	555.1	18	<0.0001	0.2	0.16
UK-Ireland	9	20	[16–25]	92.6%	121.6	8	<0.0001	0.3	0.35
USA-Canada	7	25	[16–35]	97.5%	265.7	6	<0.0001	0.4	0.23
Australia	7	18	[10–26]	98.3%	63.4	6	<0.0001	0.2	0.56
Year of the study									
(1995–2006)	22	17	[13–21]	98.1%	645.3	21	<0.0001	0.2	0.31
(2007–2018)	20	18	[13–23]	99.0%	1015.1	19	<0.0001	0.2	0.28
Quality score									
<3	5	17	[7–28]	97.3%	78.1	4	<0.0001	0.4	0.48
≥3	37	17	[14–21]	98.8%	1645.6	36	<0.0001	0.2	0.19
Measurement tool									
MOAS-SOAS-OAS	23	16	[12–20]	99.2%	1389.2	22	<0.0001	0.2	0.22
Other tools	19	20	[16–25]	96.4%	215.1	18	<0.0001	0.4	0.01
Study setting									
Single	21	14	[11–17]	97.9%	652.3	20	<0.0001	0.1	0.53
Multicenter	21	21	[16–26]	98.2%	1002.4	20	<0.0001	0.2	0.24

Table 10.4 Meta-regression results: univariate and multivariate models

Models	Risk factor	Type of data	Coefficient	Coefficient p-value	Explained heterogeneity R^2 (%)	Test for residual heterogeneity Q_E	df	p-value	Begg's test Tau	p-value
Univariate	**Gender**	**(N. of male/total sample)**	**0.3726**	**0.0035**	**17.9%**	**1195.5**	**36**	**<0.0001**	**0.2**	**0.10**
	Age	(Mean age)	−0.0054	0.3513	0.0%	1208.8	34	0.3513	0.2	0.12
	Ward size	**(Average N. of bed)**	**0.0012**	**0.0217**	**16.4%**	**679.5**	**26**	**<0.0001**	**0.3**	**0.04**
	Length of stay	(Average days)	0.0044	0.0695	12.5%	599.5	18	<0.0001	0.2	0.16
	Admissions	(N. of admissions/total sample)	0.0172	0.4651	0.0%	1654.2	39	<0.0001	0.2	0.10
	Involuntary admissions	**(N. of involuntary admissions/total sample)**	**0.0978**	**0.0225**	**12.8%**	**1018.5**	**24**	**<0.0001**	**0.3**	**0.07**
	Bipolar disorder	(N. of bipolar/total sample)	−0.1011	0.5996	0.0%	1318.6	25	<0.0001	0.2	0.07
	Schizophrenia disorder	(N. of schizophrenia/total sample)	0.1483	0.1379	2.3%	1307.6	34	<0.0001	0.2	0.11
	Personality disorder	(N. of personality disorder/total sample)	0.3218	0.1879	3.7%	1129.0	23	<0.0001	0.2	0.11
	Alcohol abuse	**(N. of alcohol abusers/total sample)**	**0.3238**	**0.0007**	**36.1%**	**573.8**	**20**	**<0.0001**	**0.2**	**0.19**
	History of violence	(N. of patients with history of violence/total sample)	0.1880	0.1295	19.2%	40.9	7	<0.0001	0.4	0.11
Multivariable model					73.5%	143.0	12	<0.0001	0.4	0.06
Variables	**Gender**	**(N. of male/total sample)**	**0.5315**	**0.0074**						
	Ward size	**(Average N. of bed)**	**0.0018**	**<0.0001**						
	Involuntary admissions	**(N. of invol. admiss/total sample)**	**0.1027**	**0.0019**						

10.5 Discussion

This updated study of violence committed by inpatients within acute psychiatric ward, including a further seven studies with a total of 5331 hospital admissions, confirms the results of our previous study regarding the prevalence of violence by psychiatric inpatients. We found the overall prevalence to be 18%, meaning that almost 1 out of 5 patients committed a violent act while admitted to an acute psychiatric ward. Moreover, the combined results of studies published since 2015 were similar to those of the 34 earlier studies, which suggests that the management and prevention of violence by inpatients have not changed much in recent years. The reason the rate of violence may not have declined, despite the greatly increased awareness of the potential for violence and focus on containing violent patients, may be due to the increased stress on mental health services required to contain acute patients for shorter periods with fewer beds, and the growing proportion of involuntary patients, which is itself associated with a higher prevalence of violence.

Not surprisingly, the proportion of male inpatients was associated with the prevalence of violence in acute wards. While males are known to be more likely to commit acts of violence than individual women, this might not fully explain why wards with a higher proportion of males have more violence. Other possible explanations include that men with a history of violence are more likely to be admitted, that threatening male patients are more likely to be restrained and segregated than female patients, or even that the absence of women and the increased interaction between mentally ill males increased the likelihood of violence between male patients.

The proportion of involuntary patients was also associated with the proportion of violent patients. While violent patients are more likely to be admitted on an involuntary basis, it also may be the case that patients who are involuntary are more likely to become violent because of their attitude to detention in hospital and treatment with medication. While other clinical reasons might have also influenced the proportion of violent subjects, we did not find that the major disorders detected (e.g., schizophrenia, bipolar, or personality disorders) influenced the overall incidence of violence.

The proportion of patients with alcohol-use disorder was associated with the prevalence of violence, but this is unlikely to be a result of the disinhibition associated with alcohol use, as those patients were unlikely to have been affected by alcohol by the time of the act of violence. The proportion of patients with other forms of substance-use disorder was not found to be associated with the prevalence of violence, possibly because substance-use disorders alone are not usually the reason for admission to hospital, and are instead comorbid with other conditions, typically psychotic illness and severe personality disorder.

We did not find that the proportion of patients with a history of violence was associated with the prevalence of violence. At an individual patient level a history of violence is often reported as a main predictor of future violence [20, 27, 33, 58, 61] but in our study this did not translate to increased levels of violence at the level of ward or study. This is not to suggest that people with a history of personal violence in the studies we include were not more violent—but simply suggests that having more potentially violent patients on a ward paradoxically might not increase the overall prevalence of violent episodes. While the reasons for this can only be guessed at, it may be that the presence of a greater number of potentially violent patients on a ward has an inhibiting effect on the behavior of other patients.

The high overall rate of violence is not entirely surprising considering the effect of manifestations of mental illness and mental disorder on the perception of threat, social judgement, and inhibition, and that admission to hospital is increasingly based on the protection of the patients and others from serious harm. However, it is a continuing irony of psychiatric hospital care that the admission of many patients for their own protection instead exposes them to a significant risk of violence at the hands of other patients, as well as the often terrifying experience of sharing an enclosed space with irrational and threatening fellow patients.

10.6 Conclusion

This updated meta-analysis of the prevalence of violence by acute psychiatric inpatients confirms the continuing prevalence of acts of violence by inpatients in first world countries, and the factors contributing to the probability of violence at a ward level. The results of this study can guide strategies for reducing acts of violence, including in the design of wards to reduce the likelihood of violence arising from between-patient interactions, and increased treatment for males, those with alcohol-use disorder, and those detained on an involuntary basis.

References

1. Olofsson B, Jacobsson L. A plea for respect: involuntarily hospitalized psychiatric patients' narratives about being subjected to coercion. J Psychiatr Ment Health Nurs. 2001;8(4):357–66.
2. Daffern M, Mayer M, Martin T. Staff gender ratio and aggression in a forensic psychiatric hospital. Int J Ment Health Nurs. 2006;15(2):93–9.
3. Fisher WA. Elements of successful restraint and seclusion reduction programs and their application in a large, urban, state psychiatric hospital. J Psychiatr Pract. 2003;9(1):7–15.
4. Needham I, Abderhalden C, Halfens RJ, Dassen T, Haug HJ, Fischer JE. The effect of a training course in aggression management on mental health nurses' perceptions of aggression: a cluster randomised controlled trial. Int J Nurs Stud. 2005;42(6):649–55.
5. Bowers L, Simpson A, Alexander J, Hackney D, Nijman H, Grange A, et al. The nature and purpose of acute psychiatric wards: the Tompkins Acute Ward Study. J Ment Health. 2005;14(6):625–35.
6. Authorities ACfL, England tNHSi. Change here!: managing change to improve local services: Audit Commission for Local Authorities & the NHS in England & Wales; 2001.
7. Caldwell MF. Incidence of PTSD among staff victims of patient violence. Hosp Community Psychiatry. 1992;43(8):838–9.
8. Hatch-Maillette MA, Scalora MJ, Bader SM, Bornstein BH. A gender-based incidence study of workplace violence in psychiatric and forensic settings. Violence Vict. 2007;22(4):449–62.
9. Cornaggia CM, Beghi M, Pavone F, Barale F. Aggression in psychiatry wards: a systematic review. Psychiatry Res. 2011;189(1):10–20.

10. Di Giacomo E, Clerici M. Violence in psychiatric inpatients. Riv Psichiatr. 2010;45(6):361–4.
11. Dack C, Ross J, Papadopoulos C, Stewart D, Bowers L. A review and meta-analysis of the patient factors associated with psychiatric in-patient aggression. Acta Psychiatr Scand. 2013;127(4):255–68.
12. Iozzino L, Ferrari C, Large M, Nielssen O, de Girolamo G. Prevalence and risk factors of violence by psychiatric acute inpatients: a systematic review and meta-analysis. PLoS One. 2015;10(6):e0128536.
13. Podubinski T, Lee S, Hollander Y, Daffern M. An examination of the stability of interpersonal hostile-dominance and its relationship with psychiatric symptomatology and post-discharge aggression. Aggress Behav. 2016;42(4):324–32.
14. Eriksen BMS, Bjorkly S, Lockertsen O, Faerden A, Roaldset JO. Low cholesterol level as a risk marker of inpatient and post-discharge violence in acute psychiatry—a prospective study with a focus on gender differences. Psychiatry Res. 2017;255:1–7.
15. Cullen AE, Bowers L, Khondoker M, Pettit S, Achilla E, Koeser L, et al. Factors associated with use of psychiatric intensive care and seclusion in adult inpatient mental health services. Epidemiol Psychiatr Sci. 2018;27(1):51–61.
16. Lockertsen O, Procter N, Vatnar SKB, Faerden A, Eriksen BMS, Roaldset JO, et al. Screening for risk of violence using service users' self-perceptions: a prospective study from an acute mental health unit. Int J Ment Health Nurs. 2018;27(3):1055–65.
17. Shafi A, Gallagher P, Stewart N, Martinotti G, Corazza O. The risk of violence associated with novel psychoactive substance misuse in patients presenting to acute mental health services. Hum Psychopharmacol. 2017;32(3) https://doi.org/10.1002/hup.2606.
18. Sanghani SN, Marsh AN, John M, Soman A, Lopez LV, Young YA, et al. Characteristics of patients involved in physical assault in an acute inpatient psychiatric setting. J Psychiatr Pract. 2017;23(4):260–9.
19. Renwick L, Stewart D, Richardson M, Lavelle M, James K, Hardy C, et al. Aggression on inpatient units: clinical characteristics and consequences. Int J Ment Health Nurs. 2016;25(4):308–18.
20. von Elm E, Altman DG, Egger M, Pocock SJ, Gotzsche PC, Vandenbroucke JP. The Strengthening the Reporting of Observational Studies in Epidemiology (STROBE) statement: guidelines for reporting observational studies. Lancet. 2007;370(9596):1453–7.
21. Higgins JP, Thompson SG, Deeks JJ, Altman DG. Measuring inconsistency in meta-analyses. BMJ. 2003;327(7414):557–60.
22. Begg CB, Mazumdar M. Operating characteristics of a rank correlation test for publication bias. Biometrics. 1994;50(4):1088–101.
23. Duval S, Tweedie R. Trim and fill: a simple funnel-plot-based method of testing and adjusting for publication bias in meta-analysis. Biometrics. 2000;56(2):455–63.
24. Gilbody SM, Song F, Eastwood AJ, Sutton A. The causes, consequences and detection of publication bias in psychiatry. Acta Psychiatr Scand. 2000;102(4):241–9.
25. Abderhalden C, Needham I, Dassen T, Halfens R, Haug HJ, Fischer J. Predicting inpatient violence using an extended version of the Broset-Violence-Checklist: instrument development and clinical application. BMC Psychiatry. 2006;6:17.
26. Abderhalden C, Needham I, Dassen T, Halfens R, Haug HJ, Fischer JE. Structured risk assessment and violence in acute psychiatric wards: randomised controlled trial. Br J Psychiatry. 2008;193(1):44–50.
27. Amore M, Menchetti M, Tonti C, Scarlatti F, Lundgren E, Esposito W, et al. Predictors of violent behavior among acute psychiatric patients: clinical study. Psychiatry Clin Neurosci. 2008;62(3):247–55.
28. Ash D, Galletly C, Haynes J, Braben P. Violence, self-harm, victimisation and homelessness in patients admitted to an acute inpatient unit in South Australia. Int J Soc Psychiatry. 2003;49(2):112–8.
29. Barlow K, Grenyer B, Ilkiw-Lavalle O. Prevalence and precipitants of aggression in psychiatric inpatient units. Aust N Z J Psychiatry. 2000;34(6):967–74.
30. Beauford JE, McNiel DE, Binder RL. Utility of the initial therapeutic alliance in evaluating psychiatric patients' risk of violence. Am J Psychiatry. 1997;154(9):1272–6.

31. Biancosino B, Delmonte S, Grassi L, Santone G, Preti A, Miglio R, et al. Violent behavior in acute psychiatric inpatient facilities: a national survey in Italy. J Nerv Ment Dis. 2009;197(10):772–82.
32. Bjorkdahl A, Olsson D, Palmstierna T. Nurses' short-term prediction of violence in acute psychiatric intensive care. Acta Psychiatr Scand. 2006;113(3):224–9.
33. Boggild AK, Heisel MJ, Links PS. Social, demographic, and clinical factors related to disruptive behaviour in hospital. Can J Psychiatry. 2004;49(2):114–8.
34. Bowers L, Simpson A, Alexander J. Patient-staff conflict: results of a survey on acute psychiatric wards. Soc Psychiatry Psychiatr Epidemiol. 2003;38(7):402–8.
35. Carr VJ, Lewin TJ, Sly KA, Conrad AM, Tirupati S, Cohen M, et al. Adverse incidents in acute psychiatric inpatient units: rates, correlates and pressures. Aust N Z J Psychiatry. 2008;42(4):267–82.
36. Cookson A, Daffern M, Foley F. Relationship between aggression, interpersonal style, and therapeutic alliance during short-term psychiatric hospitalization. Int J Ment Health Nurs. 2012;21(1):20–9.
37. Dumais A, Larue C, Michaud C, Goulet MH. Predictive validity and psychiatric nursing staff's perception of the clinical usefulness of the French version of the Dynamic Appraisal of Situational Aggression. Issues Ment Health Nurs. 2012;33(10):670–5.
38. Eaton S, Ghannam M, Hunt N. Prediction of violence on a psychiatric intensive care unit. Med Sci Law. 2000;40(2):143–6.
39. Ehmann TS, Smith GN, Yamamoto A, McCarthy N, Ross D, Au T, et al. Violence in treatment resistant psychotic inpatients. J Nerv Ment Dis. 2001;189(10):716–21.
40. Grassi L, Peron L, Marangoni C, Zanchi P, Vanni A. Characteristics of violent behaviour in acute psychiatric in-patients: a 5-year Italian study. Acta Psychiatr Scand. 2001;104(4):273–9.
41. Hartvig P, Roaldset JO, Moger TA, Ostberg B, Bjorkly S. The first step in the validation of a new screen for violence risk in acute psychiatry: the inpatient context. Eur Psychiatry. 2011;26(2):92–9.
42. Ketelsen R, Staude A, Godejohann F, Driesen M. The advisor team in the psychiatric hospital: assignments and experiences in coping with aggression and compulsion. Psychiatr Prax. 2007;34(6):306–10.
43. Krakowski MI, Czobor P. Psychosocial risk factors associated with suicide attempts and violence among psychiatric inpatients. Psychiatr Serv. 2004;55(12):1414–9.
44. Lam JN, McNiel DE, Binder RL. The relationship between patients' gender and violence leading to staff injuries. Psychiatr Serv. 2000;51(9):1167–70.
45. Mauri MC, Rovera C, Paletta S, De Gaspari IF, Maffini M, Altamura AC. Aggression and psychopharmacological treatments in major psychosis and personality disorders during hospitalisation. Prog Neuropsychopharmacol Biol Psychiatry. 2011;35(7):1631–5.
46. Nijman HL, Merckelbach HL, Allertz WF, à Campo JM. Prevention of aggressive incidents on a closed psychiatric ward. Psychiatr Serv. 1997;48(5):694–8.
47. Nijman H, Merckelbach H, Evers C, Palmstierna T, à Campo J. Prediction of aggression on a locked psychiatric admissions ward. Acta Psychiatr Scand. 2002;105(5):390–5.
48. Oulis P, Lykouras L, Dascalopoulou E, Psarros C. Aggression among psychiatric inpatients in Greece. Psychopathology. 1996;29(3):174–80.
49. Raja M, Azzoni A, Lubich L. Aggressive and violent behavior in a population of psychiatric inpatients. Soc Psychiatry Psychiatr Epidemiol. 1997;32(7):428–34.
50. Raja M, Azzoni A. Hostility and violence of acute psychiatric inpatients. Clin Pract Epidemiol Ment Health. 2005;1:11.
51. Saverimuttu A, Lowe T. Aggressive incidents on a psychiatric intensive care unit. Nurs Stand. 2000;14(35):33–6.
52. Troisi A, Kustermann S, Di Genio M, Siracusano A. Hostility during admission interview as a short-term predictor of aggression in acute psychiatric male inpatients. J Clin Psychiatry. 2003;64(12):1460–4.
53. Cohen DP, Akhtar MS, Siddiqui A, Shelley C, Larkin C, Kinsella A, et al. Aggressive incidents on a psychiatric intensive care unit. Psychiatr Bull. 2008;32:455–8.

54. Daffern MTS, Ferguson M, Podubinski T, Hollander Y, Kulkhani J, et al. The impact of psychiatric symptoms, interpersonal style, and coercion on aggression and self-harm during psychiatric hospitalization. Psychiatry. 2010;73(4):365–81.
55. L. M. Aggression on a psychiatric acute ward: a three-year prospective study. Psychol Rep. 2003;92:1229–48.
56. Owen CTC, Jones M, Tennant C. Violence and aggression in psychiatric units. Psychiatr Serv. 1998;49(11):1452–7.
57. Ross JBL, Stewart D. Conflict and containment events in inpatient psychiatric units. J Clin Nurs. 2012;21:2306–15.
58. Soliman AE, Reza H. Risk factors and correlates of violence among acutely ill adult psychiatric inpatients. Psychiatr Serv. 2001;52(1):75–80.
59. Vaaler AE, Iversen VC, Morken G, Fløvig JC, Palmstierna T, Linaker OM. Short-term prediction of threatening and violent behaviour in an Acute Psychiatric Intensive Care Unit based on patient and environment characteristics. BMC Psychiatry. 2011;11:44.
60. Podubinski TLS, Hollander Y, Daffern M. Patient characteristics associated with aggression in mental health units. Psychiatry Res. 2017;250:141–5.
61. Blomhoff S, Seim S, Friis S. Can prediction of violence among psychiatric inpatients be improved? Hosp Community Psychiatry. 1990;41(7):771–5.

Violence and Mental Disorders in Jails

Ester di Giacomo and Massimo Clerici

Mentally ill patients are entering the criminal justice system at alarming rates, representing a significant percentage of those incarcerated [1]. Persons with mental illness and co-occurring substance-abuse disorders are incarcerated at disproportionately high rates in comparison to the general population [2]. Diagnoses are predominantly in the schizophrenia spectrum with 70% also actively abusing substances at the time of incarceration [3].

Nearly two-thirds (65.0%) of inmates had a DSM-IV Axis I or Axis II disorder. Personality disorders were the most common disorders (51.9%), followed by anxiety (25.3%) and substance-use disorders (24.9%). Over one-third of inmates (36.6%) had comorbid types of disorder. The most common comorbid types of disorders were substance-use disorders plus personality disorders (20.1%) and anxiety disorders plus personality disorders (18.0%) [4, 5].

Generally speaking, those affected by severe mental illness who are incarcerated (I-SMI) have less schooling; they more often reported suicide attempts and violent and nonviolent crimes; and they had a higher level of comorbidity involving Cluster B personality disorders and substance-use disorders [6]. Moreover, they more often suffer victimization within the prison system [7].

Psychiatric illnesses show different connotations among general inpatients, and forensic and incarcerated patients. For example, compared to schizophrenics, forensic schizophrenics are more severely clinically impaired showing higher rates of comorbid alcohol and substance disorder and more suicide attempts, had more previous hospitalizations, and were younger at disease onset [8].

Furthermore, psychiatric pathologies seem to mediate the type of offence. The relevance that the rate of sexual crimes among individuals with schizophrenia is

E. di Giacomo · M. Clerici (✉)
School of Medicine and Surgery, University of Milano Bicocca, Milan, Italy

Psychiatric Department, ASST Monza, Monza, Italy
e-mail: massimo.clerici@unimib.it

relatively low is illustrative. Studies indicate significant differences distinguishing schizophrenia sex offenders from schizophrenia non-sex offenders, the former of whom were more likely to be married, employed, and non-heterosexual (homosexual and bisexual orientations) and demonstrated less hospitalization, antisocial personality, substance abuse, negative symptoms, and overall illness severity [9].

An appropriate psychiatric follow-up seems effective in reducing psychiatric relapses as well as re-incarceration, with a useful integration between pharmacotherapy and psychosocial interventions. In fact, patients whose first service after release from incarceration was outpatient or case management were less likely to receive subsequent emergency services or to be re-incarcerated within 90 days [10].

11.1   Schizophrenia and Other Psychosis

One of the largest systematic reviews about mental health in prisoners, led by Fazel and colleagues [11], documented an average prevalence of psychosis around 4%. Both the genders showed the same value, women with a wider interval of confidence (3–5 vs. 3–4 in men).

Prisoners affected by psychosis are those at higher risk of victimization [7]. Positive psychotic symptoms are the most associated with hostility and violent behaviors, alone or when associated with manic symptoms [12].

Many prisoners may experience first psychotic episode once incarcerated. For those patients, behavior associated with psychotic symptoms may have led to their arrest, but correctional facilities are poorly equipped to identify their needs and to provide the type of comprehensive treatment needed to improve functional status, quality of life, and illness recovery [13].

The prevalence of psychosis among prisoners is higher than that in the general psychiatric population, especially for delusional disorder that shows a prevalence eight times higher than expected in the community [14].

11.2   Dual Diagnosis

Dual diagnosis, a term representing a comorbidity between mental illness and substance abuse, is really frequent among inmates.

Substance and alcohol dependence is high among incarcerates with a general prevalence of about 56% for alcohol dependence, 49% for opiate dependence, and 61% for cocaine dependence [15]. Fazel and colleagues attested a gender-mediated difference in the prevalence of substance abuse, more common in males, and alcohol abuse that has higher prevalence in females.

Dual diagnosis influences both psychiatric and criminal history. In fact, having a substance-use disorder appeared to be the key factor contributing to poorer correctional outcomes for offenders with mental disorders [16].

Furthermore, inmates with dual diagnoses were more likely to be homeless and to be charged with violent crimes than other inmates [17].

An engagement in substance use treatment during incarceration seems a protective factor linked to a reduction of re-incarceration rate in addicted prisoners (OR = .60) [18].

Another aspect to care about is the higher rate of health problems and greater rates of chronic health (HIV, hepatitis, infectious diseases) problems exhibited by drug-involved prisoners compared to prisoners who have not used drugs [19].

Detoxification might be problematic within the prison context—particularly during the first days—and the provision of such treatment services is variable. Alcohol and opiates are the two most common and problematic substances for detoxification management in prisons. A poor offering of such treatment might imply serious adverse outcomes, for example the management of withdrawal. It has been attested that only 34% of US jails offer any detoxification treatment [20], implying that about one million arrestees annually are at risk of untreated withdrawal from alcohol, including delirium tremens and its associated high mortality [21].

Opiate substitution and CBT-based relapse prevention therapies should be made available to all prisoners. Evidence supports their efficacy and long-lasting effects after release.

The management of opiate withdrawal in prison is generally symptomatic, and mostly based on detoxification rather than maintenance. Some systematic reviews [22] confirm the efficacy in reducing withdrawal severity using long-acting opioids [23]. Further evidence highlighted an equivalent clinical effectiveness for detoxification between methadone and buprenorphine (Leeds Evaluation of Efficacy of Detoxification Study—LEEDS). A further study compared dihydrocodeine and buprenorphine demonstrating comparable effectiveness for acute opiate detoxification [24]. On the basis of this evidence, all prisoners should be offered acute detoxification on arrival.

11.3   Personality Disorders

Studies reporting the prevalence of personality disorders among prisoners may face some bias. Large high-quality studies using clinically based diagnoses have reported a prevalence of 7–10% [25–27] compared with 65% found in reviews of studies that have used diagnostic instruments [27]. The discrepancy could be partly explained by the inclusion of antisocial personality disorder, the most common personality disorder in prisoners, for which diagnostic criteria overlap with the reasons for entering prison. Three of these criteria (disregard of norms and rules, low threshold for aggression or violence, and inability to profit from experience) are together highly correlated with criminogenic factors.

Personality disorders belonging to cluster B are, in general, the most represented. Together with antisocial PD, borderline and narcissistic PDs play an important part in composing inmate percentages [28]. Even if they represent a minority among PDs in prisoners, Cluster A PDs are significantly associated with incarceration for violent crimes and prostitution [28].

Borderline PD is more represented in incarcerated women, with a prevalence of slightly more than 10% [29].

A comorbidity between antisocial and borderline PDs is common and complicates the profile. Emotional dysregulation is one of their key features and it is central in driving acts of violence [30, 31].

11.4 Suicide and Attempted Suicide

Suicide and self-harm are more common in prisoners than community-based persons of similar age and gender [11]. The relative risks of suicide in male prisoners are around 3–6 compared to the general population, with a higher risk in women prisoners (relative risk typically more than 6).

Common stressors preceding the suicide were inmate-to-inmate conflict (50%), recent disciplinary action (42%), fear (40%), physical illness (42%), and adverse information (65%) such as loss of good time or disruption of family/friendship relationships in the community. Forty-one percent had received a mental health service within 3 days of the suicide [32]. The highest overall risk was present in those inmates with a non-schizophrenic psychotic disorder (RR = 13.8, CI = 5.8–32.9), but an elevated risk of suicide was also observed among inmates with major depressive disorder (relative risk [RR] = 5.1, 95% confidence interval [CI] = 1.9–13.8), bipolar disorder (RR = 4.6, CI = 1.3–15.9), and schizophrenia (RR = 7.3, CI = 1.7–15.9) [33].

Similarly to difficulties with drug addiction, the risk of suicide is particularly severe in the first days after incarceration, needing timely preventive actions.

11.5 Violence

Violence and aggressions in the prison context are challenging problems. Psychopathy is considered one of the best predictors of violence and prison misconducts and is arguably an important clinical construct in the correctional setting [34]. A previous violent criminal history and callous and antisocial psychopathic traits were predictors of violent misconducts, whereas antisocial psychopathic traits and impulsivity best predicted nonviolent misconducts [34]. Drug abuse is often associated with violent behavior and aggressions for impulse dyscontrol due to drug effects or increased bullying due to drug debts [35].

As reported above, some psychiatric disorders, independently from a dual diagnosis, are more often involved with aggressions.

Emotional dysregulation appears fundamental in understanding such behavior as well as a greater and deserved attention to psychopathy that is better detailed and described in Sect. 11.3 alternative model's trait-based conception of the antisocial PD of the DSM 5 [36–38].

11.6 Historical Hints About the Closure of Italian Forensic and Criminal Hospitals

In 1978, Italy enacted the "Basaglia Law," which closed all the state mental health hospitals and reformed Italian mental health legislation and organization. In 2013, a new law closed all the 6 state hospitals for the criminally insane and substituted them with some "Residenze per l'Esecuzione delle Misure di Sicurezza (REMS-Residential Facilities for the Application of Security Measures)," deeply changing the treatment of psychiatric patients who committed a crime while mentally insane. Unfortunately, the 2013 law drastically reduced the number of beds dedicated to such patients with a gradual setting change characterized by a greater rate of their incarceration. Contemporary, the Ministry of Health allocated health assistance within prisons with the creation of mental health teams from local mental health services and departments. The establishment of those prison mental health teams guarantees care and treatment of the main psychiatric pathologies, dual diagnosis, and an indispensable treatment continuity after inmate release. Efficacy and efficiency of this new system are still under evaluation [39].

References

1. Collins TN, Avondoglio JB, Terry LM. Correctional psychopharmacology: pitfalls, challenges, and victories of prescribing in a correctional setting. Int Rev Psychiatry. 2017;29(1):34–44.
2. Rock M. Emerging issues with mentally ill offenders: causes and social consequences. Adm Policy Ment Health. 2001;28(3):165–80.
3. Munetz MR, Grande TP, Chambers MR. The incarceration of individuals with severe mental disorders. Community Ment Health J. 2001;37(4):361–72.
4. Chen CC, Tsai SY, Su LW, Yang TW, Tsai CJ, Hwu HG. Psychiatric co-morbidity among male heroin addicts: differences between hospital and incarcerated subjects in Taiwan. Addiction. 1999;94(6):825–32.
5. Piselli M, Attademo L, Garinella R, Rella A, Antinarelli S, Tamantini A, et al. Psychiatric needs of male prison inmates in Italy. Int J Law Psychiatry. 2015;41:82–8.
6. Dumais A, Cote G, Larue C, Goulet MH, Pelletier JF. Clinical characteristics and service use of incarcerated males with severe mental disorders: a comparative case-control study with patients found not criminally responsible. Issues Ment Health Nurs. 2014;35(8):597–603.
7. Daquin JC, Daigle LE. Mental disorder and victimisation in prison: examining the role of mental health treatment. Crim Behav Ment Health. 2018;28(2):141–51.
8. Landgraf S, Blumenauer K, Osterheider M, Eisenbarth H. A clinical and demographic comparison between a forensic and a general sample of female patients with schizophrenia. Psychiatry Res. 2013;210(3):1176–83.
9. Alish Y, Birger M, Manor N, Kertzman S, Zerzion M, Kotler M, et al. Schizophrenia sex offenders: a clinical and epidemiological comparison study. Int J Law Psychiatry. 2007;30(6):459–66.
10. Hawthorne WB, Folsom DP, Sommerfeld DH, Lanouette NM, Lewis M, Aarons GA, et al. Incarceration among adults who are in the public mental health system: rates, risk factors, and short-term outcomes. Psychiatr Serv. 2012;63(1):26–32.
11. Fazel S, Hayes AJ, Bartellas K, Clerici M, Trestman R. Mental health of prisoners: prevalence, adverse outcomes, and interventions. Lancet Psychiatry. 2016;3(9):871–81.

12. van Beek J, Vuijk PJ, Harte JM, Scherder EJA. Symptom profile of psychiatric patients with psychosis or psychotic mood disorder in prison. Int J Offender Ther Comp Criminol. 2018;62(13):4158–73.
13. Ford E. First-episode psychosis in the criminal justice system: identifying a critical intercept for early intervention. Harv Rev Psychiatry. 2015;23(3):167–75.
14. Tamburello AC, Bajgier J, Reeves R. The prevalence of delusional disorder in prison. J Am Acad Psychiatry Law. 2015;43(1):82–6.
15. Lewis CF. Substance use and violent behavior in women with antisocial personality disorder. Behav Sci Law. 2011;29(5):667–76.
16. Wilton G, Stewart LA. Outcomes of offenders with co-occurring substance use disorders and mental disorders. Psychiatr Serv. 2017;68(7):704–9.
17. McNiel DE, Binder RL, Robinson JC. Incarceration associated with homelessness, mental disorder, and co-occurring substance abuse. Psychiatr Serv. 2005;56(7):840–6.
18. Luciano A, Belstock J, Malmberg P, McHugo GJ, Drake RE, Xie H, et al. Predictors of incarceration among urban adults with co-occurring severe mental illness and a substance use disorder. Psychiatr Serv. 2014;65(11):1325–31.
19. Leukefeld CG, Staton M, Hiller ML, Logan TK, Warner B, Shaw K, et al. A descriptive profile of health problems, health services utilization, and HIV serostatus among incarcerated male drug abusers. J Behav Health Serv Res. 2002;29(2):167–75.
20. Oser CB, Knudsen HK, Staton-Tindall M, Taxman F, Leukefeld C. Organizational-level correlates of the provision of detoxification services and medication-based treatments for substance abuse in correctional institutions. Drug Alcohol Depend. 2009;103(Suppl 1):S73–81.
21. Hasin DS, Stinson FS, Ogburn E, Grant BF. Prevalence, correlates, disability, and comorbidity of DSM-IV alcohol abuse and dependence in the United States: results from the National Epidemiologic Survey on Alcohol and Related Conditions. Arch Gen Psychiatry. 2007;64(7):830–42.
22. Duthe G, Hazard A, Kensey A, Shon JL. Suicide among male prisoners in France: a prospective population-based study. Forensic Sci Int. 2013;233(1-3):273–7.
23. Amato L, Davoli M, Minozzi S, Ferroni E, Ali R, Ferri M. Methadone at tapered doses for the management of opioid withdrawal. Cochrane Database Syst Rev. 2013;(2):Cd003409. https://doi.org/10.1002/14651858.
24. Sheard L, Wright NM, El-Sayeh HG, Adams CE, Li R, Tompkins CN. The Leeds Evaluation of Efficacy of Detoxification Study (LEEDS) prisons project: a randomised controlled trial comparing dihydrocodeine and buprenorphine for opiate detoxification. Subst Abuse Treat Prev Policy. 2009;4:1.
25. Gunn J, Maden A, Swinton M. Treatment needs of prisoners with psychiatric disorders. BMJ. 1991;303(6798):338–41.
26. Birmingham L, Mason D, Grubin D. Prevalence of mental disorder in remand prisoners: consecutive case study. BMJ. 1996;313(7071):1521–4.
27. Fazel S, Danesh J. Serious mental disorder in 23000 prisoners: a systematic review of 62 surveys. Lancet. 2002;359(9306):545–50.
28. Warren JI, Burnette M, South SC, Chauhan P, Bale R, Friend R. Personality disorders and violence among female prison inmates. J Am Acad Psychiatry Law. 2002;30(4):502–9.
29. Zhu XM, Zhou JS, Chen C, Peng WL, Li W, Ungvari GS, et al. Prevalence of borderline personality disorder and its risk factors in female prison inmates in China. Psychiatry Res. 2017;250:200–3.
30. Falcus C, Johnson D. The violent accounts of men diagnosed with comorbid antisocial and borderline personality disorders. Int J Offender Ther Comp Criminol. 2018;62(9):2817–30.
31. Moore KE, Gobin RL, McCauley HL, Kao CW, Anthony SM, Kubiak S, et al. The relation of borderline personality disorder to aggression, victimization, and institutional misconduct among prisoners. Compr Psychiatry. 2018;84:15–21.
32. Way BB, Miraglia R, Sawyer DA, Beer R, Eddy J. Factors related to suicide in New York state prisons. Int J Law Psychiatry. 2005;28(3):207–21.

33. Baillargeon J, Penn JV, Thomas CR, Temple JR, Baillargeon G, Murray OJ. Psychiatric disorders and suicide in the nation's largest state prison system. J Am Acad Psychiatry Law. 2009;37(2):188–93.
34. Thomson ND, Towl GJ, Centifanti LC. The habitual female offender inside: How psychopathic traits predict chronic prison violence. Law Hum Behav. 2016;40(3):257–69.
35. di Giacomo E, Clerici M. Psychiatric illness in incarcerated population. Rassegna Italiana di Criminologia. 2018;3:225–30.
36. Wygant DB, Sellbom M, Sleep CE, Wall TD, Applegate KC, Krueger RF, et al. Examining the DSM-5 alternative personality disorder model operationalization of antisocial personality disorder and psychopathy in a male correctional sample. Personal Disord. 2016;7(3):229–39.
37. APA. Diagnostic and statistical manual of mental disorders. 5th ed. Washington, DC: American Psychiatric Association; 2013.
38. di Giacomo E, Aspesi F, Colmegna F, Clerici M. Narcissistic Personality Disorder: clinical challenges and burden, diagnostic improvement and need of in-depth research (under review).
39. Bani M, Travagin G, Monticelli M, Valsecchi M, Truisi E, Zorzi F, et al. Pattern of self-injurious behavior and suicide attempts in Italian custodial inmates: a cluster analysis approach. Int J Law Psychiatry. 2019;64:1–7.

Violent Behavior in Forensic Residential Facilities: The Italian Experience After the Closure of Forensic Psychiatric Hospitals

12

Enrico Zanalda, David De Cori, Grazia Ala, Alessandro Jaretti Sodano, and Marco Zuffranieri

12.1 Introduction

The final closing of forensic psychiatric hospitals (Ospedali Psichiatrici Giudiziari—OPG) in Italy and the transitioning to the new model of care, the psychiatric residential community, were completed in January, 2017, more than 40 years after the passage of the Basaglia Law. To substitute some of the OPG's functions, the majority of Italian regions built secure, residential units, which we will refer to as REMS [1, 2] (*Residenze per l'Esecuzione delle Misure di Sicurezza*—Residences for the Execution of Security Measures). Italy is the first and perhaps the only country in the world to have embraced the principals of deinstitutionalization to the point where the hospital-based model of forensic mental care was replaced by residential units, staffed only by healthcare personnel [3]. However, the reform cannot be considered complete without a total revision of the penal code and a new model for the treatment of people detained in prisons.

Globally, approximately 10 million people are confined to prison at any given time. Possibly 30 million more are in and out each year. Research has demonstrated that psychiatric disorders are very common among inmates. In many countries, there is a higher percentage of people with severe mental illness in prisons than in psychiatric hospitals. And yet, these serious mental disorders are often incorrectly diagnosed and

E. Zanalda (✉) · D. De Cori · M. Zuffranieri
Dipartimento Interaziendale di Salute Mentale ASL TO3 & AOU San Luigi Gonzaga, Collegno, TO, Italy
e-mail: ezanalda@aslto3.piemonte.it; ddecori@aslto3.piemonte.it; mzuffranieri@aslto3.piemonte.it

G. Ala
REMS San Michele, Bra, CN, Italy

A. J. Sodano
REMS Anton Martin, Fatebenefratelli Hospital, San Maurizio Canavese, TO, Italy
e-mail: jarettisodano@fatebenefratelli.eu

© Springer Nature Switzerland AG 2020   211
B. Carpiniello et al. (eds.), *Violence and Mental Disorders*, Comprehensive Approach to Psychiatry 1, https://doi.org/10.1007/978-3-030-33188-7_12

treated. A recent study [4] provides an overview of the incidence of psychiatric disorders in penal institutions, and analyzes the data on rates of suicide and violence victimization and the risk factors that these conditions generate. It also outlines evidence-based programs for mental health treatment. Using this study as a basis, the authors offer an analysis of behavior in people with mental illnesses in Italy, where psychiatric hospitals were closed 40 years ago and where there have been no forensic psychiatric hospitals since 2017. The experiences of inmates detained in prison and inpatients in REMS will be based on data from the Piedmont region.

12.2   Prevalence

There are many studies and reviews that document an elevated prevalence of psychiatric disorders in inmates. Careful scrutiny is needed to interpret these data because certain disorders can be overestimated, as in the case of ADHD. One systematic review stated that 26% of all prisoners were diagnosed with ADHD [4]. This contradicts two high-quality studies, carried out recently, that report prevalence rates of 17% and 11%, respectively.

Prevalence of personality disorders is also easily misinterpreted. Broad, precision studies using clinically based diagnoses have observed prevalence between 7% and 10%, while other studies reported a prevalence as high as 65% [4]. This discrepancy may be partially influenced by the inclusion of the antisocial personality disorder, the most widespread personality disorder among prisoners. In fact, diagnostic criteria of this disorder coincide with the causes for imprisonment at the outset. Some features of this disorder (for example, disregard for rules and regulations, a low threshold for aggressive or violent behavior, and an inability to learn from experience) are all strongly related to criminogenic factors. Despite this, many prevalence results are consistent. The most outstanding of these are depression and psychotic illnesses.

Another very important theme is the elevated prevalence of substance misuse. Recent findings have demonstrated high rates of comorbidity between mental illness and substance abuse [5]. To be noted, this comorbidity has a negative effect on the prognosis of individual psychiatric disorders and it is proven to increase the possibility of repeated offending as well as premature mortality.

Below, we will review adverse outcomes that are associated with psychiatric disorders.

12.3   Suicide and Self-Harm

Little attention has been paid to suicide events in prisons and in forensic psychiatric hospitals, on a national as well as international level. In these two high-risk areas, prisons and hospitals, a retrospective study was conducted in state institutions to monitor completed suicide attempts over a 5-year period from 2000 to 2004 [6]. The study concludes that the difference between the average suicide rate in forensic psychiatric hospitals and in the prison system was statistically comparable. Usually the difference between patients who committed suicide in a forensic psychiatric hospital and those who committed suicide in prison was the following: inpatients in psychiatric hospitals more commonly committed violent offenses and had a record of suicide attempts. To be noted, the length of time that passed between entering the institution and the suicide attempt was markedly shorter in the prison group than in the hospital group. Finally, younger inmates in both facilities committed suicide sooner after admission [6].

An observational study was carried out in Italy to monitor the rate of suicides and attempted suicides, based on gender, age, place of birth, and security level in northeastern Italian prisons from 2010 to 2016. The study also investigated the effects of overcrowding, the kind of offenses committed, and previous attempts at self-inflicted injuries and suicide. More than 90% of suicides and attempted suicides were committed by men between the ages of 21 and 49 years. Most of these men had previously perpetrated violent offenses. It should be noted that 14% of suicides and 19% of attempted suicides had a record of self-inflicted injury and attempts to commit suicide. The predictors for suicidal behavior were male, on average, 30 years of age [7].

12.4   Violence

Other events that occur in a prison as a result of psychiatric disorders are violence and victimization. Violence is very common in prison but little is known about its prevalence. Studies have been made that show physical assault to be 13–27 times higher in correctional institutions than it is in the population at large [8, 9]. Prisoner-to-prisoner, nonfatal physical aggression is the most common brand of violence in prison; unfortunately, homicides also occur [8].

A broad meta-analysis of 90 studies revealed that strong predictors of violations fall into four categories: (1) higher levels of gang involvement, (2) higher numbers of inmates in the institution, (3) a higher security level in the institution, and (4) higher proportion of high-security inmates. The most pronounced sociodemographic predictor of prison misconduct was youth. On the other hand, being black, being single, and a low level of education were less significant as predictors. Regarding criminal characteristics, the existence of prior offenses was the strongest predictor; while conviction for a violent offense was not considered a notable predictor [10]. Deviant behavior at an early age (i.e., a longer criminal record, arrest at a younger age, and prior imprisonment) has also been linked to problems of management during incarceration. Lastly, infractions in penal institutions can also be strongly predicted by clinical variables such as aggressiveness, impulsivity, antisocial behavior, and psychopathy [11, 12].

Mental disorders raised the risks of physical victimization. Imprisoned males with mental disorders were more vulnerable to physical victimization: 1.6 times higher (prisoner-on-prisoner) and 1.2 times higher (staff-on-prisoner) than prisoners without mental disorders. Female inmates with mental disorders reported physical victimization by other prisoners 1.7 times more than their fellow inmates who did not have mental disorders [9].

Moreover, a disorder of considerable prevalence, often underestimated, is posttraumatic stress disorder (PTSD). People caught in the cogs of the criminal justice system are frequently subjected to violent and traumatic experiences. These experiences can spark PTSD in prisoners.

A very recent systematic review and meta-analysis, the first to date, tried to gauge the prevalence of PTSD in prisoners. The study monitored 21,099 incarcerated men and women in 20 countries. The point prevalence of PTSD was revealed as follows: 0.1–27% for men, and 12–38% for women. Female prisoners demonstrated a higher prevalence of PTSD; currently high levels of PTSD are shown in the prison population, more commonly in women [13].

12.5   Substance-Use Disorders

A very recent study [14] evaluated the connection between substance abuse and category of crimes committed by prisoners with substance-use problems; more specifically, the study questions whether substance-use habits vary in prisoners who have committed violent crimes.

The use of illegal drugs and homelessness had a lower prevalence in violent offenders; but binge drinking and use of sedatives had a higher prevalence, more than patients who were sentenced for drug crimes. Patients who had committed violent crimes had lower prevalence of injected drug use. Instead, binge drinking and use of sedatives were positively associated with violent crime. However, use of heroin, cocaine, amphetamines, and injected drugs was negatively associated with violent crime. Within the group of violent offenders, fatal violence was linked to sedatives; instead homelessness, age, and use of amphetamines and heroin were negatively linked to fatal violence.

Finally, in this sampling of inmates who suffer from substance-use disorders, it was shown that the violent perpetrators' use of conventional, illegal drugs may be less common than in patients sentenced for other criminal violations. In contrast, these same violent perpetrators were found to manifest a more prevalent consumption of sedatives and alcohol in excess. In the subgroup of violent perpetrators with problems of substance abuse, sedatives are positively connected, while illegal drugs are negatively connected, to fatal violence [14].

Another recent review study [15] estimated the prevalence of alcohol- and drug-abuse disorders in the prison population. The study included 18,388 prisoners in 10 countries. It was estimated that the prevalence of alcohol abuse was 24%. In males the percentages ran from 16% to 51% and in females from 10% to 30%. There was evidence of heterogeneity by sex for drug-use disorders: in particular, in male prisoners it averaged 30% (range 10–61%) and in female prisoners 51% (range 30–69%).

In conclusion, disorders caused by substance use are highly prevalent in the prison population. Roughly 25% of newly incarcerated males and females manifested an alcohol-abuse disorder; the presence of a drug-use disorder was shown to be at least as high in men and yet higher in women [15].

12.6 Three Aspects of Security

Physical security: This includes all facets of the physical environment, from architectural considerations for safety and security (i.e., walls, safety windows) to locks, alarm systems, etc.

Relational security: It considers the quality of the human component, i.e., the patient-professional relationship, familiarity with the patients' histories, and level of general knowledge of the forensic patient population. Relational security seems to be, above all else, the most important factor in delivering a safe and secure setting for therapeutic treatment and for insuring the patients' therapeutic progress. It should be noted that the quality of the physical environment significantly affects the quality of relational security.

Procedural security: This focuses on policies and procedures put in place to guarantee safety and security, e.g., search protocols and surveillance of prohibited objects [16].

Forensic psychiatric hospitals, which must necessarily provide a secure physical as well as a safe therapeutic environment, are of high cost as they implement state-of-the-art features of medical architecture. Even though the evidence base within forensic psychiatry remains sketchy regarding many areas of intervention, these hospitals are nonetheless able to provide solid, specialized treatment to offenders with mental disorders and to others with similar profiles, insuring medical care and lowering the risk of re-offending [15, 17].

More research is needed on an international level, and more interaction between clinicians, scientists, architects, legislators, and medical/legal representatives to continue to improve the quality of institutions and services.

12.7 The Italian Situation

On March 31, 2015, in accordance with Law 81/2014, Italy made a historical step to close the existing forensic psychiatric hospitals (Ospedali Psichiatrici Giudiziari—OPG). This law delineated a new roadmap for care that provided small-scale, therapy-intense facilities called REMS to replace the old forensic psychiatric hospitals [18, 19]. The law promotes innovative, recovery-oriented, rehabilitative treatment for people with mental disorders who have committed a criminal offense, without criminal intention, but who are, nonetheless, regarded as socially dangerous.

Moreover, an important innovation was in the shifting of responsibility and pathway management from the Ministry of Justice to the Ministry of Health. This shift brought to light the contradictions, previously obscured, on which the Supreme Court (section I, Sentence of 30/01/81) and the Constitutional Court (Sentence 253/2003 and 367/2004) had passed judgment in order to avoid automatic hospitalization in OPGs for patients considered socially dangerous.

It is important to remember that the OPGs were untouched through numerous reforms:

- The laws 180 and 833 of 1978.
- "Project Objective Protection of Mental Health 1994–1996" and "1998–2000").
- "Reform of Penitentiary Medicine," article 5 of Law of 30 November 1998, n.419.
- D.P.R. n. 230/00 ("Regulations of the statutes of penitentiary bylaws on measures used to limit and restrict freedom") in which it was established that, while the OPG still remained under the jurisdiction of the Penitentiary Administration, the care of the inmates was increasingly more important than their confinement.

In any case, following the closing of civil psychiatric asylums, the OPG often became the receptacle of all problematic and difficult-to-manage individuals [20]. Today, with the closing of the OPGs, it is possible to hypothesize that the role once filled by the OPG has gone back to the prisons which, with no change in the penal code, is once again leaning on the National Health System, also for the purpose of relocating certain inmates (Sentence of the Constitutional Court n. 99/2019). In this regard, it must be noted that the condition of patients who pose a danger to society, not attributable to mental disorders, was not modified. It is perhaps because this does not have direct consequences on the reduction of inmates in penal institutions, becoming in some way an obstruction for the concession of benefits outside the prison walls.

The Italian Penal Code provides a mediation between the classical and positivistic approaches by the creation of what is called the "dual track" (doppio binario) [21], under which offenders who were judged capable of free will would be directed to the penal track (i.e., trial, sentence, imprisonment); offenders who were mentally incapacitated and considered a danger to society would be admitted to the forensic psychiatric hospital track [22].

Therefore, the reform provides the closing of the judicial version of the facility where security detention measures were in place, whereas for the cases that did not require detention, the National Health System was already operative, in accordance with the Sentence of the Constitutional Court n. 253/2003. This subdivision created by the dual track does not have clinical effectiveness and remains unchanged, even though the enforcement of security measures is now the responsibility of the National Health System.

In particular, the aftermath of the dual track is that psychiatric care cannot be provided to patients in prison who are "not guilty for reasons of insanity." This mandatory situation is an obstacle to the creation of a psychiatric care unit in the prisons. In this manner, the National Health System is compelled to guarantee care and assistance to sentenced individuals even when the correctional aspect is greater than the therapeutic one.

The Italian Supreme Court (SSUU 9163/2005) extended the insanity claim to severe personality-disordered defendants, determining an overlapping of two groups: inmates with psychiatric diagnoses and mentally ill patients who committed crimes. As long as detention institutions, prisons and forensic psychiatric hospitals both were under the auspices of the Department of Penitentiary Administration (DAP); the governance was assigned to the penal system; the health services were then involved only marginally in the program of treatment. After the reform, the health system was called into action and had to accept the artificial subdivision. This led to the present contradictory situation.

More complications were determined by the reform of Title V of the Constitution, in 2001, which assigned the organization of health services to the regions of Italy [23]. In this manner, the responsibility went from the national DAP to 20 different regional health authorities. In 2015, a joint decree from the Ministries of Health and Justice defined the organizational and structural characteristics of the "Residences for the Execution of Security Measures" (REMS). According to Law 81/2014, only a limited number of patients who committed crimes could be treated in a REMS, and only when it was not possible to treat them in any other local facility. The REMS are healthcare structures, built by the regions with a number of beds proportionate to the local resident population but markedly inferior to the number of beds in the old OPGs, because they were not considered a substitute for them. The REMS are structures that must guarantee admission to patients who are not yet able to be discharged into society, referring to people who have already been sentenced and are in the custody of local services. Unfortunately, they were also used not only as places to enforce detention security measures but also to enforce cautionary detention measures.

Each REMS is a healthcare structure with a maximum of 20 beds; it can be either public or private and, in either case, is managed by the regional healthcare system. Its location is decided by the Commission for Public Safety and its structural requisites must be approved by the Penitentiary Administration. It is also necessary to follow the protocols of intervention with law enforcement officials and with the competent surveillance courts. The director of the REMS is a medical doctor and it is responsible for the health of the patients within the structure. Fortunately, he/she will not accept any patients over the number of available beds. This *proviso* is very different from OPGs and their satellite structures that were often overcrowded. The decision on the part of the directors, to consider the REMS as places of treatment, was the object of bitter controversy with some judges, who could not conceive of a refusal of entry.

The way in which the process of closing the OPGs was initiated was often ideological, reiterating some themes that had previously emerged at the time when civil psychiatric asylums were closed (confusion between the effects of serious psychoses and institutionalization) [20]. The topic of violence was neglected, minimizing the need to verify episodes of violence within the healthcare structure. In the debate, more attention was paid to violence done to the patients by the institution than to violent outbursts perpetrated by the patients themselves. The violent behavior of the inmates was often attributed to hostile living conditions in the OPG [24]. This translated into inefficient planning that concentrated solely on the number of beds guaranteed in the REMS by the regions. "This is particularly serious since Staff assaults also have implications for prisoners and patients as client care is dependent on a physically, psychologically and emotionally fit staff" [25]. "Violence can also pose a significant barrier to discharge into the community and can result in periods of longer incarceration. Research indicates that it can take several months for nursing staff to recover emotionally from an assault" [26].

The peculiarities regarding the management of problematic patients, with a high potential for antisocial behavior, were never sufficiently examined, limiting their analysis to how many, among the patients in the OPG, were considered unfit for discharge, as if this subgroup was left over and would eventually disappear, a product of the past organization rather than a category that would present itself in new cases in the new facilities.

On the whole, we could say that the challenge was met [27], but not without consequences. It must be decided whether these consequences, that impact patients, staff, and regional health service system, were handled in the most effective way.

Presumably, in the past, the level of security that characterized treatment of patients responsible for crimes in the OPG must have been, on an average, higher than necessary. In fact, the treatments, at least in the Piedmont region, were managed in structures with a lower level of security on a physical and procedural level and many people on the waiting list for the REMS were managed in their homes without significant problems. On this front, one might say that the reform offers the possibility to develop guidelines to "provide psychiatric care in the *least restrictive* setting or manner" [28]. In Italy, this procedure, unlike other countries, was never formally established. It would seem that the judicial system is waiting for a sign from the healthcare system regarding these guidelines in order to arrive at an empirical definition of this concept [29]. The reason for excessive restriction, in the past, can probably be found in the ample heterogeneity of inmates subject to confinement. In fact, the present code establishes that security measures are not only intended for people deemed socially dangerous due to mental illness. The characteristics to be considered dangerous are more related to the possibility of recurrence of the crime rather than its violence. In this situation, a patient who never committed a violent crime but has a high probability to repeat similar nonviolent crimes is also considered socially dangerous. The discriminating factor, therefore, is not the type of crime or the seriousness of its consequences; it is the probability of recurrence. It should not be surprising that the danger posed by some individuals can be contained in situations even less restrictive than a REMS.

To our knowledge only two studies have analyzed the problem in an empirical fashion in Italy [30, 31]. The purpose of the first study is to describe the progressive process of surpassing the forensic hospitals in Italy (OPGs) and to identify the necessary care and rehabilitation pathways in this process, in the experience of the community health service in Salerno, Italy. The authors made an analysis of the recent laws related to the ongoing process and an analysis of epidemiological and structural data referring to the period between 2010 and 2017 concerning the OPGs/ Residential Services for the Execution of Security Measures (REMS)/mental health system in Campania, Italy, and in the territory of Salerno. The authors show that a thorough restructuring of the National Health Service is required. A substantial path in Campania has been completed, with the closure of OPGs, and the realization of definitive REMS, the Departments for Mental Health Care in prison, the Regional Technical Group, and the territorial services to replace the OPGs. The result of these transformations is a profound change in the healthcare approach, as evidenced by current ongoing changes in indicative parameters of care pathways and their outcomes. In conclusion, this new approach highlights both improvement features and totally or partially unaddressed problematic features. As for actual management issues, communication between mental healthcare services and the judicial system has been improved. The overall evaluation of the transformations in progress is positive [30].

Another Italian study [31] proposes to compare sociodemographic clinical and treatment-related characteristics of long-term patients (139 in the study) who have a long record of serious, violent behavior with controls. The purpose is to identify the predictors of verbal as well as physical aggressiveness in the span of a 1-year follow-up, in a prospective cohort study, during which time the patients are living in residential facilities. The authors concluded that, if treatment and clinical supervision are provided, patients with a long history of violence, living in residential facilities, do not manifest higher levels of aggressiveness than patients with no significant record of violent behavior. Given that verbal aggression is linked to more aggravated forms of aggression, rapid intervention is advisable to reduce the risks of escalation [31].

12.8   Definitive Closure of Forensic Psychiatric Hospitals (OPG) and Activation of Community Treatment of Forensic Patients in Piedmont

In the Piedmont region, two REMS are in operation: "Anton Martin" in San Maurizio Canavese (TO) with 20 beds, an average of 2 reserved for women, and "San Michele" in Bra (CN) with 18 beds, all reserved for men.

The project in the Piedmont region, the closing of the OPG and taking responsibility for psychiatric patients guilty of crimes, has assigned a highly relevant role to the healthcare agencies, requiring their directors to nominate a representative to the psychiatric forensic unit (UPF). These UPF agencies employ a variety of professionals and should be made up of representatives of local services (addiction services, child and adolescent neuropsychiatry, assistance for the elderly and disabled) which, in the Piedmont region, are not part of the mental health department. The representatives of the UPF agencies convene monthly with regional representatives, the directors of the REMS, and the Head of Services of Psychiatric Observation of the Region located at the detention center in Torino.

In this way, we tried to keep the various components of the network of treatment in close contact, to facilitate the implementation of local assistance and treatment for the benefit of patients who committed crimes. In the case of persons incarcerated with measures of security, the UPF agencies work alongside the teams in the REMS to organize projects that favor discharge and follow-up assistance on a local level.

The focal point is to stimulate timely, responsible assistance for the patient by specialized local services, even in cases of patients scheduled to enter the REMS, but who have not yet been admitted, with the hope of revealing possible incongruities. Also important is the collaboration with the judges' psychiatric consultants, who should be informed of the possibility of treatment outside the REMS, in cases that pose a lower level of danger to society. The function of the regional network, therefore, is to monitor the waiting list for entrance into REMS, singling out the high-priority cases and suggesting alternative treatment where possible.

This network operates in the area that the legal system and the participation of a large number of magistrates leave open to the discretion of the clinicians, but the results obtained, while promising, are stunted, as already described, by the inadequacy of the reform, particularly where norms and funding are concerned.

12.9 Aim of the Study

This chapter has the objective to present a retroactive study on the episodes of violence in the two REMS in Piedmont region during the year 2018.

12.10 Materials and Methods

The retrospective study was conducted by analyzing the episodes of violence reported in the clinical files of patients hospitalized in the two REMS in Piedmont from January to December 2018, using a validated scale to gauge violent acts: to this end, the Modified Overt Aggression Scale (MOAS) was used [32].

This scale has been designed, tested, and used in numerous studies to measure acts of violence and in the current study we propose to measure the following areas:

- Verbal aggression
- Aggression against property
- Aggression against self
- Physical aggression

In addition, sociodemographic data was analyzed and also the average time of hospital stays in the two REMS in Piedmont, Anton Martin in San Maurizio

Canavese (TO) with 20 beds, 2 of which are for women, and San Michele in Bra (CN) with 18 beds for men only.

The prospective study, still being conducted, also uses the MOAS scale, gauging the acts of violence verified in the two REMS in Piedmont region. At present, data is available for the first 3 months of observation, February–April 2019.

12.11   Results

Overall, during the course of 2018, in the two REMS 70 treatments were managed for patients, who had committed crimes, respectively, 34 in the REMS "Anton Martin" and 36 in the REMS "San Michele." The sociodemographic and clinical diagnosis of patients are presented in Table 12.1.

(a) REMS "Anton Martin": In the course of the year 2018, there were 34 programs for treatment that had an average hospitalization time of 358 days (±204.64 SD); the episodes of violence measured on the MOAS scale for the year 2018 in the course of 34 projects of treatment are shown in Table 12.2.

(b) REMS "San Michele": In the course of the year 2018, 36 projects of treatment were managed and had an average hospitalization time of 201 days. The episodes of violence registered on the MOAS scale for the year 2018 during the execution of the 36 projects of treatment are represented in Table 12.2.

Table 12.1 Demographic and clinical characteristics

	Anton Martin		San Michele	
	N	(%)	N	(%)
Males	32	(94.1)	24	(100)
Age (Mean ± st.dev)	42.47	±13.5	37.63	±11.3
Marital status				
Unmarried	25	(73.5)	23	(95.8)
Divorced	4	(11.8)	1	(4.2)
Married	2	(5.9)	–	
Widow/er	3	(8.8)	–	
Diagnosis				
Personality disorders	13	(38.2)	16	(66.7)
Psychosis[a]	23	(64.7)	13	(54.2)
Bipolar disorders	2	(5.9)	–	
Intellectual disabilities[b]	3	(8.8)	7	(29.2)
Substance-use disorders[b]	7	(20.6)	6	(25.0)

[a]Includes schizophrenia, psychosis not otherwise specified, and delusional disorder
[b]Always in comorbidity

Table 12.2 Episodes of violence according to MOAS scale

	Anton Martin		San Michele	
	N	(% of projects)	N	(% of projects)
Episodes of violence				
Against objects	6	(17.6)	7	(29.2)
Against other patients	11	(32.4)	3	(12.5)
Against staff	4	(11.8)	–	
Suicide attempts	1	(2.9)	–	
Suicides	–		–	
Self-inflicted injuries	–		–	
Projects 2018	34	(100)	24	(100)

12.12 Discussion

Among the final objectives of the REMS are both cure of the pathology of the patients and control of their violent behavior; both can be treated in an environment that guarantees the safety of the hospitalized patients and the staff. Even though security is not the primary objective of healthcare activity, in these structures it is an absolutely necessary factor in daily procedures.

The staff in the REMS guarantees that the patients are assisted as medical patients. This assistance encompasses professional experience and a code of professional ethics, as well as the application of pre-established operational protocols. Control and safety are intended as protection for the patient and are requisites for the rehabilitation process. One of the safety indicators is bound to the professionalism of the staff, who are specifically schooled and trained. In any case, only with direct experience can the staff acquire the serenity needed to handle the more complex cases. Unfortunately, in the course of the year 2017, the turnover of healthcare staff was significantly influenced by five incidents in the workplace that resulted in injuries with prognoses of over 30 days. In 2018, thanks to the security measures put in place and with greater experience, the aggressions against personnel diminished and there were no significant injuries on the job. After each injury a clinical audit is performed and the people involved analyze the possibility of a miscalculation of the risks that may have contributed to the episode. For example, it emerged that verbal aggression is a very important prelude to physical aggression by the patients.

In the study, it emerged that verbal aggression is very frequent and is managed quickly with an interpersonal approach to avoid possible aggressive behavior of a nonverbal nature. However, aggression is not always preceded by a warning posturing or behavior of the patients that can be easily interpreted by the staff. Especially in the early stages, when patients are new to the community and find themselves confronted with the rules of the REMS and with problems of "fitting in," they can demonstrate unexpected aggression. The low tolerance for frustration, psychopathological problems (often accompanied by low intellect), and angry outbursts often decline into passive-aggressive behavior, in provocative, argumentative, or polemic posturing. More frequently, however, they manifest themselves in sudden outbursts of anger with swearing, insults, and, at times, explicit threats.

The circumstances that most often unleash aggressive behavior in the patients regard the difficulty of adapting to the rules of the structure and the absence of a course of treatment for the rehabilitation process for the period following their stay in the REMS. Often the patient shows little self-criticism regarding the crime committed and intolerance of the judicial restrictions imposed. The rules of the REMS presented to the patients aim to establish a therapeutic and rehabilitative roadmap, to recuperate the patients' self-awareness and improve their interpersonal and social skills.

The rehabilitation treatments are personalized, based on the observation of the capabilities of each subject, and carried out by a multidisciplinary team. The activities that appear most appropriate are first discussed by the team and then with the patients themselves. The patients are stimulated periodically to review their participation in activities, their skill in interpersonal relations, and their behavior with other patients and staff. This is also done to prevent antagonistic situations from which episodes of violence can develop. A solid knowledge of the patients' problems on the part of the staff can help to prevent and manage hostile behavior when it appears. The therapeutic program and rehabilitation program also aim to improve the capability of the patients to manage their own anger when it arises.

Much of the staff's activity is dedicated not only to the observation of the single patient but also to the dynamics of the group, with the purpose of monitoring the interpersonal environment and to prevent, as far as is possible, aggressive outbursts, either verbal or behavioral. For example, in 2018, cases of aggressive episodes among inpatients involved 32%. The constant interaction of patients in a restricted communal environment offers an elevated number of occasions for contrast on a daily basis.

From our observations, aggressive behavior, especially of a physical nature, is mostly initiated by a limited group of patients who are difficult to manage. These are the so-called "difficult patients": they are often people with psychopathic criminal connotations (antisocial personality disorder), often with low intelligence levels and a history of substance abuse. They also manifest the absence of awareness of their sickness and the absence of compliance to pharmaceutical treatment, combined with a low response to pharmaceuticals, which are only administered to reduce impulsivity. Uncontrolled behavior, in fact, is generally impulsive and short-circuited and therefore unexpected. Or better said, it is expected that "difficult patients" will demonstrate uncontrolled behavior but it is impossible to predict when that will happen.

When they demonstrate a superficial adhesion to the treatment program, with a relative improvement in behavior, an insignificant daily occurrence could ignite an impulsive act of violence which was not predictable until that moment. This type of patient is the most difficult to treat and to live with. Underestimating this small group of "difficult patients," their defiance, and their possible aggressive behavior could put the positive outcome of the entire project of the REMS at serious risk. And in a larger sense, it could compromise the model for communal treatment of patients who have committed crimes. The presence of these "difficult patients" in the REMS creates significant organizational problems that seriously impact the rehabilitation programs of their fellow patients. The "difficult patients" who cannot take advantage of the therapeutic care offered in the REMS, because of their antisocial or criminal behavior, sap the energy and the resources of the staff and worsen the situation for the other patients, whose resources and health they affect negatively. It is not possible in a REMS to guarantee management of violent, uncooperative persons whose defiant behavior does stem from not only a psychopathological condition but also a desire to be delinquent and to rebel against any rules of communal life. These patients do not have the requisites to be treated in the REMS as they necessitate custody and not cure. Only if they show the desire to collaborate and to participate in the therapeutic treatment can they attempt a program in REMS, which—in our opinion—should not be considered the only place where they could be helped.

Recently, it was necessary to add a new figure to the staff at the REMS, who is not a healthcare representative but one assigned to security (internal security operator/OPSI). The presence and duties of the OPSI make an important contribution to the rehabilitation program; these professionals are complementary to the presence and to the duties of healthcare personnel, whom they support by reducing the risk of injury in the community. The job of the OPSI is the prevention of aggressive acts, with the objective of improving safety inside the REMS, through active collaboration with the healthcare staff. An OPSI is an extra, unarmed guard, in addition to the one at the main entrance. During the day, the OPSI helps to welcome the patients who enter the REMS from the outside. He/she is present in the delicate procedure of admission of patients into the structure, of admitting their visiting relatives and lawyers, and of the patients' reentry after trials, hearings, special permissions, and extramural activities. The OPSI is responsible for the management of the control room, the switchboard, and the reception area of the REMS and it is his/her job to support the personnel in an active manner. He/she interacts directly with the staff and keeps informed of situations that might require added surveillance with the objective of preventing a crisis. He/she does not handle any type of health procedure but is called upon if the staff requires his/her help to accompany patients on extramural excursions or in activities within the REMS that require additional surveillance. The inclusion of the OPSI as a permanent fixture, in 2018, reduced episodes of violence, reduced injury to healthcare personnel, and therefore reduced the turnover of the same. It increased the safety of the patients and the staff and increased the possibility to execute clinical practices and rehabilitation programs in the REMS. As mentioned above, another condition that intensifies aggressiveness in the patients is the lack of a tangible program for the period following treatment in the REMS. A solid interaction with local services, not only psychiatric services but the entire area of mental health services that include addiction services and the services for the aged and disabled, is indispensable. In any case, these services, besides having limited resources for at-home treatment, are based on the residence of the patient. In the case of patients who committed crimes, their residences are often unknown. The homeless or noncitizens without documents are the people who have most difficulty finding adequate care. The rules are not always clear; in order to verify a date of birth which is inconsistent on various documents, bureaucratic procedures often overlap. Sometimes there are no documents at all. Without a tax number (Social Security Card) or healthcare card, it is impossible to program any course of treatment outside the REMS.

Another complication is the rapport with judges and parole officers. Many judges do not accept the idea that there is a waiting list to enter in a REMS and do very little to find alternative courses through their consultants; the parole officers show little sensitivity to the rehabilitation program in the REMS. In the case of rehabilitation activities outside the REMS, they often take divergent action with respect to different patients. For example, at Christmas, it was planned that a theater group perform a play outside the REMS at San Michele di Bra. However, several "actor/patients" were not given permission to perform in the public theater, without a clear reason given to the healthcare workers. Therefore, the play had to be performed within the confines of the REMS. There is a wide spectrum of options that vary from judge to judge, and it is not always the same throughout the rehabilitation process, in spite of the protocols agreed on by the region and the local court of appeals, in place since 2015.

The lack of revision of the penal code and penal procedures has resulted in a difficult situation for the judges as well, as they must often make immediate decisions without the benefit of a continuous dialogue with healthcare workers. These same healthcare workers also find it difficult to supply the magistrates with adequate information. We stress these aspects because the difficulty in providing the patient with a clear roadmap of a therapeutic program is one of the main reasons for frustration, anger, and aggressiveness.

In conclusion, the episodes of violence in REMS can be prevented by knowing the patients well and selecting those with a diagnosis that would benefit from therapeutic and rehabilitative treatment in a community facility. It is recommended that these patients have already been sentenced. One factor that helps to guarantee security in the facility is that patients are not "in transit." It is also necessary to increase the interaction between the judicial and the healthcare sectors to organize the best possible programs inside and outside the REMS. While we wait to achieve these goals, we underline the positive experience of reducing injuries to the staff in the REMS, Anton Martin, thanks to the addition of an unarmed guard to manage internal security. Lastly, we hope to see a revision of the penal code in all articles that mention the OPG-forensic psychiatric hospitals; generally speaking, the dual track should be abolished. It is a system for which a person with a mental disorder who has been acquitted cannot remain in custody inside a correctional facility even if he/she has proven to be unmanageable in the REMS. It is absolutely necessary to avoid that the REMS become the receptacle for difficult and uncooperative patients, who may continue to manifest violent and uncontrollable behavior. It is our opinion that the course of treatment for patients who have committed crimes should begin in mental health services in correctional facilities, continue in the REMS, and proceed to follow-up assistance by services on a local level, proportionate to the patients' level of cooperation and response to treatment. Further prospective studies on the functioning of Italian REMS are needed to increase the knowledge of patient characteristics related to violent behavior in order to prevent it.

Acknowledgments The authors thank Marina Gentile and Antonella Maffioletti of the Health Regional Authority and Martina Ciminiello for technical editing.

References

1. Margara A. Il lungo processo di superamento degli ospedali psichiatrici giudiziari. Riv Sper Fren. 2011;1:53–74.
2. Crepet P, De Plato G. Psychiatry without asylums: origins and prospects in Italy. Int J Health Serv. 1983;13(1):119–29.
3. Carabellese F, Felthous AR. Closing Italian forensic psychiatry hospitals in favor of treating insanity acquittees in the community. Behav Sci Law. 2016;34(2–3):444–59.
4. Fazel S, Hayes AJ, Bartellas K, Clerici M, Trestman R. The mental health of prisoners: a review of prevalence, adverse outcomes and interventions. Lancent Psychiatry. 2016;3(9):871–81.
5. Butler T, Indig D, Allnutt S, Mamoon H. Co-occurring mental illness and substance use disorder among Australian prisoners. Drug Alcohol Rev. 2011;30:188–94.
6. Voulgaris A, Kose N, Konrad N, Opitz-Welke A. Prison suicide in comparison to suicide events in forensic psychiatric hospitals in Germany. Front Psychol. 2018;9:398.
7. Castelpietra G, Egidi L, Caneva M, Gambino S, Feresin T, Mariotto A, et al. Suicide and suicides attempts in Italian prison epidemiological findings from the "Triveneto" area, 2010–2016. Int J Law Psychiatry. 2018;61:6–12.
8. Blitz CL, Wolff N, Shi J. Physical victimization in prison: the role of mental illness. Int J Law Psychiatry. 2008;31:385–93.
9. Teplin LA, McClelland GM, Abram KM, Weiner DA. Crime victimization in adults with severe mental illness—comparison with the national crime victimization survey. Arch Gen Psychiatry. 2005;62:911–21.
10. Goncalves LC, Goncalves RA, Martins C, Dirkzwager AJE. Predicting infractions and health care utilization in prison: a meta-analysis. Crim Justice Behav. 2014;41:921–42.
11. Campbell MA, French S, Gendreau P. The prediction of violence in adult offenders: a meta-analytic comparison of instruments and methods of assessment. Crim Justice Behav. 2009;36:567–90.
12. Schenk AM, Fremouw WJ. Individual characteristics related to prison violence: a critical review of the literature. Aggress Violent Behav. 2012;17:430–42.
13. Baranyi G, Cassidy M, Fazel S, Priebe S, Mundt AP. Prevalence of posttraumatic stress disorder in prisoners. Epidemiol Rev. 2018;40:134–45.
14. Håkansson A, Jesionowska V. Associations between substance use and type of crime in prisoners with substance use problems—a focus on violence and fatal violence. Subst Abuse Rehabil. 2018;9:1–9.
15. Fazel S, Yoon IA, Hayes AJ. Substance use disorders in prisoners: an updated systematic review and meta-regression analysis in recently incarcerated men and women. Addiction. 2017;112:1725–39.
16. Seppanen A, Törmänen I, Shaw C, Harry Kennedy H. Modern forensic psychiatric hospital design: clinical, legal and structural aspects. Int J Ment Health Syst. 2018;12:58.
17. Casacchia M, Malavolta M, Bianchini V, Di Michele V, Giosuè P. Closing forensic psychiatric hospitals in Italy: a new deal for mental health care? Riv Psichiatr. 2015;50(5):199–209.
18. Ferracuti S, Biondi M. The reform of the Penitentiary Order. A cultural revolution that involves the Mental Health Services. Riv Psichiatr. 2018;53(1):1–4.
19. Yoon I, Fazel S, Slade K. Outcomes of psychological therapies for prisoners with mental health problems: a systematic review and meta-analysis. J Consult Clin Psychol. 2017;85(8):783–802.
20. Cimino L. Il superamento degli Ospedali Psichiatrici Giudiziari: un'analisi critica. Riv Crim, Vitt e Sicur. 2014;8(2):229–45.

21. Di Lorito C, Castelletti L, Lega I, Gualco B, Scarpa F, Völlm B. The closing of forensic psychiatric hospitals in Italy: determinants, current status and future perspectives. A scoping review. Int J Law Psychiatry. 2017;55:54–63.
22. Pelissero M. Pericolosità sociale e doppio binario. Vecchi e nuovi modelli di incapacitazione. Torino: Giappichelli; 2008.
23. France G, Taroni F. The evolution of health-policy making in Italy. J Health Polit Policy Law. 2005;30(1–2):169–88.
24. Gadon L, Johnstone L, Cooke D. Situational variables and institutional violence: a systematic review of the literature. Clin Psychol Rev. 2006;26:515–34.
25. Nhiwatiwa FG. The effects of single session education in reducing symptoms of distress following patient assault in nurses working in medium secure settings. J Psychiatr Ment Health Nurs. 2003;10(5):561–8.
26. Baxter E, Hafner RJ, Holme G. Assaults by patients: the experience and attitudes of psychiatric hospital nurses. Aus N Z J Psychiatry. 1992;4:567–73.
27. Sacchetti E, Mencacci C. The closing of the Italian forensic hospitals: six months later. What we have learned and we need. Evid Based Psychiatr Care. 2012–2015;1:37–9.
28. Atkinson JM, Garner HC. Least restrictive alternative–advance statements and the new mental health legislation. Psychiatr Bull. 2002;26(7):246–7.
29. Tomlin J, Bartlett P, Völlm B. Experiences of restrictiveness in forensic psychiatric care: systematic review and concept analysis. Int J Law Psychiatry. 2018;57:31–41.
30. Latte G, Avvisati L, Calandro S, Di Filippo C, Di Genio M, Di Iorio G, et al. From OPG to REMS: the role of a territorial health service in the implementation of security and non-custodial measures towards offenders with psychological problems. Riv Psichiatr. 2018;53(1):31–9.
31. De Girolamo G, Buizza C, Sisti D, Ferrari C, Bulgari V, Iozzino L, et al. Monitoring and predicting the risk of violence in residential facilities. No difference between patients with history or with no history of violence. J Psychiatr Res. 2016;80:5–13.
32. Kay SR, Wolkenfelf F, Murrill LM. Profiles of aggression among psychiatric patients: I. Nature and prevalence. J Nerv Ment Dis. 1988;176:539–48.

Part IV

Prevention and Management of Violence in Mental Health

Violence Risk Assessment in Mental Health

13

Liliana Lorettu, Alessandra M. A. Nivoli, Paolo Milia, and Giancarlo Nivoli

13.1   Introduction

In 1996, the 49th World Health Assembly adopted Resolution WHA49.25, declaring that violence is a leading worldwide public health problem and that it is increasing dramatically.

In 2000, an estimated 1.6 million people worldwide died as a result of self-inflicted, interpersonal or collective violence, for an overall age-adjusted rate of 28.8 per 100,000 individuals. Most of these deaths occurred in low- to middle-income countries. Less than 10% of all violence-related deaths occurred in high-income countries [1].

Approximately half of these deaths were suicides, one-third were murders and one-fifth were war related.

The workplace is one of the settings in which violent behaviour can occur and the healthcare sector is one of the most affected. Violence in healthcare facilities is a growing problem.

Epidemiological estimates of violent behaviour in healthcare are difficult to produce due to a number of biases.

The main biases include the lack of a clear and shared definition of violent behaviour, and the non-reporting of many violent behaviours, leading to incorrect prevalence data.

One US report calculated that every week 20 people are killed in the workplace and 18,000 are attacked [2]; these data were confirmed by European reports [3]. About 48% of non-lethal incidents of workplace violence take place in the healthcare sector [4]. About 50% of healthcare workers are victims of violence during

L. Lorettu (✉) · A. M. A. Nivoli · P. Milia · G. Nivoli
Department of Medical, Surgical and Experimental Sciences, University of Sassari-AOU, Sassari, Italy
e-mail: llorettu@uniss.it; anivoli@uniss.it; paolo.milia@aousassari.it

© Springer Nature Switzerland AG 2020   231
B. Carpiniello et al. (eds.), *Violence and Mental Disorders*, Comprehensive Approach to Psychiatry 1, https://doi.org/10.1007/978-3-030-33188-7_13

their careers [5, 6]. Healthcare workers have a 16 times greater risk of suffering from workplace violence than workers in other sectors [7]. Within the healthcare sector, nurses are the category most at risk [8, 9]. Female workers, both nurses and doctors, are exposed to an even higher risk [10]. In a sample of 1826 health professionals, about 11% had suffered from physical assault, 5% on more than one occasion, while 64% had received threats and verbal abuse [11]. Saeki et al. [12] report a prevalence of 15%.

Incidents of workplace violence are strongly under-reported, especially in mental health services [13, 14]. Many factors contribute to this situation, including the belief that the violence suffered is the result of a personal inability to manage the patient, and the belief that violent behaviour is inherent in the patient's complex mental health condition and hence in the profession [15].

One particular form of violence, murder, is not very frequent but extremely disturbing. Research in the USA shows that between 1980 and 1990 106 health workers were killed [16]. The US BLS (Bureau of Labour Statistics) [4] reported that 69 health workers were killed between 1996 and 2000. In Italy, between 1988 and 2010, 17 doctors were killed in workplace-related circumstances [17]. Lorettu et al. [17] have identified four categories of situations at risk: one category includes murders committed in the context of doctor-patient conflict; the second and largest group consists of murders committed by psychiatric patients; the third group consists of murders committed in an unsafe workplace; and the fourth and last group comprises murder in the context of stalking behaviour.

A study on homicide in psychiatric hospitals in Australia and New Zealand identified three categories: homicides by acutely ill patients soon after admission, homicides by forensic patients in low-security settings, and homicides in which vulnerable and elderly patients were victims. The study concludes that 'An important task in any psychiatric hospital is to protect patients and staff from physical violence' [18].

Despite the high prevalence of violent behaviour in healthcare settings, not all healthcare facilities have developed a specific policy against violence, including specific risk assessment and targeted training of healthcare professionals. In the UK only 435 of the hospitals have drawn up and implemented a specific workplace violence prevention policy and only 3% of hospitals provide targeted training to their staff, even though 87% of healthcare workers continue to fear being attacked in the workplace [19].

The services of the Royal College of Psychiatrists, UK, have considered violence risk assessment an integral part of the profession since 1996.

The European Risk Observatory of the European Agency for Safety and Health at Work (EU-OSHA) has identified violence and harassment among the emerging psychosocial risks in occupational safety and health (OSH).

In Italy, the Ministry of Health's Quality Department has identified violence against health workers as a sentinel event and in November 2007 issued the 'Recommendations for preventing acts of violence against health workers', which in 2012 were included by the Ministry of Health in the Training Manual on Clinical Governance for patient and worker safety, which includes a whole chapter on 'Violence against health workers'. The Joint Commission on Accreditation of Healthcare Organizations, which currently also operates in Italy on behalf of various public hospitals, considers risk assessment in healthcare settings a quality indicator for preventing and reducing the number of violent incidents.

All healthcare sectors are at risk of workplace violence; however a number of studies have found that the risk is higher in emergency and psychiatric departments [11, 12].

One review of 424 studies on violent behaviour by hospitalised patients found that the incidence of violent behaviour in psychiatric hospitals was 32.4% [20]. Dickens et al. [21] found that 42.9% of the violent episodes had been reported in the forensic setting. This violent behaviour by patients occurs across the various clinical settings, including psychiatric wards, residential care and community psychiatry and can affect all the operators involved in the management of psychiatric patients.

The social alarm caused by news reports of serious acts of violence by psychiatric patients has led some countries to introduce mandatory risk assessment in emergency services: see for example the so-called Kendra Law of the State of New York or the British Care Programme Approach.

In addition to clinical risk assessment, which aims to reduce workplace violence, there are other conditions in which risk assessment is required.

Psychiatric risk assessments are also used in the forensic field. In forensic psychiatric evaluations, the expert is asked to produce a risk assessment which, together with other elements, is used to make important decisions. For instance, in criminal proceedings, the assessment can support the decision to commit a patient to secure psychiatric facilities with restriction of their personal freedom (in Italy until 2015 patients could be committed to judicial psychiatric hospitals, since replaced by Residences for the Execution of Security Measures). In civil proceedings, risk assessment plays a role, for example, in decisions on awarding the custody of children. In criminal cases, mental health assessments influence the conviction, severity of the sentence, involuntary commitment to mental institutions and time spent in such facilities.

Many studies have explored the relationship between mental illness and violent behaviour. This relationship has long been characterised by many prejudices which have often prevented correct understanding and management of the problem.

One very common prejudice is to automatically link mental illness with violent behaviour. This increases the stigma against mental illness and supports the demand for or the maintenance of ideological and indiscriminate freedom-restricting social and healthcare policies.

Although multiple factors are involved in the occurrence of violent behaviour, severe mental illness remains a risk factor and as such it requires risk assessment, in clinical and forensic settings, as well as operator training on violence risk assessment and risk management.

13.2 Risk Assessment

Risk is defined as the possibility that a given action or inaction may lead to a loss or a bad consequence. The concept of risk is often used as a synonym for the probability of a loss or a hazard/threat. Risk assessment is the systematic collection of information to determine the degree to which harm (to self or others) is likely at some future point in time.

Risk assessment must take into account both risk factors and protective factors and must be usable in the short term [22].

Assessing the risk of aggressive or violent behaviours linked to mental disorders has become a requirement in several mental health settings serving very different patient populations: psychiatric units (with acute inpatients), community psychiatry (with outpatients) and forensic psychiatry (with psychiatric offenders), which require different risk assessments. For acute patients admitted to psychiatric units, risk assessment is aimed at preventing violent behaviour in the short term. For patients of community mental health services (and in forensic settings) the purpose of risk assessment is to prevent violent behaviour in the short to medium term.

In Italy, the mental healthcare model has evolved over the years: before the 1970s the dominant paradigm was one of involuntary institutionalisation, with emphasis on protecting society, rather than treating patients. This was followed by a shift towards a community-based mental health service, centred on patient care and respecting the freedom and dignity of the individual. The detention model was mainly based on the equation mental illness—violent behaviour: under this approach risk assessment was by and large unnecessary, given the blanket association of mental illness with violent behaviour and the consequent indiscriminate restriction of personal freedom.

In the current mental healthcare model, the rationale for risk assessment lies in the focus on the patient's treatment, is primarily aimed at the patient's safety and is a cornerstone of the success of the therapeutic process. The aim of risk assessment is to identify patients who present a risk of violence, and to plan for them specific interventions and programs to prevent violent behaviour, distinguishing them from patients who do not present such risk and do not require specific programmes [23, 24]. One important objective and challenge is the need to balance appropriate patient care respecting their autonomy, dignity and safety, with the safety of health professionals and the community.

Over the years, a number of assessment tools have been developed to improve risk assessment and its outcomes, with different origins, purposes and uses in different settings.

Risk assessment is followed by clinical measures with different levels of care, but also by risk management aimed at reducing the risk.

The link between risk assessment and risk management is a complex process that must provide answers to the problem identified, by applying the knowledge derived from scientific evidence and designing a specific treatment plan.

Making a risk assessment without following it up with risk management actions is not good clinical practice.

The link between risk assessment and risk management entails several complexities.

The first complexity stems from the dynamism of the phenomenon: risk assessment is a dynamic process (just as the patients, their mental disorder, their life circumstances, the resources available are dynamic). Consequently the response, i.e. risk management, must be equally dynamic and readily adaptable to needs.

Secondly, risk management requires periodic verification of its implementation, feasibility, effectiveness and available tools.

A further key element of the risk assessment-risk management process is the circulation of information: the two systems must be closely linked, and information must flow smoothly, with continuous feedback enabling constant adaptation of the strategy in response to changes in risk assessment.

Finally, the circulation of information must be checked.

The NICE Guideline on Violence and Aggression [25] places violence risk assessment and management measures at the heart of the organisation of psychiatric and emergency services and requires their knowledge and observation by all staff with specific training courses, as well as the information and involvement of service users, to protect patients' rights. The following table (Table 13.1) lists the clinical risk management recommendations from the UK Department of Health [26].

The Functional Analysis of Care Environments (FACE) [27] is a portfolio of risk assessment tools based on a multidisciplinary assessment of needs and of possible strategies, and includes the evaluation of outcomes. It is an effective risk management tool.

Risk management responses cannot be indiscriminate and generalised: they should provide individual, personalised responses to the real need identified. Table 13.2 shows the different responses to different risk levels according to the response customisation principle [23, 27].

The validity and usefulness of risk assessment and of the tools used depend on two variables: calibration, i.e. adjustment of the tool to improve its accuracy, and discrimination, i.e. the tool's actual ability to identify individuals who present a real risk of violence (the real positives) and to respond with specific treatment actions. The discrimination variable is measured by reference to specificity (a test is specific for a given aspect and not for others) and sensitivity (the ability of the test to capture even minimal elements). In this specific case, an ideal evaluation should have high sensitivity, making it possible to identify violent individuals as true positives, and a high specificity to identify non-violent individuals as true negatives. However, even where specificity and sensitivity criteria are respected, operational limits remain linked to the basic prevalence, since an evaluation tool with good sensitivity and specificity works well in the case of a high prevalence of violence, but less so in the case of a low prevalence of violence.

A number of risk assessment tools are available, with different origins and purposes and for use in different contexts.

For all evaluation tools, the following elements are also important: the ability to determine the probability of occurrence of a given event (relative risk), the time frame in which it may occur and the type of event (violence against others, self-harm/suicidal behaviour).

The factors measured by violence risk assessment tools can be divided into static and dynamic. Static factors are those that are part of the patient's history and cannot be changed.

Table 13.1 Best Practice in Managing Risk 2007 UK Department of Health, National Risk Management Programme 16 best practice points for effective risk management (RM)

1.	Best practice involves making decisions based on knowledge of the research evidence, knowledge of the individual service user and their social context, knowledge of the service user's own experience, and clinical judgement.
2.	Positive risk management as part of a carefully constructed plan is a required competence for all mental health practitioners.
3.	Risk management should be conducted in a spirit of collaboration and based on a relationship between the service user and their careers that is as trusting as possible.
4.	Risk management must be built on a recognition of the service user's strenghts and should emphasise recovery.
5.	Risk management requires an organisational strategy as well as efforts by the individual practitioner.
6.	Risk management involves developing flexible strategies aimed at preventing any negative event from occurring or, if this is not possible, minimising the harm caused.
7.	Risk management should take into account that risk can be both general and specific, and that good management can reduce and prevent harm.
8.	Knowledge and understanding of mental health legislation is an important component of risk management.
9.	The risk management plan should include a summary of all risks identified, formulations of the situations in which identified risks may occur, and actions to be taken by practitioners and service user in response to crisis.
10.	Where suitable tools are available, risk management should be based on assessment using the structured clinical judgement approach.
11.	Risk assessment is integral to deciding on the most appropriate level of risk management and the right kind of intervention for a service user.
12.	All staff involved in risk management must be capable of demonstrating sensitivity and competence in relation to diversity in race, faith, age, gender, disability and sexual orientation.
13.	Risk management must always be based on awareness of the capacity for the service user's risk level to change over time, and a recognition that each service user requires a consistent and individualised approach.
14.	Risk management plan should be developed by multidisciplinary and multi-agency teamsoperating in an open, democratic and transparent culture that embrace reflective practice.
15.	All staff involved in risk management should receive relevant training, which is updated at least every 3 years.
16.	A risk management plan is only as good as the time and effort put into communicating its findings to others.

Dynamic factors are those that refer to the individual, their environment and their social and family setting, and can change over time.

Static factors are elements such as having suffered violence or having committed violent acts in the past. Dynamic factors are the use of drugs and alcohol, the presence of mental health conditions and the presence of drug therapy.

Risk assessment tools can be classified into three types: the clinical, the actuarial and the structured clinical model.

The *clinical model* was used in past years. Under this model, risk assessment was mainly based on the clinician's experience and judgment. This approach was not structured as a method and left wide discretion to the clinician to collect and assess

Table 13.2 FACE risk assessment

0	1	2	3	4
No apparent risk	Small apparent risk	Significant apparent risk	Serious apparent risk	Serious and imminent apparent risk
No history of risk or premonitory signs suggesting risk	There are currently no behaviours suggesting risk, but the patient's history or premonitory signs indicate probable risk. The standard treatment ensures necessary supervision or control. No specific risk prevention plans or measures are in place.	The patient's medical history and clinical conditions suggest the presence of risk and this is considered a major problem. A specific plan must be drawn up in addition to the treatment plan.	In view of the circumstances a risk management plan should be developed and implemented.	The patient's history and condition indicate the presence of risk, e.g. the patient is preparing to act. The risk prevention plan has the highest priority.

information arbitrarily, lacked transparency and was highly vulnerable to cognitive biases. Over the years, clinical risk assessments have been found to be poorly accurate, very close to the randomness of the coin toss [28], and have been heavily criticised because decisions restricting the personal liberty of individuals were made on the basis of non-objective evaluations, giving rise to significant ethical, professional and clinical problems [29].

The *actuarial model* uses an algorithm to produce a risk score derived from statistical data. It targets static risk factors for which statistical analysis has shown a correlation with an increased risk of violence. The risk is expressed with a score and is referred to a specific period of time.

Various authors have highlighted the limitations inherent in actuarial methods, in particular the fact that they derive from retrospective studies on specific populations that do not lend themselves well to more general extrapolation [30].

Firstly, actuarial assessments are of a statistical nature and have limited clinical relevance, with poor applicability for specific interventions; secondly, they only examine static factors, leaving out all those dynamic factors that enable individual and contextualised assessment of each patient; thirdly, actuarial models concern the long-term perspective and are not practically and operationally usable in the short term; lastly, since they are based on static elements, they do not allow changes to the risk assessment which remains always the same for a given individual, and are not useful for treatment follow-up purposes.

While actuarial risk assessment models are statistically useful, they should not be used alone, but should be flanked by other tools [31].

Table 13.3 List of the most common risk assessment tools

Name	Type	Setting	Type of risk	Evidence
Clinical Risk Management Tool/ Working with Risk *CRMT*	Clinical	All	V, S, SC	Not available
Functional Analysis of Care Environment	Clinical	All	V, S, SC	Good
Risk Assessment Management and Audit System RAMAS	Clinical	All	All	Modest
Generic Integrated Risk Ass. for Forensic Env. *GIRAFE*	Clinical	Forensic	All	Not available
Classification of Violent Risk *COVR*	Actuarial	Forensic	V	Good
Short Term Assessment of Risk and Treatability *START*	Clinical	All	V, S, SC	Good
Historical Clinical Risk 20 *HCR 20*	Clinical	All	V	Very good
Psychopathy Checklist Revisited PCL R	Actuarial	All	V	Very good
Static 99	Actuarial	Forensic	V	Modest
Sexual Violence Risk 20 SVR 20	Clinical	Forensic	V	Good
Violence Risk Appraisal Guide VRAG	Actuarial	Forensic	V	Very good
Interactive Classification Tree	Actuarial	Forensic	V	Good

The *structured clinical approach* is based on dynamic factors and is aimed at risk management. The structured clinical approach is based on specific factors derived from scientific evidence, on the examiner's experience and on the direct involvement of the people around the patient (the resources available to the patient examined). Apart from the risk of violence, this approach is often used to assess the risk of suicide and of serious carelessness. The limitations of this approach are poor inter-rater reliability, the strong dependence on clinical judgment and the ease of use in defensive medicine as it makes it possible to assign more value to false positives.

See the study by Singh and Fazel [32], which examined 128 risk assessment tools providing an overview of the most commonly used tools and their characteristics.

Table 13.3 shows the most common risk assessment tools, their type, the clinical evidence available and their use settings.

In a more general context, in addition to the schematism of a structured evaluation, and for the purposes of a more comprehensive forensic psychiatric evaluation, it is useful to consider both the risk factors for violent behaviour and the protective factors.

The following *risk factors* have been identified:

Socio-demographic factors: These include gender, age, marital status, economic status and exposure to violent subcultures of violence.

Personal factors: These include coming from physically and mentally abusive families [33, 34], previous violent behaviour and early juvenile delinquency [35–37].

Factors related to substance abuse: Several studies point out that the use and abuse of alcohol and drugs increase the risk of violent behaviour [38–40]; it should be noted that the comorbidity of severe mental illness and alcohol and drug use increases the risk of violent behaviour almost twofold compared to violent behaviour related to serious mental disorder alone [41, 42].

Factors related to mental disorder: Although this topic has been addressed by numerous studies and reflections, it is still the subject of debate. Some takeaway messages are highlighted in the literature: not all mental disorders increase the risk of violent behaviour [43]; in serious mental disorders the risk of violent behaviour is moderately higher than in the general population [40, 44–47]; mental disorders alone are not sufficient for predicting violent behaviour, since other concurrent risk factors are necessary, such as past predictors (previous violent behaviour, previous victimisation), clinical factors (substance abuse), bio-psychosocial factors (age, sex) and contextual factors (stressful life events) [48]; different mental disorders are associated with a different risk of violent behaviour [43, 49, 50]; the concurrent presence of several symptoms and their severity, in combination with other risk factors such as substance abuse and criminal history, increase the risk of violent behaviour [51].

Treatment factors: Many treatment factors are linked to an increased risk of violent behaviour, such as non-compliance with medication [52], abrupt interruption of medication [53, 54], non-compliance or pseudo-compliance of the patient's inability to seek help [55], and conflict or violence with the environment or with caregivers [56].

Situational factors act as environmental stressors (breakup with partner, job loss, money problems) [57].

Factors related to recidivism: Assessing the elements relevant to violence recidivism is another important element for violence risk assessment. Some studies highlight the presence of individuals with specific clinical features such as a triple diagnosis (schizophrenia, alcohol abuse, antisocial personality disorder). Others have highlighted the most frequent factors in criminal recidivism by identifying the big eight: criminal history, antisocial personality, antisocial cognition, antisocial associates, family problems, employment instability, lack of prosocial leisure pursuits, and alcohol and drug abuse.

As to *protective factors*, some can be deduced from risk factors (biopsychosocial factors, personal factors, factors related to alcohol and drug abuse, factors related to mental disorder, factors related to treatment, circumstantial factors, factors related to recidivism). Another protective factor is the availability of psychosocial interventions for managing crisis situations that might result in violent acts. Great emphasis is given to factors related to the treatment of the mental disorder (such as compliance with medication and psychotherapy, insight, ability to seek help, building a therapeutic alliance) and the ability to self-manage violence with a focus on the ability to recognise one's own violence and triggers.

Another specific protection factor in the forensic field is the presence of adequate social support.

Protective factors have also been included in assessment scales. The Structured Assessment of Protective Factors for violence risk (SAPROF) [58] identifies the following factors:

- *Internal factors* (such as good intelligence, secure attachment in childhood, empathy, coping skills)
- *Motivational factors* (such as work, leisure activities, financial management, motivation for treatment)
- *External factors* (e.g. social network, intimate relationship)

This assessment tool for protective factors, which is useful in association with clinical examination, assesses protective factors by assigning them the following scores: low, low-moderate, moderate, moderate-high and high.

Consequently, again in the more general context and with a view to a broader forensic psychiatric evaluation, an assessment of the risk of violent behaviour in mental illness may be made on a broader basis of general knowledge encompassing at least four areas involved in violence risk:

- The patient
- The context/environment
- The victim
- Emotional reactions

In each of these areas there are risk factors and protective factors. The information obtained from the investigation must be cross-checked in order to obtain elements as close as possible to real-world data and to enable adequate risk management without recourse to indiscriminate interventions.

13.3   Risk Assessment: The Patient

Assessing the risk of violent behaviour in psychiatric patients is increasingly considered an integral part of good clinical practice. Risk assessment must meet different needs at different times. While mental illness should not always be equated with violent behaviour, it is equally important not to deny the possible risks posed by psychiatric patients or even the existence of the mental disorder.

Acute psychiatric patients admitted to a psychiatric unit need a risk assessment covering some specific parameters.

It is important to carry out a clinical evaluation that, through a diagnostic filter, is able to rule out or identify organic causes for the violent behaviour. It is particularly useful to follow the acronym FIND ME (functional, infectious, neurological, drugs, metabolic, endocrine) in order to investigate possible organic causes of violent behaviour [59].

In addition, as part of a short-term assessment, Simon and Tardiff's Checklist [60] is an unstructured tool for the clinical risk assessment of violence risk approved by a consensus of experts and tested in clinical practice (Table 13.4).

However, for the purposes of broader reflection, more specifically for forensic psychiatric purposes, we suggest assessing the violent behaviour of a psychiatric

Table 13.4 Factors that must be evaluated in the assessment of the short-term risk of violence

1.	Appearance of the patient
2.	Presence of violent ideation and degree of formulation and/or planning
3.	Intent to be violent
4.	Available means to harm and access to the potential victim
5.	Past history of violence and other impulsive behaviours
6.	Alcohol or drug use
7.	Presence of psychosis
8.	Presence of certain personality disorders
9.	History of non-compliance with treatment
10.	Demographic and socio-economic characteristics

patient through three progressive stages implying very different kinds of scientific and clinical knowledge that can be usefully integrated:

1. Examination of the psychiatric disorder
2. Examination of violent behaviour
3. Assessment of a treatment plan

1. Examination of the mental disorder includes the search for symptoms and signs to enable diagnosis in a specific category. In addition to making a categorical diagnosis, it is essential to examine the dimensions that may be present, such as impulsiveness and/or anger, which may have played a role in the violent behaviour and which contribute to formulation of a dimensional diagnosis; finally, the dynamic aspects must also be examined, including examination of the defence mechanisms in order to formulate a dynamic diagnosis as well [61].
2. The examination of violent behaviour is essential for good knowledge of the case, for risk assessment and for establishing a treatment plan. It can include at least two stages of investigation from the aetiological diagnosis of violent behaviour (i.e. the social, cultural, subcultural and cross-generational learning of violent behaviour) to the victimological diagnosis (i.e. the link between author and victim, the victim's role).
3. Assessment and formulation of the treatment plan: To make an assessment and design a treatment plan it is essential to have a two-pronged approach: the first prong is to assess and treat the mental disorder, with a feasible and monitorable treatment plan aimed at controlling the mental condition. The second prong is treatment of the violent behaviour, which must be combined with the medication for the mental illness, and which starts from the individual's level of insight into their violent behaviour, its triggers and the underlying relational dynamics.

13.4 Risk Assessment: The Setting

The setting in which the risk assessment is carried out can be very different, with different implications.

A clinical setting for acute patients (psychiatric units and emergency units) requires a risk assessment focused on avoiding violent behaviour in the short term (usually the hospitalisation period), ensuring patient and caregiver safety.

In a forensic setting, in facilities for mentally disordered offenders, the risk assessment is aimed at preventing violent behaviour in the short term (during stay in the facility and in the medium term (after discharge from the facility).

In addition, the setting itself requires specific assessments that go beyond the patient's examination, since each setting may present specific risk elements. Some workplaces have characteristics that may be related to a high risk of violent behaviour. Some examples are environments with poor lighting, without alarm systems, facilities that are isolated and/or not easily and quickly reachable in case of emergency, places where the influx of visitors is not monitored and facilities without security personnel. Other possible triggers are linked to operational arrangements of the work environment; for example, long waiting times may be a critical issue especially for frontline staff [62]. In addition to being poorly prepared and trained for risk assessment, medical staff are often also poorly protected. A telephone survey in the emergency departments in the USA found that 63% of the facilities do not have 24/7 security personnel; visitor access is controlled only in 21% of facilities; in high-risk areas 39% use a security code; 46% have alarm buttons, 14% have an isolation room, 36% use a CCTV system and 1.6% use a metal detector for detecting weapons [63].

Setting-related protection measures often coincide with risk management. One example is that of a large urban hospital in the USA [64, 65] with a high incidence of violent behaviour; the hospital adopted a series of measures which have drastically reduced violent behaviour, such as the deployment of security personnel, metal detectors, plexiglass in the triage rooms, keypad security system, monitoring of inflows into emergency departments and use of vehicle barriers. Risk management in the workplace is carried out by security personnel who are assigned a key role in the security system. However, employing security personnel is expensive and this often limits their use significantly. Appropriate training of security personnel is commonly considered to be a key factor. However, the decision on whether they should be able to use or even carry firearms remains a controversial topic. Other systems such as the use of tasers or pepper sprays are often suggested, although these systems too are not entirely risk free. Alarm systems are a valuable risk management tool in emergency departments and acute psychiatric units. The presence of an alarm system makes it possible to activate immediate response to an incident. Where needed, the various responders can consider different levels of response to an alarm signal. An emergency department should also have a direct alarm line to the nearest police station. Access control and regulation in the evening and night hours is also a useful element in preventing violence.

13.5   Risk Assessment: The Victim

A full risk assessment should also include the assessment of the risk factors relating to potential victims.

It is important to point out that victims often play a specific role in the dynamics leading to the violent incident. Recognising this should in no way be construed as victim-blaming. It means identifying the role played by the victim in order to identify the factors conducive to a person being victimised, and to act on these, especially for treatment purposes.

Some biopsychosocial data are classically recognised as being victimisation risk factors. Being a female is widely recognised as a specific victimisation risk in all contexts [66].

In violence risk assessment several risk factors for victimisation are found across different settings.

In emergency units and/or psychiatric units, many studies have found that the victims of workplace violence are more often women and young (bibliography). Young age is also associated with less work experience. The lack of experience, the difficulty in managing the relationship and the inability to decode their own defence mechanisms and those of patients are among the risk factors for victimisation. A study by Erkol [67] describes the profile of the victim. The professionals at risk are individuals with limited work experience (newly hired professionals and/or recent graduates), individuals without specific training on risk assessment and management and individuals with duties involving frequent and prolonged direct contact with the patient or also with the patient's family.

Another victim assessment setting is the patient's cohabiting family. Many studies on the violent behaviour of the mentally ill have shown that violent behaviour often occurs in the family [68]. The dynamics are numerous and complex, linked to the emotions expressed in the families of psychiatric patients that feed the 'family tension', to the presence of complex and intricate defence mechanisms by which family members tend to underestimate the risk of violence (by resorting to minimisation and/or denial), or to an overestimation of violence risk leading to violent behaviour towards the patient, which in turn generates more violence. Other dynamics can be associated to a general and widespread feeling of guilt towards the family member-patient, leading to tolerance of the family member's violent behaviour beyond the acceptable risk. There may also be poor violent behaviour management skills, e.g. failure to apply talk-down and de-escalation techniques. Lastly, there is lack of information and education of family members about available resources such as social services and the police.

Protective factors include psycho-educational interventions for family members of patients with serious mental illnesses aimed at the knowledge of the elements of psychopathology, role of therapy and recommended ways of dealing with the patient's violent behaviour (including holding the patient accountable, even by reporting the incident to the police). The purpose is to prevent what is often termed 'a violent incident that could be seen coming'.

13.6 Risk Assessment: Emotional Reactions

Correct risk assessment includes careful evaluation of the healthcare providers' emotional reactions.

The therapeutic relationship with a psychiatric patient who engages in violent behaviours can be beset by problems that can undermine the correctness and adequacy of the diagnostic process and the consequent treatment plan. Violent behaviour, just like mental illness, may have a number of recurrences, some of which may be seemingly unpredictable, unexpected and incomprehensible. This entails further clinical, ethical and legal responsibilities and poses additional difficulties for professionals. Emotional reactions, in the form of defence mechanisms, are triggered to manage the emotional burden caused by violent behaviour. The possible defence mechanisms are many: they may occur in combination, and they are affected by many variables such as the type of patient and the therapist's specific training, psychological profile and workplace setting. The positive function of the defence mechanism is to protect the professional against the anxiety that can be induced by a violent patient. However, the inadequate use of defence mechanisms may hinder the understanding of the complexity of a violent psychiatric patient. This is the case when the operation of defence mechanisms and the consequences of such operations are not adequately recognised. It follows that the inadequate use of defence mechanisms can constitute an 'interpretative shield', an 'iatrogenic' resistance to understanding the patient and thus wrong decisions [69].

The therapist's inability to manage anxiety and the consequent use of defence mechanisms influence inappropriately the therapist's behaviour and relationship with the patient and can be perceived by the patient who, despite being psychotic, is able to test their therapist and assess their limitations and weaknesses. As the patient perceives the therapist's defence mechanisms and thereby the therapist's own fear and anxiety in respect of the mental illness and violent behaviour, he/she finds confirmation of his/her own anxiety, mental illness and violence. Moreover, therapists who are not trained to detect the inadequate use of defence mechanisms will find it increasingly difficult to manage the violent patient because they will progressively lose some professional skills and because the inadequate management of violent behaviour breeds further violence [69].

For example, the psychiatrist should avoid acting on the basis of their feeling of omnipotence, reactive to the fear caused by an agitated patient in the manic phase, as this feeling may lead the psychiatrist to face the patient alone, thus exposing themselves to the risk of violent behaviour by the patient.

Equally wrong is the inappropriate recourse to restraint, dictated by the psychiatrist's fear of the patient and modulated by the defence mechanism of projection, through which the psychiatrist overestimates the patient's potential for violence because they attribute their own hostility and anger to the patient. Inappropriate and/or indiscriminate use of restraint feeds the climate of violence in the unit and contributes to the escalation of violent behaviour.

A psychiatrist who has to assess the risk of violence of a psychiatric patient who has committed violent acts against children may, by using the defence mechanism of identification of the aggressor and minimising the mental illness elements, overestimate the risk of violence with very different clinical and legal consequences, such as sending the patient to prison rather than to a treatment centre.

See the literature for an in-depth analysis of the subject and a detailed description of the many defence mechanisms used with psychiatric patients who commit violent acts [14, 69].

In addition to the operators' defence mechanisms, it is useful to point out the collective defence mechanisms, widely applied to relieve the anxiety caused by the patient's violent behaviour in the population. For example, in news reports on particularly violent and cruel incidents that affect the public's sensitivity, mental illness is often invoked as the cause of the violent behaviour. The use of the misleading link between the mental disease and the violent behaviour in these media reports acts as a collective defence mechanism, because it is reassuring to attribute a frightening violent and cruel behaviour to the 'other', to someone who is different from us, to a sick person, and to draw a clear line separating normal individuals (who are assumed to be unable of such cruel violent behaviour) from sick persons, different from us, who committed the violent act 'in a fit of madness'. Such collective defence mechanisms have a number of consequences. Firstly, they reinforce the automatic stereotypical link between mental illness and violent behaviour (from which they also stem); secondly, they increase the demand for a reactive and detention-focused response by the institutions, assigning to psychiatry the task of social control and defence; lastly, they constitute a cognitive distortion by focusing the violent behaviour issue exclusively on mental illness, by preventing reflection of the role of other causal factors of violent behaviour which require specific assessment and management strategies (use of drugs, social exclusion, poverty, lack of moral compass, etc.) and, above all, by allowing society not to question itself.

In this sector, *protective factors* are many and varied according to whether the defence mechanisms are individual (of the professionals involved in the risk assessment) or collective, as expressed by society.

Individual protection factors include the supervision of the professionals dealing with difficult cases and ongoing training. The supervision of professionals enables them to become aware of their own emotional reactions, decode them and recognise their influence on the relationship with the patient and on the professionals' own consequent behaviour. Professionals may find themselves 'stuck' in certain defence mechanisms and be unable to recognise their dysfunctional reaction on their own, because the defence mechanism itself hinders appropriate understanding of such reaction, as it serves to manage anxiety. Supervision, especially in the management of difficult cases, makes it possible to assess the situation objectively, from an external viewpoint. Nivoli et al. propose possible different levels of intervention on professionals based on the level of introspection achieved [14] (Table 13.5).

Ongoing training allows mental health professionals to be constantly aware of the possible 'pitfalls' of defence mechanisms, recognise them and avoid behavioural conditioning.

As regards the *protective factors* against the collective defence mechanisms used in society, it is important to step up the campaign against stigmatisation by the media. It is necessary to work with the media to reduce the use of the stereotypic association of mental illness-violence and analyse correctly the violent acts by

Table 13.5 Level of introspection of the mental health professional and psychotherapeutic intervention on emotional transference reactions

Level of introspection (of the mental health professional)	Level of intervention (on the mental health professional)
Insight is present and appropriate (into one's own emotional and behavioural reactions)	No intervention (recognition, acceptance, therapeutic use of one's own emotions)
Limited introspection and presence of anxiety (with strong feelings of fear, anger, frustration, etc.)	Group therapy (with the group of colleagues and staff)
Limited introspection and presence of stereotyped use of anxiety defence mechanisms (denial, projection, splitting, identification, etc.)	Individual therapy (with the group therapy supervisor of the treatment unit)
Lack of introspection and counter-aggressive action towards the patient and staff (feelings of guilt, low self-esteem, etc.)	Individual therapy (with a therapist not necessarily from the same treatment unit)

individuals with serious mental disorders. In Italy, the Italian Society of Psychiatry has launched an awareness and collaboration campaign with the media that includes 'training' on the use of psychiatric terminology ('using the right words') with the correct use of terms such as psychosis, psychopathy, paranoia and fit of madness, to ensure that media reports are accurate and not marred by preconceptions or assumptions that contribute to the stigmatisation of mental health patients.

13.7 Risk Assessment: Open Questions

Violence risk assessment in psychiatry still involves several open questions.

While a number of studies have confirmed the effectiveness of certain risk assessment tools in detecting true positives, there are few studies on outcome indicators and consequently we lack reliable evidence about the effectiveness of response interventions after violence risk has been identified and about the consequences of failing to spot individuals at risk of violent behaviour (false negatives) [18]. Possible preventive measures cannot be applied indiscriminately to all patients. Some elements must necessarily be present: the risk must be effective, current and real; the choice of preventive strategy must be appropriate to the severity of the risk.

The measurement of risk factors continues to have a mainly statistical value (especially for actuarial tools) for large populations but it is difficult to apply in individual cases and when there is low prevalence.

The simultaneous presence of risk factors and protective factors, and their sheer number, risk spreading risk assessment over such a broad 'clinical space' that its validity is impaired. Moreover, it should be borne in mind that risk factors are not themselves the causes of violent behaviour; therefore, confusing them with actual causes can be extremely risky for the consequent intervention choices.

The applicability of risk assessment in mental health services is hindered by the long-standing difficulty of translating scientific research into real-world clinical practice. Although the need to perform risk assessment is widely accepted, its actual implementation may be hampered by several difficulties, such as inadequate motivation and personal interest by mental health professionals, their workload and time constraints, the frequent lack of specific training and the belief that violent behaviour goes hand in hand with mental illness. However, it is good clinical practice for psychiatrists whose patients exhibit violent behaviour to assess both risk factors and protective factors and how they interact with each other.

Risk assessment, intended as risk formulation, should be promptly recorded in the patient's medical record in order to achieve two important aims:

- To benefit the patient whose situation is evaluated in terms of risk factors and protective factors
- To document objectively the good clinical practice of the psychiatrist, who worked with professional competence, diligence and prudence

Recording the risk assessment and the consequent risk management in the patient's record is always advisable in view of possible professional liability claims and disputes.

Risk assessment can be a source of legal liability for the psychiatrist because of the scrutiny to which the psychiatrist's decisions are subjected and of their consequences in terms of patient restraint and/or other restrictions on the patient's freedom, or, where no risk management plan was implemented, in the event of patient violence or suicidal behaviour. The increasing attention of the media and the judiciary to cases of malpractice, the many malpractice court cases related to the violent or suicidal behaviour of the psychiatric patient and the continuous changes in the legislation on psychiatric care increasingly create professional liability concerns for psychiatrists in the field of risk assessment and risk management.

Risk assessment also involves ethical and professional conduct issues. The psychiatrist, like any other doctor, owes a duty of care and professional confidentiality to the patient. Risk assessment is beneficial for the patient to the extent that it helps to draw up a patient-specific treatment plan, particularly in the clinical setting. In the context of forensic psychiatry, in which risk assessment may result in a restriction of the patient's freedom, or a decision on the custody of children, the patient's benefit risks being sacrificed to social protection concerns. This raises questions about the psychiatrist's ethical and professional conduct position.

In forensic psychiatry, professional confidentiality, which is another ethical cornerstone of the patient-doctor relationship, may also be called into question when psychiatrists have to answer questions on risk assessment and share information with the justice system while continuing to provide patient care. Risk assessment, which in legal settings meets the needs of courts, can pose specific ethical challenges to psychiatrists, different from those encountered in other areas of psychiatric practice and which deserve in-depth reflection covering legal, theoretical and organisational aspects.

Other aspects of the patient's and the psychiatrist's liability need to be addressed. Patients have the right to refuse treatment and they are not automatically liable for violent behaviour following such refusal. On the other hand, psychiatrists have historically been given a social mandate to protect and monitor patients, and have been held responsible for the patient's behaviour; thus they must attempt to balance this mandate and responsibility with the patient's freedom of choice.

Lastly, a few more concerns in the field of risk assessment are worth noting. Variables such as the use of substances can play a highly misleading role in a risk assessment and subsequent risk management. Every day, the literature and, especially, clinical practice confirm that the use of substances increases the risk of violent behaviour in individuals with or without mental illness [70, 71]. Therefore, these individuals are those in greatest need of risk assessment, but they are also those most resistant to evaluation and treatment and who often steer well clear of the healthcare system.

Another important group are psychiatric patients who drop out of pharmacotherapy [22]. The literature highlights the protective role of pharmacotherapy and compliance with treatment and the importance of the therapeutic relationship. However, mental health professionals often have no effective means to retrieve drop-out patients, especially when the dilemma is between the patient's freedom of choice and need for care.

Lastly, in the specific field of psychiatry, it is important to point out that the stigma on mental illness often delays or prevents access to treatment by psychiatric patients. Although scientific evidence has disproved the automatic association between mental disorder and violent behaviour, in the public's perception this association still persists and is often fuelled by inaccurate media reporting of violent incidents.

13.8   Conclusions

Violence remains a multicausal phenomenon, in which many very different factors come together, having different influences and different consequences. Thinking that we can focus on a small number of causal factors, or just on one, such as mental illness, as a way of preventing and managing violence successfully does not correspond to clinical reality, epidemiological data and literature, and is a very naïve assumption.

For a broader and more correct understanding, it is far more appropriate to see violence as part of a *continuum*, with, at one end, multiple factors that contribute to causing violent behaviour, whose assessment and management cannot be left exclusively to mental health practitioners, given the many variables involved. Intervention in this field must cover various aspects: political, economic, financial, cultural and subcultural, to address the many causal factors that contribute to violent behaviour. At the other end of the scale, to a much smaller extent, we find mental illness and its contribution to violent behaviour, which requires specific risk assessment and management. In between, we should not forget the significant contribution of substance use to violent behaviour both in clinical terms, in so far as it increases the risk of violent behaviour in individuals with and without mental illness, and in social terms, in so far as substance use supports criminal networks linked to drug trafficking and distribution. Response in this area must include political, organisational, economic and health policies.

The WHO has highlighted that 'The public health approach also emphasises collective action. It has proved time and again that cooperative efforts from such diverse sectors as health, education, social services, justice and policy are necessary to solve what are usually assumed to be purely 'medical' problems. Each sector has an important role to play in addressing the problem of violence and, collectively, the approaches taken by each have the potential to produce important reductions in violence' (WHO).

Predicting human behaviour is a difficult endeavour in many areas, and predicting violent behaviour is certainly no exception.

Therefore, in the context of violent behaviour, it is appropriate to be able to 'see' beyond mental illness, to avoid the risk of focusing attention on a part and missing the whole picture.

References

1. O.M.S. Violenza e Salute nel Mondo. Rapporto dell'Organizzazione Mondiale della Sanità. In Quaderni di Sanità Pubblica, CIS Editore; 2002.
2. The National Institute for Occupational Safety and health (NIOSH). Violence in the workplace risk factors and prevention strategies. Current Intelligence Bulletin 57, DHHS, N. 96; 1996.
3. Paoli P, Merllié D. Third European survey on working conditions. European foundation for the improvement of living and working conditions; 2000.
4. Occupational Safety and Health Administration (OSHA) guidelines for preventing workplace violence for health care & social service workers. www.osha.gov. US Department of Labor; 2004.
5. Schulte JM, Nolt BJ, Williams RL, et al. Violence and threats of violence experienced by public health field-workers. JAMA. 1998;280:439.
6. Al-Sahlawi KS, Zahid MA, Shahid AA, et al. Violence against doctors: 1. A study of violence against doctors in accident and emergency departments. Eur J Emerg Med. 1999;6:301.
7. Elliott PP. Violence in health care. What nurse managers need to know. Nurs Manage. 1997;28(12):38–41.
8. Kingma M. Workplace violence in the health sector: a problem of epidemic proportion. Int Nurs Rev. 2001;48:129–30.
9. Lee DT. Violence in the health care workplace. Hong Kong Med J. 2006;12(1):4–5.
10. Boyle M, Koritsas S, Coles J, Stanley J. A pilot study of workplace violence towards paramedics. Emerg Med J. 2007;24(11):760–3.
11. Gascón S, Martínez-Jarreta B, González-Andrade JF, Santed MA, Casalod Y, Rueda MA. Aggression towards health care workers in Spain: a multi-facility study to evaluate the distribution of growing violence among professionals, health facilities and departments. Int J Occup Environ Health. 2009;15(1):29–35.
12. Saeki K, Okamoto N, Tomioka K, Obayashi K, Nishioka H, Ohara K, Kurumatani N. Work-related aggression and violence committed by patients and its psychological influence on doctors. J Occup Health. 2011;53(5):356–64.
13. Dubin WR, Lion JR. Clinician safety. Washington: American Psychiatric Association; 1993.
14. Nivoli GC, Lorettu L, Sanna MN. Valutazione e trattamento del paziente violento. In: Trattato Italiano di Psichiatria. Masson; 1999.
15. Bruns D, Disorbio JM, Hanks R. Chronic pain and violent ideation: testing a model of patient violence. Pain Med. 2007;8(3):207–15.

16. Goodman RA, Jenkins EL, Mercy JA. Workplace-related homicide among health care workers in the United States, 1980 through 1990. JAMA. 1994;272:1686–8.
17. Lorettu L, Falchi L, Nivoli F, Milia P, Nivoli GC, Nivoli AM. L'omicidio del medico. Riv Psichiatr. 2015;50(4):175–80.
18. Nielssen O, Large MM. Homicide in psychiatric hospitals in Australia and New Zealand. Psychiatr Serv. 2012;63(5):500–3.
19. National Union of Public Employees. Violence in the NHS. Hlth Serv News; 1991.
20. Bowers L, Stewart D, Papadopoulos C, Dack C, Ross J, Khanom H. Inpatient violence and aggression: a literature review. Report from the Conflict and Containment Reduction Research Programme. London: Institute of Psychiatry, Kings College London; 2011.
21. Dickens G, Picchioni M, Long C. Aggression in specialist secure and forensic inpatient mental health care: incidence across care pathways. J Forensic Pract. 2013;15(3):206–17.
22. O'Rourke M, Wrigley C, Hammond S. Violence within mental health services: how to enhance risk management. Risk Manag Health Policy. 2018;11:159–67.
23. Spinogatti F. La predittività dei comportamenti dannosi. In: Psichiatria Oggi, Anno XXVIII, 1; 2015.
24. Large M, Nielssen O. The limitations and future of violence risk assessment. World Psychiatry. 2017;16(1)
25. National Institute for Health and Care Excellance (NICE). Violence and aggression short term management in mental health, health and community settings. Update edition The British Psychological Society and The Royal College of Psychiatrists, 2015.
26. Department of Health, National Risk Management Programme. Best practice in managing risk. London: National Risk Management Programme; 2007.
27. Clifford PI. The FACE Recording and Measurement System: a scientific approach to person-based information. Bull Menninger Clin. 1999;63(3):305–31. [cited 2013 Sep 21]. http://www.ncbi.nlm.nih.gov/pubmed/10452193.
28. Ennis BJ, Litwack TR. Psychiatry and the presumption of expertise: flipping a coin in the courtyard. Calif Law Rev. 1974;62:693–752.
29. Appelbaum PS. Ethics in evolution: the incompatibility of clinical and forensic functions. Am J Psychiatry. 1997;154(4):445–6.
30. Dernevik M. Structured clinical assessment and management of risk of violent recidivism in mentally disordered offenders [Internet]; 2004. http://publications.ki.se/xmlui/handle/10616/39264.
31. Buchanan A, Binder R, Norko M, Swartz M. Resource document on psychiatric violence risk assessment. Am J Psychiatry. 2011;169(3):340.
32. Singh JP, Fazel S. Forensic risk assessment: a metareview. Crim Justice Behav. 2010;67:965–8.
33. Monahan J, Steadman H, editors. Violence and mental disorder. Chicago, IL: Chicago University Press; 1994.
34. Walsh EL, Gilvarry C, Samele C, Harvey K, Manley C, Tattan T, Tyrer P, Creed F, Murray R, Fahy T. UK700 Group predicting violence in schizophrenia: a prospective study. Schizophr Res. 2004;67(2–3):247–52.
35. Klassen D, O'Connor WA. Demographic and case history variables in risk assessment deidre. In: Monahan J, Steadman H, editors. Violence and mental disorder. Chicago, IL: Chicago University Press. p. 1994.
36. Connor DF. Aggression and antisocial behavior in children and adolescent: research and treatment. New York: Guilford; 2002.
37. Millaud F, Roy R, Gendron P, Aubut J. Un inventaire pour l'evaluation de la dangerositè de patient psiquiatrique. Rev Can Psychiatry. 1992;37:608–11.
38. Taylor PJ, Gunn J. Homicides by people with mental illness: myth and reality. Br J Psychiatry. 1999;174:9–14.
39. Brennan PA, Mednick SA, Hodgins S. Mayor mental disorders and criminal violence in a Danish birth cohort. Arch Gen Psychiatry. 2000;57(5):494–500.

40. Wallace C, Mullen P, Burgess P, Palmer S, Ruschena D, Browne C. Serious criminal offending and mental disorder. Case linkage study. Br J Psychiatry. 1998;172:477–84.
41. Dubreucq JL, Joyal C, Millaud F. Risque de violence et troubles mentaux graves. Ann Med Psychol. 2005;163:852–65.
42. Senon JL, Manzanera C, Humeau M, Gotzamanis L. Les maladies mentaux sont-ils plus violents que les citoiens ordinaries? Inf Psychiatr. 2006;82:645–52.
43. Nivoli GC, Lorettu L, Milia P, Nivoli A: Psichiatria Forense. Piccin; 2019.
44. Fazel S, et al. Schizophrenia, substance abuse, and violent crime. JAMA. 2009; 301(19):2016–23.
45. Hodgins S. Mental disorder, intellectual deficiency and crime. Evidence from a birth cohort. Arch Gen Psychiatry. 1992;49(6):476–83.
46. Lewis ME, Scott DC, Baranoski MV, Buchanan JA, Grilith EE. Prototypes of intrafamily homicide and serious assault among insanity acquittees. J Am Acad Psychiatry Law. 1998;26:37–48.
47. Lindqvist P, Allebeck P. Schizophrenia and crime. A longitudinal follow-up of 644 schizophrenics in Stockholm. Br J Psychiatry. 1990;157:345–50.
48. Elbogen B, Johnson SC. The intricate link between violence and mental disorders. Arch Gen Psychiatry. 2009;66:152–61.
49. Pinna F, Tusconi M, Dessi C, Pittaliga G, Fiorillo A, Carpiniello B. Violence and mental disorders. A retrospective study of people in charge of a community mental health center. Int J Law Psychiatry. 2016;47:122–8.
50. Brennan PA, Mednick SA, Hodgins S. Major mental disorders and criminal violence in a Danish birth cohort. Arch Gen Psychiatry. 2000;57(5):494–500.
51. Benezee M, Lebihan P, Burgos ML. Criminologie et psychiatrie. EMC. 2002 37-906-A-10:1–15.
52. Erb M, Hodgins S, Freese R, Moller Isberner R, Jockel D. Homicide and schizophrenia: maybe treatment does have a preventive effect. Crim Behav Ment Health. 2001;11(1):6–26.
53. Appelbaum PS, Robbins PC, Monahan J. Violence and delusions data from the MacArthur Violence Risk Assessment Study. Am J Psychiatry. 2000;157(4):566–72.
54. Marleau JD, Millaud F, Auclair N. A comparison of parricide and attempted parricide: a study of 3 psychotic adults. Int J Law Psychiatry. 2003;26(3):269–79.
55. Millaud F, Dubreucq JL. Evaluation de la dangerositè du malad mental psicotique. Ann Med Psychol. 2005;163:846–51. Dangerousness evaluation of psychotic patient: introduction.
56. Voyer M, Senon JL, Paillard C, Jaafari N. Dangerosite psiquiatrique et predictivite. Inf Psychiatr. 2009;85(8):745–52.
57. Esteve D. Y a-t-il une prévention du parricide psicotique? Perspectives Psiquiatriques. 2003;42(1):56–62.
58. de Vogel V, de Vries Robbé M, de Ruiter C, Bouman YH. Assessing protective factors in forensic psychiatric practice: introducing the SAPROF. Int J Forensic Ment Health. 2011;10:171–7.
59. Moore G, Plaff J. Assessment and emergency management of the acutely agitated or violent adult; 2017. https://www.upresearchgate.net >publication.
60. Simon R, Tardiff K. Textbook of violence assessment and management. Arlington, VA: American Psychiatric Publishing, Inc.; 2008.
61. Nivoli G, Lorettu L, Milia P, Nivoli A. La valutazione clinica del paziente con disturbo mentale e comportamento violento sulle persone. Giornale Italiano di Psicopatologia. 2008;14(4):396–412. ISSN:1592-1107.
62. Hobbs FDR, Keane UM. Aggression against doctors: a review. J Med. 1996;89:69–72.
63. Ellis GL, Dehart DA, Black C, et al. ED security: a national telephone survey. Am J Emerg Med. 1994;12:155.
64. Ordog GJ, Wasserberger J, Ordog C, et al. Weapon carriage among major trauma victims in the emergency department. Acad Emerg Med. 1995;2:109.
65. Preventing workplace violence. Tips for safety in emergency departments and psychiatric hospitals. Environment of Care News, published by Joint Commission Resources 2008;11:4.
66. Nivoli GC, Lorettu L, Milia P, et al. Vittimologia e Psichiatria Ediermes CSE Torino; 2010.

67. Erkol H, Gökdoğan MR, Erkol Z, Boz B. Aggression and violence towards health care providers—a problem in Turkey? J Forensic Leg Med. 2007;14(7):423–8.
68. Lorettu L, Sanna N, Nivoli GC. Le passage a l'acte, homicide du schizophrène. In: Millaud F, editor. Le passage a l'acte. Masson Papis; 2009.
69. Lorettu L. Le reazioni emotive al paziente violento: difficoltà diagnostiche e terapeutiche. CSE Torino; 2000.
70. Van Dorn R, Volavka J, Johnson N. Mental disorder and violence: is there a relationship beyond substance use? Soc Psychiatry Psychiatr Epidemiol. 2011;47:487–503. https://doi.org/10.1007/s00127-011-0356-x.
71. Friedman RA. Violence and mental illness—how strong is the link? N Engl J Med. 2006;355(20):2064–6.

Psychopharmacology of Violent Behavior Among People with Severe Mental Disorders

14

Leslie Citrome and Jan Volavka

14.1 Introduction

The psychopharmacological management of violent behavior among persons with psychosis involves several steps. Of immediate clinical concern is the acute management of agitation and aggression, followed by the long-term prevention of agitation and aggression. The acute management of agitation and aggression is simple to understand and the psychopharmacological interventions available span a wide array of different agents and formulations. Long-term management is complicated by the heterogenous nature of the causes of aggressive behavior [1, 2]. For example, a person who is psychotic may be aggressive in direct reaction to their delusions and hallucinations, or they may be suffering from poor impulse control and responding to a relatively minor stressor such as being told not to smoke in a nonsmoking area. In addition, despite being psychotic, a person with psychopathy may use violence instrumentally for personal or financial gain.

The terms aggression and violence, although similar, are not entirely synonymous [3]. Aggression has been described as overt noxious or destructive behavior and has been studied in both animals and humans. Violence denotes aggression among humans. Hostility is another matter; in addition to overt aggression, it may include temper tantrums, irritability, refusal to cooperate, jealousy, suspicion, and many other attitudes and behaviors. Rating scales such as the Positive and Negative Syndrome Scale (PANSS) define hostility as "verbal and nonverbal expressions of

L. Citrome (✉)
Department of Psychiatry and Behavioral Sciences, New York Medical College,
Valhalla, NY, USA
e-mail: citrome@cnsconsultant.com

J. Volavka
Department of Psychiatry, Faculty of Medicine and University Hospital in Pilsen, Charles University, Pilsen, Czech Republic

Department of Psychiatry, New York University School of Medicine, New York, NY, USA

© Springer Nature Switzerland AG 2020
B. Carpiniello et al. (eds.), *Violence and Mental Disorders*, Comprehensive
Approach to Psychiatry 1, https://doi.org/10.1007/978-3-030-33188-7_14

anger and resentment, including sarcasm, passive-aggressive behavior, verbal abuse, and assaultiveness" and is evaluated by "interpersonal behavior observed during the interview and reports by primary care workers or family" [4]. Moreover, the PANSS Hostility item can be rated as high as 6 (maximum score is 7) and yet the patient may not be physically assaultive toward others. These definitions will affect how we can interpret the studies done regarding the pharmacological management of violent behavior among people with severe mental disorders. The bulk of available data relates to people with schizophrenia.

14.2 Short-Term Pharmacotherapy of Agitation and Aggression

Agitation is a heterogeneous syndrome with varying causations and presentations and is responsible for almost 2 million annual visits to emergency departments in the USA alone [5]. Broadly, agitation can be defined as abnormal, excessive motor and verbal activity [6]. When agitation evolves into aggression, it can result in patient and staff injury, and should be considered a medical and psychiatric emergency [7]. Agitation is common during the acute phase of treatment of schizophrenia and bipolar disorder and can be a significant obstacle to care in the emergency department and on an inpatient unit [8]. As such, pharmacological interventions specifically indicated for the treatment of agitation associated with schizophrenia or bipolar mania have become available and will be the focus of this section of the chapter.

Pharmacological options to manage agitation have mainly consisted of antipsychotic medications, with or without benzodiazepines. However, somatic causes of agitation may preclude the use of antipsychotic medication such as acute withdrawal from alcohol or benzodiazepines (which can be comorbid with an exacerbation of schizophrenia or bipolar mania), for which the preferred medication intervention would be a benzodiazepine alone because administration of an antipsychotic may induce a seizure. It is assumed that non-pharmacological techniques are also being utilized, such as verbal de-escalation [9]. Routes of administration include oral, parenteral (principally intramuscular but in some situations intravenous), and more recently available inhalation [10]. Treatment goals include calming the agitated patient as rapidly as possible (without excessive sedation), decreasing the likelihood of harm to self or others, allowing the performance of diagnostic tests and procedures, attenuating psychosis, and decreasing the need for seclusion or restraint (a time where staff and patient injury can occur) [11]. Table 14.1 outlines the characteristics of selected anti-agitation medications.

When offered and accepted by the patient, oral medications have the benefit of being noninvasive but can be slow in onset of action. This is mitigated in part by the patient feeling cared for and engaged in treatment. Concern over covert nonadherence by not swallowing the pill can be addressed by using liquid or orally disintegrating tablets which have been available for many different antipsychotic medications as well as some benzodiazepines, with access differing across countries. An orally administered option that deserves special mention is sublingual

Table 14.1 Characteristics of selected oral, intramuscular, intravenous, and inhaled medications used for agitation [adapted with permission from Faden J, Citrome L. Examining the safety, efficacy, and patient acceptability of inhaled loxapine for the acute treatment of agitation associated with schizophrenia or bipolar I disorder in adults. Neuropsychiatr Dis Treat. 2019;15:2273–2283]

Medication	Dosage (mg)	T_{max}^a	Advantages	Disadvantages
Oral				
Lorazepam	0.5–2	20–30	No active metabolites. Can treat comorbid alcohol/benzodiazepine withdrawal. Can be combined with antipsychotic for synergistic effects	No antipsychotic effect. Can cause respiratory depression. Can be misused by persons with addictive disorders. In the presence of physiological tolerance, diminished efficacy may be observed. Paradoxical behavioral disinhibition risk
Haloperidol	5–10	2–6 h	Reduces and treats psychosis. Can be given with benzodiazepines. Inexpensive	Risk of akathisia and dystonic reactions
Risperidone	2	60	Reduces and treats psychosis. Also available as an ODT and liquid formulation. Low risk of EPS compared to FGAs. Can be given with benzodiazepines	Higher rate of dystonic reactions than other SGAs
Olanzapine	5–10	5–8 h	Reduces and treats psychosis. Also available as an ODT. Low risk of EPS compared to FGAs	Can cause excess sedation and adverse effects when given concurrently with benzodiazepines—combination should be avoided
Asenapine	10	30–90	Sublingual administration. Absorbed in the oral mucosa. Low risk of diversion. Low risk of EPS compared to FGAs	Low bioavailability if swallowed. Side effects of oral hypoesthesia and dysgeusia. No food or fluids for 2–10 min after administration
Intramuscular				
Lorazepam	0.5–2	20–30	No active metabolites. Can treat comorbid alcohol/benzodiazepine withdrawal. Can be combined with antipsychotic for synergistic effects	No antipsychotic effect. Can cause respiratory depression. Can be abused in addiction. Paradoxical behavioral disinhibition risk
Haloperidol	2–10	20–60	Reduces and treats psychosis. Can be given with benzodiazepines. Inexpensive	Risk of akathisia and dystonic reactions

(continued)

Table 14.1 (continued)

Medication	Dosage (mg)	T_{max}[a]	Advantages	Disadvantages
Ziprasidone	10–20	15–60	Reduces and treats psychosis. Low risk of EPS compared to FGAs. Can be given with benzodiazepines	QTc prolongation. Caution in patients with impaired renal function because the excipient is cleared by renal filtration
Olanzapine	10	15–45	Reduces and treats psychosis. Low risk of EPS compared to FGAs	Concomitant administration with a benzodiazepine can result in excessive sedation and cardiorespiratory depression
Aripiprazole	9.75	1–3 h	Reduces and treats psychosis. Low risk of EPS compared to FGAs	Rates of sedation and orthostatic hypotension are greater when administered with benzodiazepines. No longer available in the USA
Intravenous				
Haloperidol	2–5 or higher	Immediate	Near-immediate onset of action	Requires venous access. Increases risk of QT prolongation and torsades de pointes. Requires cardiac monitoring
Inhaled				
Loxapine	10	2	Fast onset. High patient acceptability	Can't be given in the presence of airway/lung disease. Dysgeusia. Requires cooperation. Cost

EPS Acute extrapyramidal symptoms, *FGA* First-generation antipsychotic, *GI* Gastrointestinal, *ODT* Orally disintegrating tablet, *SGA* Second-generation antipsychotic

[a]Time to maximum concentration in minutes unless stated otherwise

asenapine; in contrast to all other orally disintegrating tablets, sublingual asenapine is absorbed in the oral mucosa and thus has a more rapid uptake into the blood than the other agents that are absorbed further on in the gastrointestinal tract and subject to first-pass metabolism [12]. When assessed in a randomized placebo-controlled clinical trial at a single study site, one dose of asenapine 10 mg resulted in reduction of agitation with an effect size similar to what can be observed with intramuscular options [13].

Intramuscular administration results in reliable absorption into the systemic circulation, thus bypassing the gastrointestinal system. When necessary, intramuscular medications can be administered over the patient's objections; however, without adequate staff and training, needlestick injuries may occur. The principal disadvantages of this route of administration are that it is invasive, can be perceived as coercive, and can be painful. Patient rapport and therapeutic alliance can be damaged. Nonetheless, by entering the systemic circulation through the muscle's vasculature, these formulations provide faster absorption, bioavailability, and a more rapid onset of action when compared with oral medications [14–16]. Of clinical importance, injections of antipsychotics into the muscle can lead to higher rates of acute extrapyramidal symptoms such as acute dystonia and acute akathisia; these adverse reactions are more common with first-generation antipsychotics such as haloperidol compared to second-generation antipsychotics [17, 18]. The experience of an acute dystonic reaction may result in the patient being unwilling to take antipsychotic medications in the future [14]. A caveat regarding the use of intramuscular benzodiazepines such as lorazepam and diazepam is that they can lead to respiratory depression, especially in those with lung disease or sleep apnea. Despite the long list of potential problems with intramuscular administration of anti-agitation agents, this intervention remains generally effective in rapidly reducing agitation and consequently reduces the immediate risk of further escalation to aggressive behavior.

Combining intramuscular agents has long been commonly employed, such as the combination of haloperidol and lorazepam, which is supported in part by clinical trial evidence reported over 20 years ago [19]. Of interest when oral medications are being considered, liquid risperidone 2 mg combined with oral lorazepam 2 mg had a comparable therapeutic effect when compared with combined intramuscularly administered haloperidol 5 mg with lorazepam 2 mg in a convenience sample of willing participants [20] and in a larger prospective randomized study [21].

Inhalation is a newer means of delivering an anti-agitation agent and inhalation to the deep lung is how inhaled loxapine results in very rapid absorption, reaching a peak plasma concentration in 2 min [22]. Inhaled loxapine is administered using a handheld, single-use, breath-activated device and no special breathing or hand/breath coordination is required [23]. Inhaled loxapine has a prominent warning for bronchospasm, and in the USA it requires a Risk Evaluation and Mitigation Strategy (REMS) as mandated by the US Food and Drug Administration [10]. Inhaled loxapine requires patient cooperation to administer and thus it may not be an appropriate choice for persons exhibiting severe levels of agitation.

On the horizon is an intranasal formulation of powdered olanzapine that is in development for the treatment of agitation. The delivery of olanzapine is to the vascular rich upper nasal space rather than the deep lung, resulting in a pharmaco-kinetic profile somewhat faster than that observed with intramuscular injection [24].

14.3 Long-Term Pharmacotherapy of Violence in Psychosis

In most cases, one or more of the pharmacological treatments for acute agitation and aggression described in the preceding segment of this chapter will be effective. However, in a minority of patients, aggressive behavior will persist. The pharmaco-therapy options in that situation have recently been reviewed elsewhere [11]; here we provide a brief update and a reconsideration of several issues.

14.3.1 Clozapine

In 1993, clozapine was found to reduce hostility and aggression in an observa-tional study of 223 treatment-resistant schizophrenia patients [25]. Since that time, randomized controlled trials have demonstrated clozapine's superior effects against hostility [26] and aggression [27] in comparison with several other antipsychotics.

A recent report compared the effects of clozapine and olanzapine on violent offending. Swedish registries were used to study 1004 patients treated with clozap-ine and 2258 patients treated with olanzapine [28]. All patients were diagnosed with a psychotic disorder (F20-F29, *ICD-10*). A within-person mirror image approach was used to compare offending before and after initiation of clozapine or olanzapine treatment. The results showed that clozapine treatment led to greater reduction in violent offending than olanzapine. This was not true for nonviolent offending.

Clozapine has adverse effects that limit its use. *Agranulocytosis* poses the prin-cipal risk of clozapine use, developing in approximately 1% of the treated patients [29]. *Metabolic abnormalities* and *weight gain* are well-known adverse effects of clozapine.

Myocarditis is a dangerous and difficult-to-diagnose adverse effect developing mostly in the first month of clozapine treatment [30]. A study reported 231 cases of combined clozapine-induced myocarditis and cardiomyopathy out of 24,730 patients on clozapine (0.93%) [31]. A recent review has identified 23 case reports of clozapine-associated *pulmonary embolism* [32]. This complication developed mostly during the first 6–7 weeks of treatment, and it appeared independent of the clozapine dose. It is well known that in some patients, clozapine causes *orthostatic hypotension* at the beginning of treatment; this may necessitate a slower dose esca-lation rate. However, rarely it may cause *hypertension*.

Constipation is a frequent adverse effect of clozapine. In a recent record review study, 4 of 188 patients who were prescribed clozapine developed ileus requiring hospital admission, and 2 of these needed a permanent stoma. In 154 patients who had complete records, 41% either had laxatives prescribed or had constipation doc-umented in medical records [33]. Clozapine may cause tonic-clonic *seizures*, which develop in approximately 0.2% of the treated patients [34]. The risk increases with clozapine dose.

Thus, clozapine is the most effective treatment of violence in psychosis, but its use is limited by adverse effects. Some of these adverse effects are potentially lethal. However, appropriate blood (and other) monitoring makes the treatment quite safe. When treating a persistently violent psychotic patient, one should weigh the danger of adverse effects of clozapine against the danger of potentially less effective treatment with another medication instead of clozapine. The prescriber should keep in mind that clozapine treatment was associated with *lower* mortality rate than any other antipsychotic in a large epidemiological study [35].

14.3.2 Olanzapine

In post hoc analyses of the European First-Episode Schizophrenia Trial (EUFEST), olanzapine showed significantly superior effects against hostility in comparison with haloperidol, quetiapine, and amisulpride in early phases of treatment [36]. Similar results were demonstrated by post hoc analyses of the Clinical Antipsychotic Trials of Intervention Effectiveness (CATIE) [37]. Olanzapine exhibited significantly superior effects against hostility in comparisons with perphenazine, quetiapine, ziprasidone, and risperidone at various time points during the first 18 months (Phase 1) of the CATIE. In both EUFEST and CATIE, hostility was assessed using the eponymous PANSS item. In general, PANSS Hostility has a significant relationship to overt physical aggression [38], and is sometimes used as its proxy measure.

Patients participating in the EUFEST and CATIE studies were not selected for being hostile or aggressive. This limits their usefulness for examining such problems. However, another study did specifically study aggression and enrolled violent patients diagnosed with schizophrenia and schizoaffective disorder [27]. Clozapine showed greater efficacy than olanzapine and olanzapine demonstrated greater efficacy than haloperidol in reducing overt aggressive behavior.

Olanzapine can cause weight gain and metabolic abnormalities. A recent review of second-generation antipsychotics focused on population metabolic outcomes such as type 2 diabetes mellitus, dyslipidemia, obesity, hypertension, or metabolic outcome [39]. Both clozapine and olanzapine were strongly associated with the risk of developing type 2 diabetes. Thus, superiority of olanzapine's efficacy needs to be weighed against its metabolic consequences in treating individual patients.

14.3.3 Other Atypical Antipsychotics

Risperidone effects on hostility and aggression were tested in several studies with inconsistent results [40–42]. Efficacy of *aripiprazole* against hostility was superior to placebo and not significantly different from haloperidol in combined post hoc analyses of several short-term, double-blind studies [43]. *Aripiprazole lauroxil*, a long-acting injectable (LAI) formulation, was effective against agitation and hostility in comparison with placebo [44]. This antihostility effect appeared independent of a general antipsychotic effect. *Ziprasidone* was superior to haloperidol in its effect against hostility only in the first week of a 6-week trial [45]. Effects of *olanzapine, quetiapine, risperidone, and perphenazine* against overt physical aggression were compared during the first 6 months of the CATIE study mentioned above. No difference between the medications was found, except that *perphenazine* showed greater aggression reduction than quetiapine [46]. Effects of lurasidone on hostility were examined in patients with an acute exacerbation of schizophrenia in a pooled post hoc analysis of five short-term studies.

Lurasidone provided rapid improvement of hostility that was superior to placebo. The effect was independent of other positive symptoms and the presence of somnolence and akathisia [47]. Effects of *cariprazine* on the PANSS Hostility item in schizophrenia patients were significantly superior to placebo, and this superiority appeared independent of positive symptoms and sedation [48]. Interestingly, the magnitude of improvement increased with greater baseline hostility, suggesting that cariprazine may be particularly appropriate for very hostile patients. *Brexpiprazole* was significantly superior to placebo in reducing agitation and hostility in patients with schizophrenia in two 6-week, randomized, double-blind, placebo-controlled studies [49]. These were followed by a 52-week, open-label, extension study, during which the improvements were maintained [49]. The effect on hostility was statistically independent of other positive symptoms.

Most of the above studies share certain limitations. The studies were post hoc, having been designed to study general antipsychotic efficacy rather than specifically agitation and hostility. Their goal was to prove efficacy in comparison to placebo rather than an active comparator. Furthermore, participants were not selected for aggressive and hostile behavior. Some of the studies also excluded patients with substance-use disorder. This represents a serious limit to the generalizability of their results, since alcohol and substance use are well known to increase risk for hostility and aggression. Nevertheless, the repeated demonstrations of the specificity of antihostility effect (in terms of statistical independence of effects on other positive symptoms and of somnolence) are of potential clinical importance and worthy of future basic research to study the mechanism(s) underlying this specificity. We do not know yet how these newer atypical antipsychotics will be positioned in the armamentarium of treatments for hostility and aggression in psychosis. To answer that question, studies using active comparators are urgently needed.

14.3.4 Augmentation Strategies

Nadolol, pindolol, and other beta-adrenergic blockers have antiaggressive properties, but their use is limited because they considerably lower blood pressure and pulse rate [50–52]. Anticonvulsants or lithium is sometimes prescribed as an augmentation treatment of aggressive behavior in schizophrenia despite weak evidence of effectiveness [53].

Recent evidence suggests that augmentation of clozapine with other medications, particularly aripiprazole, enhances clozapine's effect on reducing rehospitalization in patients with schizophrenia. The evidence was based on a nationwide cohort study conducted in Finland [54]. The cohort included 62,250 patients. The hazard ratio (HR) for rehospitalization with clozapine monotherapy was 0.49 (0.47–0.51), and for clozapine with aripiprazole HR = 0.42 (0.39–0.46). The difference between the two HRs is statistically significant. Statistical significance does not necessarily imply clinical importance, and the effect on rehospitalization may be different than an effect on aggression. The effect of clozapine-aripiprazole combination should be studied in violent schizophrenia patients.

14.3.5 Asenapine in Bipolar I Manic or Mixed Episodes

In bipolar I patients with manic or mixed episodes, asenapine significantly reduced hostility and agitation in comparison with placebo [55]. These effects were at least partially independent of overall improvement of manic symptoms.

14.4   Limitations of Long-Term Pharmacotherapy of Violence

14.4.1 Limited Effectiveness of Any Pharmacotherapy of Violence in Psychosis

Psychosis is a principal problem. The effectiveness of clozapine, the most effective medication for this indication, varies widely, with some patients failing to respond. Such variation of response can be observed even in studies of inpatients where adherence to treatment and other environmental effects are relatively well controlled, such as the Krakowski study [27]. As noted in the introduction, this variation may be partly due to heterogeneity of the origins of violence. There may be at least two alternative pathways to violence in schizophrenia—one associated with

Table 14.2 Univariate logistic regression models predicting aggressive behavior among patients with 0–2 positive symptoms ($N = 163$) and with more than two positive symptoms ($N = 88$)[a]

	0–2 positive symptoms		>2 positive symptoms	
	Odds ratio (95% CI)	Z (P-value)	Odds ratio (95% CI)	Z (P-value)
Clozapine	0.83 (0.32–2.13)	−0.38 (0.704)	**0.11 (0.01-0.89)**	**−2.06 (0.039)**
Medication nonadherence	1.65 (0.65–4.19)	1.06 (0.287)	**2.79 (1.08–7.25)**	**2.11 (0.035)**
Illicit drug use	**10.25 (3.97–26.47)**	**4.81 (0.000)**	1.65(0.61–4.47)	0.99 (0.322)
Conduct disorder symptoms	**1.26 (1.09–1.46)**	**3.14 (0.002)**	1.12 (0.92–1.37)	1.19 (0.232)

P-values < 0.05 were considered statistically significant
[a]Data abstracted from [57]

premorbid antisocial conduct, and another associated with acute psychopathology of schizophrenia [56]. Interestingly, adherence to antipsychotics significantly reduced violence only in the group without a history of conduct problems [46]. These findings were replicated in an observational study of patients with schizophrenia and schizoaffective disorder examined prior to discharge and 2 years later when they were living in the community [57]. As seen in Table 14.2, neither prescription of clozapine nor medication nonadherence had any significant effect on aggressive behavior in the subset of patients who had a low level of positive symptoms and history of conduct disorder that was associated with increased aggressive behavior. Conversely, patients with high level of positive symptoms responded to clozapine and nonadherence was associated with more aggressive behavior. Conduct disorder had no effect on aggressive behavior in this group.

Collectively, these findings [46, 56, 57] suggest that developmental history should become a part of clinical evaluation and treatment planning for psychotic patients who are violent. Psychosocial approaches should complement medication treatment for adult patients with a history of conduct disorder. Future research might reveal whether such approaches could lead to modification or perhaps even replacement of medication treatment for certain patients.

14.4.2 Comorbid Personality Disorders

Evidence of conduct disorder with onset before age 15 years is a DSM-5 diagnostic criterion of antisocial personality disorder (ASP). The diagnosis cannot be made before the individual is at least 18 years old. Thus, conduct disorder (discussed above) may develop into ASP. Repeated physical fights or assaults comprise one of the diagnostic criteria of ASP. In general, ASP is characterized by a pervasive pattern of disregard for the life of others.

Psychopathy is a narrower concept than ASP; most psychopaths meet the diagnostic criteria for ASP, but most individuals with ASP are not psychopaths. The current concept of psychopathy differs from ASP in its emphasis on psychological processes and personality traits [3]. Psychopathy is operationally defined by a checklist [58]. Psychopathy checklist features are related to violence in patients with schizophrenia spectrum disorders [59]. Comorbidity between schizophrenia and psychopathy is higher in violent than in nonviolent patients [60].

Management of comorbid psychopathy relies primarily on psychosocial interventions, including cognitive behavioral therapy [61]. Other methods are available [62].

14.4.3 Comorbid Substance-Use Disorders

Comorbidity between substance use and severe psychotic disorders was assessed in the genomic psychiatric cohort comprising 9142 individuals with psychotic disorders and 101,095 population controls [63]. Data on alcohol and substance use were obtained by interviewing the participating individuals. This case–control study estimated the OR for heavy alcohol use at 4.0 (CI 3.6–4.4), and for recreational drugs (except marijuana) at 4.62 (CI 4.27–4.99).

A review and meta-analysis of 20 studies reporting data from 18,423 individuals with schizophrenia and other psychoses compared with general population controls examined the effect of comorbid substance abuse on violence [64]. The effect of substance-abuse comorbidity was marked, with OR of 2.1 (CI 1.7–2.7) without comorbidity, and an OR of 8.9 (CI 5.4–14.7) with comorbidity. Notably, the risk for homicide in individuals with psychosis (with and without comorbid substance use) compared with general population was remarkably increased (OR = 19.5) (CI 14.7–25.8).

Thus, the detection and treatment of comorbid substance-use disorders are critically important for the prevention and treatment of violence in individuals diagnosed with psychosis.

14.4.4 Nonadherence to Medication

Nonadherence in psychosis is an important limitation of pharmacotherapy. It is well known to elevate the risk of violence (including homicide) [65] and relapse of psychosis. Patient-related causes of nonadherence include lack of insight and negative attitude toward medication, as well as co-occurring substance abuse and cognitive impairment. A patient-level meta-analysis combined data from 1991 psychosis patients to show that reduced adherence to medication treatment was associated with higher levels of hostility, substance use, and impaired insight [66]. Medication-related factors include the burden of adverse effects [67] and medication cost.

A recent study explored relationships between substance use (cannabis and nicotine), poor medication adherence, and non-remission in a sample of 205 patients with first-episode psychosis [68]. A path analysis has revealed that medication adherence lies on the causal pathway between substance use and non-remission. In other words, the level of adherence mediated the relationship between substance use and non-remission of psychosis.

Adherence is a modifiable factor. It can be improved and maintained by building therapeutic alliance, sensitive management of adverse effects, and family and social support. Administration of long-acting injectable antipsychotics to non-adherent psychotic violent patients improves adherence and thus leads to reductions of hostility, number of violent incidents, and criminal offenses [69].

14.4.5 Multiplicity of Interacting Problems

The limitations of pharmacotherapy are described separately, but they frequently occur concurrently in the same patients. Such multiplicity of problems complicates clinical management. With one exception [68], the studies do not examine how the limiting factors interact with each other. Understanding such interactions would improve our ability to care effectively for multiply affected patients. Future longitudinal prospective studies may help.

14.5 Summary

The acute management of agitated and aggressive behavior is often readily addressed with the use of verbal de-escalation techniques and the emergency use of antipsychotic medications, with or without benzodiazepines. Regulatory agencies have approved several short-acting injectable second-generation antipsychotics and an inhaled formulation of loxapine specifically for the treatment of agitation in persons with schizophrenia or bipolar mania. The long-term management of aggressive behavior is more complex as the causative factors for ongoing aggressive behavior are heterogenous. Persons may become aggressive because of psychosis, poor impulse control, or psychopathy. These factors may coexist in the same patient and their importance in influencing behavior may vary over time. Comorbidity with substance use is a further complicating factor, as is nonadherence to a foundational antipsychotic medication. Thus, a multipronged approach will often be necessary to reduce the risk of aggressive behavior in at-risk patients. Although clozapine is perhaps the optimal antipsychotic for its antiaggressive effects, clozapine use can be limited by tolerability and safety issues. Poor adherence to antipsychotic medication may be addressed with the use of a long-acting injectable formulation. Non-pharmacological strategies will be required to successfully address poor impulse control (pharmacological interventions do not have robust effects) and psychopathy (effective pharmacological options do not exist at present).

Acknowledgements *Disclosures:* No funding or writing assistance was utilized in the production of this book chapter. In the past 12 months, Leslie Citrome has served as a consultant to Acadia, Alkermes, Allergan, Avanir, BioXcel, Eisai, Impel, Indivior, Intra-Cellular Therapies, Janssen, Lundbeck, Luye, Merck, Neurocrine, Noven, Osmotica, Otsuka, Pfizer, Shire, Sunovion, Takeda, Teva, Vanda. In the past 12 months, Leslie Citrome has served as a speaker for Acadia, Alkermes, Allergan, Janssen, Lundbeck, Merck, Neurocrine, Otsuka, Pfizer, Sage, Shire, Sunovion, Takeda, Teva. Other disclosures: stocks (small number of shares of common stock): Bristol-Myers Squibb, Eli Lilly, J & J, Merck, and Pfizer purchased >10 years ago; royalties: Wiley (Editor-in-Chief, International Journal of Clinical Practice), UpToDate (reviewer), and Springer Healthcare (book). In the past 12 months, Jan Volavka has received no outside funding, and has no competing interest.

References

1. Volavka J, Citrome L. Heterogeneity of violence in schizophrenia and implications for long-term treatment. Int J Clin Pract. 2008;62(8):1237–45.
2. Volavka J, Citrome L. Pathways to aggression in schizophrenia affect results of treatment. Schizophr Bull. 2011;37(5):921–9.
3. Volavka J. Neurobiology of Violence. 2nd ed. Washington, DC: American Psychiatric Publishing, Inc.; 2002.
4. Kay SR, Fiszbein A, Opler LA. The positive and negative syndrome scale (PANSS) for schizophrenia. Schizophr Bull. 1987;13:261–76.
5. Allen MH, Currier GW. Use of restraints and pharmacotherapy in academic psychiatric emergency services. Gen Hosp Psychiatry. 2004;26(1):42–9.

6. Citrome L. Addressing the need for rapid treatment of agitation in schizophrenia and bipolar disorder: focus on inhaled loxapine as an alternative to injectable agents. Ther Clin Risk Manag. 2013;9:235–45.

7. Citrome L, Volavka J. Violent patients in the emergency setting. In: Bernstein CA, editor. The psychiatric clinics of North America emergency psychiatry. Philadelphia: W.B. Saunders Company; 1999. p. 789–801.

8. Garriga M, Pacchiarotti I, Kasper S, Zeller SL, Allen MH, Vazquez G, et al. Assessment and management of agitation in psychiatry: expert consensus. World J Biol Psychiatry. 2016;17(2):86–128.

9. Richmond JS, Berlin JS, Fishkind AB, Holloman GH Jr, Zeller SL, Wilson MP, et al. Verbal de-escalation of the agitated patient: consensus statement of the American Association for Emergency Psychiatry Project BETA De-escalation Workgroup. West J Emerg Med. 2012;13(1):17–25.

10. Faden J, Citrome L. Examining the safety, efficacy, and patient acceptability of inhaled loxapine for the acute treatment of agitation associated with schizophrenia or bipolar I disorder in adults. Neuropsychiatr Dis Treat. 2019;15:2273–83.

11. Citrome L, Volavka J. Aggression in primary psychotic disorders. In: Coccaro EF, McCloskey MS, editors. Aggression clinical features and treatment across the diagnostic spectrum. Washington, D.C.: American Psychiatric Association Publishing; 2019. p. 107–30.

12. Citrome L. Asenapine review, part 1: chemistry, receptor affinity, profile, pharmacokinetics and metabolism. Expert Opin Drug Metab Toxicol. 2014;10(6):893–903.

13. Pratts M, Citrome L, Grant W, Leso L, Opler LA. A single-dose, randomized, double-blind, placebo-controlled trial of sublingual asenapine for acute agitation. Acta Psychiatr Scand. 2014;130(1):61–8.

14. Zeller SL, Citrome L. Managing agitation associated with schizophrenia and bipolar disorder in the emergency setting. West J Emerg Med. 2016;17(2):165–72.

15. Ng AT, Zeller SL, Rhoades RW. Clinical challenges in the pharmacological management of agitation. Prim Psychiatry. 2010;17(8):46–52.

16. Currier GW, Medori R. Orally versus intramuscularly administered antipsychotic drugs in psychiatric emergencies. J Psychiatr Pract. 2006;12(1):30–40.

17. Citrome L. Comparison of intramuscular ziprasidone, olanzapine, or aripiprazole for agitation: a quantitative review of efficacy and safety. J Clin Psychiatry. 2007;68(12):1876–85.

18. Satterthwaite TD, Wolf DH, Rosenheck RA, Gur RE, Caroff SN. A meta-analysis of the risk of acute extrapyramidal symptoms with intramuscular antipsychotics for the treatment of agitation. J Clin Psychiatry. 2008;69(12):1869–79.

19. Battaglia J, Moss S, Rush J, Kang J, Mendoza R, Leedom L, et al. Haloperidol, lorazepam, or both for psychotic agitation? A multicenter, prospective, double-blind, emergency department study. Am J Emerg Med. 1997;15(4):335–40.

20. Currier GW, Simpson GM. Risperidone liquid concentrate and oral lorazepam versus intramuscular haloperidol and intramuscular lorazepam for treatment of psychotic agitation. J Clin Psychiatry. 2001;62(3):153–7.

21. Currier GW, Chou JC, Feifel D, Bossie CA, Turkoz I, Mahmoud RA, et al. Acute treatment of psychotic agitation: a randomized comparison of oral treatment with risperidone and lorazepam versus intramuscular treatment with haloperidol and lorazepam. J Clin Psychiatry. 2004;65(3):386–94.

22. Spyker DA, Munzar P, Cassella JV. Pharmacokinetics of loxapine following inhalation of a thermally generated aerosol in healthy volunteers. J Clin Pharmacol. 2010;50(2):169–79.

23. Noymer P, Myers D, Glazer M. The Stacatto system: inhaler design characteristics for rapid treatment of CNS disorders. Resp Drug Deliv. 2010;1:11–20.

24. Shrewsbury SB, Swardstrom M, Satterly KH, Campbell J, Hocevar-Trnka J, Tugiono N, Gillies JD, Houekman J. SNAP 101: randomized, crossover, active placebo-controlled, safety and pharmacodynamic study of 3 ascending doses of POD olanzapine. American Psychiatric Association (APA) Annual Meeting, 18–22 May 2019, San Francisco, California, USA; 2019.

25. Volavka J, Zito JM, Vitrai J, Czobor P. Clozapine effects on hostility and aggression in schizophrenia. J Clin Psychopharmacol. 1993;13:287–9.
26. Citrome L, Volavka J, Czobor P, Sheitman B, Lindenmayer J-P, McEvoy J, et al. Effects of clozapine, olanzapine, risperidone, and haloperidol on hostility in treatment-resistant patients with schizophrenia and schizoaffective disorder. Psychiatr Serv. 2001;52:1510–4.
27. Krakowski MI, Czobor P, Citrome L, Bark N, Cooper TB. Atypical antipsychotic agents in the treatment of violent patients with schizophrenia and schizoaffective disorder. Arch Gen Psychiatry. 2006;63(6):622–9.
28. Bhavsar V, Kosidou K, Widman L, Orsini N, Hodsoll J, Dalman C, et al. Clozapine treatment and offending: a within-subject study of patients with psychotic disorders in Sweden. Schizophr Bull. 2019. pii: sbz055. [Epub ahead of print]; https://doi.org/10.1093/schbul/sbz055.
29. Citrome L, McEvoy JP, Saklad SRA. guide to the management of clozapine-related tolerability and safety concerns. Clin Schizophr Relat Psychoses. 2016;10(3):163–77.
30. Bellissima BL, Tingle MD, Cicovic A, Alawami M, Kenedi C. A systematic review of clozapine-induced myocarditis. Int J Cardiol. 2018;259:122–9.
31. Coulter DM, Bate A, Meyboom RH, Lindquist M, Edwards IR. Antipsychotic drugs and heart muscle disorder in international pharmacovigilance: data mining study. BMJ. 2001;322(7296):1207–9.
32. Sarvaiya N, Lapitskaya Y, Dima L, Manu P. Clozapine-associated pulmonary embolism: a high-mortality, dose-independent and early-onset adverse effect. Am J Ther. 2018;25(4):e434–e8.
33. Ingimarsson O, MacCabe JH, Sigurdsson E. Constipation, ileus and medication use during clozapine treatment in patients with schizophrenia in Iceland. Nord J Psychiatry. 2018;72(7):497–500.
34. Druschky K, Bleich S, Grohmann R, Engel RR, Neyazi A, Stubner S, et al. Seizure rates under treatment with antipsychotic drugs: data from the AMSP project. World J Biol Psychiatry. 2018:1–10. https://doi.org/10.1080/15622975.2018.1500030.
35. Tiihonen J, Lonnqvist J, Wahlbeck K, Klaukka T, Niskanen L, Tanskanen A, et al. 11-year follow-up of mortality in patients with schizophrenia: a population-based cohort study (FIN11 study). Lancet. 2009;374(9690):620–7.
36. Volavka J, Czobor P, Derks EM, Bitter I, Libiger J, Kahn RS, et al. Efficacy of antipsychotic drugs against hostility in the European First-Episode Schizophrenia Trial (EUFEST). J Clin Psychiatry. 2011;72(7):955–61.
37. Volavka J, Czobor P, Citrome L, Van Dorn RA. Effectiveness of antipsychotic drugs against hostility in patients with schizophrenia in the Clinical Antipsychotic Trials of Intervention Effectiveness (CATIE) study. CNS Spectr. 2014;19(5):374–81.
38. Swanson JW, Swartz MS, Van Dorn RA, Elbogen EB, Wagner HR, Rosenheck RA, et al. A national study of violent behavior in persons with schizophrenia. Arch Gen Psychiatry. 2006;63(5):490–9.
39. Hirsch L, Yang J, Bresee L, Jette N, Patten S, Pringsheim T. Second-generation antipsychotics and metabolic side effects: a systematic review of population-based studies. Drug Saf. 2017;40(9):771–81.
40. Czobor P, Volavka J, Meibach RC. Effect of risperidone on hostility in schizophrenia. J Clin Psychopharmacol. 1995;15:243–9.
41. Beck NC, Greenfield SR, Gotham H, Menditto AA, Stuve P, Hemme CA. Risperidone in the management of violent, treatment-resistant schizophrenics hospitalized in a maximum security forensic facility. J Am Acad Psychiatry Law. 1997;25:461–8.
42. Buckley PF, Ibrahim ZY, Singer B, Orr B, Donenwirth K, Brar PS. Aggression and schizophrenia: efficacy of risperidone. J Am Psychiatry Law. 1997;25:173–81.
43. Volavka J, Czobor P, Citrome L, McQuade RD, Carson WH, Kostic D, et al. Efficacy of aripiprazole against hostility in schizophrenia and schizoaffective disorder: data from 5 double-blind studies. J Clin Psychiatry. 2005;66(11):1362–6.

44. Citrome L, Du Y, Risinger R, Stankovic S, Claxton A, Zummo J, et al. Effect of aripiprazole lauroxil on agitation and hostility in patients with schizophrenia. Int Clin Psychopharmacol. 2016;31(2):69–75.
45. Citrome L, Volavka J, Czobor P, Brook S, Loebel A, Mandel FS. Efficacy of ziprasidone against hostility in schizophrenia: post hoc analysis of randomized, open-label study data. J Clin Psychiatry. 2006;67(4):638–42.
46. Swanson JW, Swartz MS, Van Dorn RA, Volavka J, Monahan J, Stroup TS, et al. Comparison of antipsychotic medication effects on reducing violence in people with schizophrenia. Br J Psychiatry. 2008;193(1):37–43.
47. Citrome L, Pikalov A, Tocco M, Hsu J, Loebel A. Effects of lurasidone on hostility in patients with an acute exacerbation of schizophrenia: a pooled post-hoc analysis of five short-term studies. Neuropsychopharmacology 2014;39(S1):5379.
48. Citrome L, Durgam S, Lu K, Ferguson P, Laszlovszky I. The effect of cariprazine on hostility associated with schizophrenia: post hoc analyses from 3 randomized controlled trials. J Clin Psychiatry. 2016;77(1):109–15.
49. Citrome L, Ouyang J, Shi L, Meehan SR, Baker RA, Weiss C. Effect of Brexpiprazole on Agitation and Hostility in Patients With Schizophrenia: Post Hoc Analysis of Short- and Long-Term Studies. J Clin Psychopharmacol. 2019;39(6):in press.
50. Alpert M, Allan ER, Citrome L, Laury G, Sison C, Sudilovsky A. A double-blind, placebo-controlled study of adjunctive nadolol in the management of violent psychiatric patients. Psychopharmacol Bull. 1990;26(3):367–71.
51. Caspi N, Modai I, Barak P, Waisbourd A, Zbarsky H, Hirschmann S, et al. Pindolol augmentation in aggressive schizophrenic patients: a double-blind crossover randomized study. Int Clin Psychopharmacol. 2001;16(2):111–5.
52. Ratey JJ, Sorgi P, O'Driscoll GA, Sands S, Daehler ML, Fletcher JR, et al. Nadolol to treat aggression and psychiatric symptomatology in chronic psychiatric inpatients: a double-blind, placebo-controlled study. J Clin Psychiatry. 1992;53(2):41–6.
53. Citrome L. Adjunctive lithium and anticonvulsants for the treatment of schizophrenia: what is the evidence? Expert Rev Neurother. 2009;9(1):55–71.
54. Tiihonen J, Taipale H, Mehtala J, Vattulainen P, Correll CU, Tanskanen A. Association of antipsychotic polypharmacy vs. monotherapy with psychiatric rehospitalization among adults with schizophrenia. JAMA Psychiat. 2019;76(5):499–507.
55. Citrome L, Landbloom R, Chang CT, Earley W. Effects of asenapine on agitation and hostility in adults with acute manic or mixed episodes associated with bipolar I disorder. Neuropsychiatr Dis Treat. 2017;13:2955–63.
56. Swanson JW, Van Dorn RA, Swartz MS, Smith A, Elbogen EB, Monahan J. Alternative pathways to violence in persons with schizophrenia: the role of childhood antisocial behavior problems. Law Hum Behav. 2008;32(3):228–40.
57. Hodgins S, Riaz M. Violence and phases of illness: differential risk and predictors. Eur Psychiatry. 2011;26(8):518–24.
58. Neumann CS, Johansson PT, Hare RD. The Psychopathy Checklist-Revised (PCL-R), low anxiety, and fearlessness: a structural equation modeling analysis. Personal Disord. 2013;4(2):129–37.
59. McGregor K, Castle D, Dolan M. Schizophrenia spectrum disorders, substance misuse, and the four-facet model of psychopathy: the relationship to violence. Schizophr Res. 2012;136(1-3):116–21.
60. Nolan KA, Volavka J, Mohr P, Czobor P. Psychopathy and violent behavior among patients with schizophrenia or schizoaffective disorder. Psychiatr Serv. 1999;50:787–92.
61. Yates KF, Kunz M, Khan A, Volavka J, Rabinowitz S. Psychiatric patients with histories of aggression and crime five years after discharge from a cognitive-behavioral program. J Forensic Psychiatry Psychol. 2010;21(2):167–88.
62. Wong SC, Olver ME. Risk reduction treatment of psychopathy and applications to mentally disordered offenders. CNS Spectr. 2015;20(3):303–10.

63. Hartz SM, Pato CN, Medeiros H, Cavazos-Rehg P, Sobell JL, Knowles JA, et al. Comorbidity of severe psychotic disorders with measures of substance use. JAMA Psychiat. 2014;71:248–54.
64. Fazel S, Gulati G, Linsell L, Geddes JR, Grann M. Schizophrenia and violence: systematic review and meta-analysis. PLoS Med. 2009;6(8):e1000120.
65. Fazel S, Buxrud P, Ruchkin V, Grann M. Homicide in discharged patients with schizophrenia and other psychoses: a national case-control study. Schizophr Res. 2010;123(2-3):263–9.
66. Czobor P, Van Dorn RA, Citrome L, Kahn RS, Fleischhacker WW, Volavka J. Treatment adherence in schizophrenia: a patient-level meta-analysis of combined CATIE and EUFEST studies. Eur Neuropsychopharmacol. 2015;25(8):1158–66.
67. Velligan DI, Weiden PJ, Sajatovic M, Scott J, Carpenter D, Ross R, et al. The expert consensus guideline series: adherence problems in patients with serious and persistent mental illness. J Clin Psychiatry. 2009;70(Suppl 4):1–46.
68. Colizzi M, Carra E, Fraietta S, Lally J, Quattrone D, Bonaccorso S, et al. Substance use, medication adherence and outcome one year following a first episode of psychosis. Schizophr Res. 2016;170(2-3):311–7.
69. Mohr P, Knytl P, Vorackova V, Bravermanova A, Melicher T. Long-acting injectable antipsychotics for prevention and management of violent behaviour in psychotic patients. Int J Clin Pract. 2017;71(9):e12997.

Non-pharmacological Approaches to Violence Among People with Severe Mental Disorders

15

Antonio Vita, Valentina Stanga, Anna Ceraso, Giacomo Deste, and Stefano Barlati

15.1 Introduction

Violence and aggression committed by patients in healthcare settings is a global health concern and a clinical challenge [1]. Mental health and medical emergency departments are most frequently involved [2]. In mental health facilities, the association between severe mental illness (SMI) and aggressive behaviour has been widely documented in a number of settings, such as acute inpatient facilities, forensic mental hospitals and outpatient services [3–6]. Different types of aggression can be identified, each one possibly requiring targeted and individualised therapeutic approaches [7]. Aggression episodes can be verbal or physical; healthcare staff most frequently experience verbal aggression [8], but about one-third of mental health personnel reported episodes of physical violence against them [9]. Violence leads to short- and long-term physical and psychological harm for victims among medical staff, and has been linked to burnout [10], increased absenteeism [11] and interrupted patient care [12]. It may also have an impact on healthcare use and costs [13]. From a patient's perspective, aggression may cause hospital readmissions, prolonged hospital stays and heightened stigmatisation [7]. It should also be noted that aggressive behaviour in persons with SMI may be caused by multiple factors, each to be addressed by different and specific treatment interventions. Violence risk

A. Vita (✉) · S. Barlati
Department of Mental Health and Addiction Services, ASST Spedali Civili of Brescia, Brescia, Italy

Department of Clinical and Experimental Sciences, University of Brescia, Brescia, Italy
e-mail: antonio.vita@unibs.it

V. Stanga · G. Deste
Department of Mental Health and Addiction Services, ASST Spedali Civili of Brescia, Brescia, Italy

A. Ceraso
Department of Clinical and Experimental Sciences, University of Brescia, Brescia, Italy

factors include static determinants (i.e. sociodemographic variables, low socioeconomic status, diagnosis of schizophrenia or psychotic disorder, comorbid antisocial personality disorder, intellectual disability, involuntary admissions, history of violence or self-destructive behaviour) and dynamic aspects (lack of insight, low control of impulsivity, current substance use, non-compliance to treatment, context of clinical practice and living conditions) [7, 14]. The presence and relative influence of each factor may be widely variable from case to case, leading to the existence of a broadly heterogeneous population of mentally ill offenders. In particular, psychopathic traits emerged among the most relevant predictors of violence. However, there still is some scepticism about the possibility to treat psychopathy, based on outdated reports of psychopaths not improving or doing worse during treatment, whereas recent literature pointed out that some components of psychopathy can be captured using appropriate risk assessment tools and may be modified with an adequate treatment [15]. Interestingly, most violence acts carried out by individuals with SMI are committed when the offender is not taking medication [16, 17]. In fact, a meta-analysis showed that non-adherence to both pharmacological and psychological therapies was one of the strongest predictors for aggression and violence in SMI [18]. Nevertheless, although pharmacological treatment is necessary, especially for handling acute violence situations, it is insufficient on its own to prevent forthcoming aggression episodes [7, 19]: the patients' perceived need of treatment should therefore be considered a target of risk management strategies [20]. The combination of medication and non-pharmacological approaches seems more effective than medication alone in improving mental state, social functioning and quality of life of SMI patients engaged in violent behaviours, as well as in treating comorbid disorders (such as substance use) and in enhancing their compliance to treatment, their self-awareness and their adoption of pro-social behaviours [19, 21]. Integrated biomedical-psychosocial treatment may lead to a reduced risk of violence over time [7, 22]. Therapies targeting cognitive function may also have an effect on the risk of re-offending, due to an indirect relationship between cognition and violence proneness [23, 24].

A wide number of non-pharmacological interventions have been adopted for offenders suffering from SMI with the aim of reducing violence outcomes, delivered in both civil and forensic settings. Many of these interventions have been borrowed from other populations of offenders, assuming that mentally healthy and mentally disordered offenders (MDOs) have comparable violence risk factors [25]. The population of MDOs fits actually "halfway" between standard prisoners, who have higher recidivism rates, and standard psychiatric patients, who are generally more insightful and have better compliance to treatment [25]. Currently, a specific evidence on the effectiveness of non-pharmacological interventions in MDOs is weak and not conclusive. Blackburn [26] conducted a literature review and concluded that the little evidence available was limited to short-term violence outcomes and open to bias due to the poor methodological quality of included studies. Another systematic review provided useful data, but was not restricted to SMI individuals, and cognitive behavioural therapy (CBT) was the only reviewed intervention [27]. The most recent systematic review, performed by Rampling et al. [25] and based on

23 studies, attempted to overcome these limitations and considered several psychological and psychosocial interventions for MDOs. The most robust evidence was for SMI patients receiving CBT or modified reasoning and rehabilitation (R&R) programme. Another review on this issue only examined the effects of treatments on patients with schizophrenia [28].

This chapter is meant to summarise the available evidence on non-pharmacological interventions (psychological and psychosocial) for reducing aggression and violence (violent attitude, verbal aggression, physical violence) in adults with SMI. We included both the interventions aimed at managing aggression in acute situations and the strategies aimed at preventing and reducing its recurrence over time. Emergency management strategies for violence (such as seclusion and restraint) were not taken into account. Among SMI, we included schizophrenia spectrum disorder, mood disorders and severe personality disorders.

15.2 Non-pharmacological Interventions in the Management of Acute Violence in SMI

15.2.1 De-Escalation Techniques

The first use of the term "de-escalation" dates back to the mid-1980s, when it is used to describe violence in the health and social care setting. De-escalation has been defined as "the main form of secondary violence prevention, occurring in the face of imminent aggression" [29] and as "a psychosocial intervention, which should be used as the first-line response to violence and aggression" [30]. This is in contrast to primary prevention, which involves steps that are taken to prevent or reduce the likelihood that violent behaviour will be initiated, and tertiary actions which instead aim to reduce the impact of violence during its occurrence and in its aftermath [31]. However, despite several conceptual and operational definitions of de-escalation in healthcare settings, currently there are no systematic descriptions about what de-escalation is [32]. In order to provide clarity for researchers, educationalists and clinicians about the issue, Hallett and Dickens [29] conducted a concept analysis of de-escalation in healthcare, with the aim of sharing the concept of de-escalation to all mental health professions, improving the prevention of violence and reducing the incidence of inadequate restrictive interventions. In their analysis authors included 79 studies finding that mental health settings were the most commonly reported environment in which de-escalation occurred, and that nursing was the mental health professional most commonly involved. Moreover, authors identified five theories about de-escalation: communication, self-regulation, assessment, actions and safety. Although each of this issue was adequate in some respects, all of them lacked empirical support. Finally authors proposed a theoretical definition of de-escalation in healthcare that is "a collective term for a range of staff-delivered interventions comprising verbal and non-verbal communication techniques, self-regulation and assessment skills, actions, and safety maintenance, with the aim to extinguish or reduce patient aggression/agitation irrespective of its cause, and to improve staff-patient relationships, eliminating or minimising coercion or restriction". This conceptual analysis could provide useful information for researchers in order to identify a theoretical model for de-escalation, an action target, its attributes and the main negative and positive consequences that should be avoided or encouraged.

Current working conditions in mental healthcare and stressful situations that are associated with aggression itself make it necessary that staff are able to cope with their own distress and anger in order to behave in a way that aggression and violence can be avoided. Therefore, stress management and anger management are the basis for applying de-escalation skills effectively. Tables 15.1 and 15.2 summarise the conflict clinical management, de-escalation rules and intervention techniques. Figure 15.1 represents the cycle of aggression (modified from [35]).

In addition the famous Hücker's law enforcement training program (1997) has been turned into indications for the mental health staff (see Table 15.3).

A very practical method is the use of instructions by self-talk. Nay [38], based on psychological researchers on anger, recommends the use of specific instructions adjusted to different stages of anger (see Table 15.4).

Table 15.1 Conflict management and de-escalation rules

General attitude towards the patient aggression	The attitude should be empathic, respect, sincerity and fairness and should be accompanied by a caring and therapeutic intention.
Assess the risks associated with each available option	Realistic expectations: Can this situation really be mastered without physical options?
Control the situation	Target is not to control the patient, but to control the situation. Conflict management within an interaction has the goal of getting the best out of the situation for both parties [33].
Share	Where it is possible, risk assessment, decision-making, responsibilities and actions should be shared with fellow colleagues.
Well timed	De-escalation works more successfully when it is done as an early intervention [34]. This is clearly illustrated by the escalation curve [35] (see Fig. 15.1).
Gain time	Very often aggressive interpersonal communication (e.g. accusations and shouting) proceeds quickly. Experimental psychological research has shown that time pressure leads to less thorough information processing and, consequently, inadequate decisions [36].
Spatial evaluation	Evaluation of the surrounding spaces and distance keeping between staff and patient has several advantages.
Attitude	De-escalation interventions have to be applied with apparent self-confidence and certainty, without being provocative. Power plays between staff and patients have to be avoided.
Safety	Staff should be aware of general safety issues. Aggressive situations often occur in ward environments where there are several other people. The safety of fellow patients or inexperienced staff should always be kept in mind.

Table 15.2 De-escalation techniques in crisis management

Phase 1 of the trigger and phase 2 of the escalation The cycle begins with a first psycho-emotional shift from the baseline (ordinary condition). Verbal and expressive behaviours make perceptible the process start.	*Interventions in the triggering phase* (1) Recognise and remove the trigger promptly, in order to avoid the rapid progress of the crisis; encourage patient movement in a neutral environment (with less stimulation). (2) Approach through a direct communication (e.g. use of the proper name), based on the existing claims, with short sentences and simple terms, positive (non-judgemental and without aggressive attitude, available for clarification), transforming the contents of violence and threat in dialectical expressions. (3) Leave the patient, in the presence of health staff and personal items (e.g. computer, books, music player) to help him/her calm down, provided that such objects do not compromise his/her or others' safety. (4) Evaluate if to modify therapy administration, for example by offering to anticipate the time, proposing to take additional therapy as needed or deciding to administer it during shift changes (in the case of potentially reactive patients the presence of more operators can be a useful strategy to better manage tension). (5) Possibility of increasing staff on duty in case if necessary (e.g. presence of complex patients).
Phase 3 of the crisis (arousal): excitement culmination point It is a phase of psychomotor activation characterised by physical, emotional and psychological changes that lead to a situation of real or presumed threat.	*Interventions in the crisis phase* (1) Clearly identify "who does what" in the staff, in particular during emergencies, in order to manage better an aggressive attack. (2) Focus the intervention on safety and the reduction of consequences, through the involvement of all the operators present. (3) Move the interaction with a patient—when possible—to a place with low stimulation, with few potentially harmful objects. (4) Move away if the simple safety distance does not guarantee security.
Phase 4 of the recovery Gradual return to the psycho-emotional baseline, but with an arousal level that is still high and potentially reactive. A particularly delicate phase, since the patient is very receptive to any new triggers.	*Interventions in the recovery phase* (1) Avoid situations that can re-trigger the arousal sequence. (2) Continue active monitoring and maintenance of the safety distance. (3) Avoid communications that are too early or inadequate, like rework and judgments, which could set off new triggers.
Phase 5 of post-critical depression Rapid return to the psycho-emotional baseline, with mood deflection, feelings of guilt, shame and remorse.	*Interventions in the post-critical phase of depression* (1) Active group discussion within the team and with the patient, supporting the review of the events also with a preventive purpose. (2) Report the event in the clinical documentation, fill in the forms relating to the episode severity and to sentinel events.

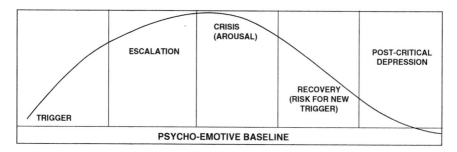

Fig. 15.1 The cycle of aggression (modified from [35])

Table 15.3 Indications for mental health staff (modified by [37])

Management of personal emotions	Avoid negative thoughts and reflections that will lead to self-fulfilling prophecies (e.g. being judging or defining a patient's behaviour or appearance "unbearable", "unacceptable").
Role distance	Mental health staff must be able to recognise situations in which the rules related to psychiatric assistance cannot be rigidly applied. In some situations it is more appropriate not to follow the professional rules (e.g. apply personal hygiene to the patient in any case or be inflexible).
Empathy/ role-taking	The ability to empathise with the patient is essential in managing critical situations, although often difficult. We may find that the patient's behaviour is explainable.
Ambiguity tolerance	Interpersonal conflict is associated with divergent opinions and point of view. In many situations, staff need to accept different attitudes and recognise the distinction between patients and themselves. Another skill is the ability to cope with hostile behaviour not emotionally.

Table 15.4 Self-talk strategy and stages of anger

Preparing for provocation	"This may upset me, but I know how to deal with it".
Impact and confrontation	"What difference will this make in a week or a month?"
Coping with arousal of anger	"My muscles are getting tight. That's my signal for a relaxation breath".
After the confrontation	"I could have used a calming phrase. Let me rethink how I could have handled it better".

15.2.2 Verbal De-escalation Techniques

Lack of trust and negative expectations are the main features of the escalation of interpersonal conflicts. This lack of trust is associated with emotional suffering, anger, tension and fear. Therefore a priority objective of verbal de-escalation is to regain the patient's trust. This can only happen when the emotional tension has run down, which in this regard is another basic goal. One skill for achieving these goals is active and empathic listening. Active and empathic listening is likely to improve mutual trust and understanding while handling the emotions. It is appropriate to use a non-judgemental and a non-critical language, in order to enhance patient's confidence. Active listening contains the following strategies (Beyondintractability. org, 2003; Changingminds.org, 2005; Conflict Resolution Network, 2005):

- Listen for both content and meaning.
- Respond to the emotional message.
- Respond honestly.
- Paraphrase the patient's message to indicate your understanding.
- Do not interrupt while the patient is talking.
- Do not give advice.
- Do not discount the patient's feelings.
- Show a real interest in the patient's opinion and acknowledge his/her position ("I see what you mean"; "I'd like to hear more about it").

In the case of strong verbal attacks, the goal is to defuse negative emotions behind discontrol (Conflict Resolution Network, 2005):

- At this point do not try to justify yourself.
- Try to face the patient's emotions (shouting occurs when the patient believe that he/she is not being heard) and verbalise how we perceive it (e.g. "I see that you are very upset", "I can see that you are very angry").

In some situations it is better to agree with the patient until the level of escalation is reduced [39]. Though a patient's claims are not justified, it is better to postpone the explanations until the crisis is over, using rhetorical techniques to re-establish an effective interaction [37] (see Table 15.5).

An intervention to avoid is the use of "Why-question", because the patient feels under pressure and perceives the operator's inability to empathise (e.g. "Why do you always behave like this?" "Why did you do this again?").

Equally, it is better to prefer open-ended questions, than closed questions. Closed questions, where the answer is only yes or no, limit the discussion. Moreover, open-ended questions allow to take time and meanwhile think about an intervention strategy (e.g. "What did you feel in this moment?" "How could we solve this situation together?").

At least it is better to avoid the following rhetorical styles, described as "roadblocks to communication" by Davidson and Wood [33] and "communication killers" by Dutschmann [40]: ordering, blaming, praising, warning, shaming, belittling, moralising, judging, probing, arguing, irony/sarcasm and name-calling.

Indeed de-escalation is not always possible. Numerous are the variables to take into consideration, such as the environmental context, the staff experience and the

Table 15.5 Verbal de-escalation techniques (modified by [37])

Talk about the initial problem	"Could we talk about … again?"
Listening without accusing	"We should talk about …"
Allow time for answer	"Take your time", "Think carefully"
Make compromises	"You have your reasons, but we should talk about together"

severity of aggressive behaviour. Different types of violence have to be managed in different ways: general cognitive behavioural interventions are appropriate for an instrumental aggression; body language or rhetoric skills are better for an episode of emotional violence [40]. Frequent but difficult-to-manage conflicts with family members or other patients lead to attacks on other people (often staff members). In these cases the trigger derives from a combination of two aversive stimulations of different people, in which a minor stimulus can lead to aggression [41].

During a de-escalation intervention even more important than what we think is what the patients might think and our ability to empathise. In the case of patients with psychotic symptoms it is much more difficult to understand how he/she feels, so it is important to have a good knowledge of the different mental disorders and specially an experienced staff in working with mentally ill people.

15.2.3 Debriefing

The debriefing is a retrospective reflection that normally should follow any adverse event, including episodes of mechanical restraints. The debriefing is an action that has both clinical and emotional-relational components and the patient must be directly involved as soon as possible. It is an adequate re-examination of the facts and emotional states experienced during the various phases of the event and can help team to define possible improvement actions and to elaborate what has happened. The main objective is to identify the triggers and those that would have prevented the escalation towards the crisis. This process allows to share and take into consideration the emotional states of the team during the crisis. The debriefing can begin immediately after the critical event through emotional support to the patient, necessary to find alternative strategies in a preventive perspective. Mechanical restraint episodes can be discussed even after the debriefing, better if with staff components and patient's territorial reference operators.

15.2.4 Mental Health Staff Training Programs

In the departments where training for effective non-violent conflict management has been implemented, staff reports that the environment changes positively. Non-violent conflict management changes the communicative style of the staff and this reflects positively on relationships. However, identifying the contents and duration of training is difficult and at the same time there is little evidence of effectiveness [42]. Only few training programs are based on evidence of the effectiveness of the training or on benefits perceived by the staff and/or users of the service [30]. Nevertheless in last years some works have been published on this topic: framework guidelines for addressing workplace violence in the healthcare sector (International Labour Conference 90th Session 2002 Report III-ILO, 2002), mental health policy implementation guide regarding developing positive practice to support the safe and therapeutic management of aggression and violence in mental health inpatient settings, and clinical guidelines for the short-term management of disturbed/violent behaviour in inpatient psychiatric and emergency settings [30]. These guidelines should be consultative, informative and regularly updated. Training staff has a positive effect on skills and increases confidence to cope with violence situations [43]. In this regard, it is suggested to schedule training courses on de-escalation techniques, shared in a widespread and continuous manner. The training should involve all medical, nursing and support staff, with the intent to change the clinical and organisational culture, supporting and encouraging internal reflection on the professional practices and providing for the revision or development of a protocol for the management of aggressive behaviour. However, training alone does not have a decisive impact on reducing episodes of aggression. Training in fact must be added to quality improvement projects at an organisational and clinical level [44].

15.3   Non-pharmacological Interventions in Preventing and Reducing Recurrent Violence in SMI

All the interventions and strategies in preventing and reducing recurrent violence in SMI are listed in Table 15.6.

15.3.1 Cognitive Behaviour Therapy

Cognitive behavioural methods are focused on modifying the distorted beliefs and cognitive processes underlying the affects and behaviours of the patients. Therefore, treatment targets are maladaptive social and coping skills, oppositional behaviours and social awareness, in order to help the patients to improve their understanding of how their feelings about self and others have an impact on their attitudes. The beneficial effect of CBT on antisocial behaviour has been described in individuals with

Table 15.6 Non-pharmacological interventions in preventing and reducing recurrent violence in SMI

Cognitive behaviour therapy
Mentalisation-based therapy
Dialectic behaviour therapy
Schema therapy
Anger/aggression-focused therapy
Reasoning and rehabilitation
Cognitive remediation
Enhanced thinking skills
Psychoeducation
Animal-assisted therapy
Supported housing
Structured risk assessment
Addressing comorbid substance-use disorders
Integrated approaches and community service programmes

antisocial personality disorder [45] and included as an established treatment strategy for these patients in NICE guidelines [46]. Evidence on the matter seems, however, rather inconclusive since many studies focus on outcomes indirectly linked to violence and aggression [47], results tend to lose their significance with longer durations of follow-up [45, 48], and in some cases CBT was not found to be more effective than treatment as usual [49]. In individuals with borderline personality disorder, there is contrasting evidence on the efficacy of CBT in reducing self-mutilation, suicidal behaviour, expression of anger and interpersonal aggressiveness, depending on study design, treatment program and duration of follow-up [50]. A small non-controlled study on forensic inpatients with personality disorders (more than 80% Cluster B) in a high-security setting found that a multidisciplinary treatment mainly based on CBT positively impacted oppositional behaviours, together with psychopathological symptoms and interpersonal functioning at a group, but not at an individual level [51]. It has been reported that patients with higher levels of psychopathy tend to benefit less from CBT, since they usually display an initial psychosocial improvement, not followed by a structural improvement in reoffending rates [51, 52]. The positive effects of CBT on anger and aggression seem to be affected by a differential response to treatment among different individuals [53]; some authors described the influence of dynamic factors (i.e. greater readiness to change) on violence outcomes [54], and then reported an influence of the pattern of Cluster B personality traits on rates of change [53].

CBT adapted to the treatment of psychosis has been described as effective in reducing positive symptoms [55], also among long-term inpatients with a forensic history [56]. The latter study was conducted in a sample of only eight patients, but seems interesting since it was the first in this kind of setting, and described potential barriers to the program implementation. The feasibility of a violence prevention program using CBT among schizophrenia inpatients at risk of violence has been investigated also in a general psychiatric ward [57]. A single-blind RCT with a more robust design compared the efficacy of CBT with that of social activation therapy in decreasing aggressive incidents (verbal and physical) in a group of violent in- and outpatients with schizophrenia [58]. The authors reported a significant improvement during treatment (probably linked to an improvement in delusional thinking), but results were no longer significant during follow-up; the importance of the mentioned study lies in the fact that violence was directly examined as an outcome using objective measures, and that social activation therapy as a comparison allowed to control for non-specific supportive aspects of the treatment [28]. Further, even though weaker, evidence on the positive effects of CBT for psychosis on clinician-rated measures of hostility and aggression in schizophrenia patients, is also available [59, 60]. Another study with a mirror-image design explored the 5-year efficacy of the Service for Treatment and Abatement of Interpersonal Risk (STAIR) programme—a CBT-based intervention originally created for nonpsychotic offenders—on 145 patients (86% of them psychotic) with a history of arrest [61]. Lower re-arrest rates, fewer hospitalisations and less days institutionalised were reported, but this can be related to violence outcomes only at an indirect level.

15.3.2 Mentalisation-Based Therapy

Mentalisation-based therapy (MBT) is a manualised intervention consisting of an integration of cognitive, relational and psychodynamic components, specifically focusing on mentalising ability, which allows the subjects to envision emotions and intentions of themselves and other people [62]. Mentalising ability is known to be associated to social functioning, and to protect individuals with violence traits against displaying aggression, violence and behavioural vulnerability in situations of interpersonal stress and perceived threats [63]. A RCT of MBT vs. treatment as usual (TAU) was conducted among 20 schizophrenia violent inpatients, demonstrating a reduction in suspiciousness, but did not directly evaluate violence as an outcome [64]. MBT was proven effective among outpatients with comorbid borderline and antisocial personality disorder in reducing symptoms related to aggression (anger, hostility, self-harm, suicidality, paranoia) and in improving social functioning indicators when compared to a CBT protocol of similar intensity but without MBT components.

15.3.3 Dialectic Behaviour Therapy

Dialectical behaviour therapy (DBT) has been derived from CBT and specifically designed for individuals with borderline personality disorder. It has also been adapted for different populations, including forensic settings [65–67], even though some authors pointed out that the effectiveness of DBT adaptations to different patients is difficult to assume [68]. DBT aims at providing therapeutic skills in managing painful feelings and decreasing interpersonal conflicts, targeting four main areas (mindfulness, distress tolerance, emotion regulation and interpersonal effectiveness). It includes both individual and group therapy sessions. Linehan et al. performed a RCT of DBT vs. TAU in subjects with borderline personality disorder and significant suicidal behaviour [69], and re-evaluated their patients 1 year after the treatment completion [70]. They found that DBT patients had reduced suicidality, trait anger and hospitalisations due to parasuicidal acts, but this effect was apparently not sustained over time. DBT appears to be effective especially in improving self-directed aggressive behaviour outcomes [50]. A case-control study evaluated the efficacy of DBT in eight patients with borderline personality disorder comparing them with nine patients with a similar personality disorder, who received standard treatment. Patients receiving DBT obtained better results in anger experiences, disposition to anger and outward experience of anger [71].

15.3.4 Schema Therapy

Schema therapy (ST) is a kind of psychotherapy comprising cognitive behavioural, psychoanalytic, gestalt therapy and attachment theory elements. Its goal is to help patients to correct maladaptive patterns of thought and behaviour ("schemas") by reducing emotions/sensations and changing cognitive patterns related to schemas and replacing them with adaptive coping mechanisms. It is primarily dedicated to patients suffering from personality disorder, and assumes that specific personality pathologies consist of specific combinations of maladaptive schemas [72]. ST has also been used among patients with high levels of psychopathy. In a small randomised trial applied in a forensic setting to patients with personality disorders, ST as a supplement to TAU was compared to TAU alone regarding the effect in reducing aggression frequency at four different follow-up times. The treatments did not reveal any statistically significant difference; however, the study has been criticised for the low quality of methodology and delivered therapy [25, 73]. A multicentre randomised clinical trial assessed the efficacy of ST among forensic patients with antisocial, borderline, paranoid and narcissistic personality disorders. According to preliminary findings, ST is superior to TAU in reducing the risk of recidivism and promoting community reintegration after 3 years of treatment, but differences in outcome measures of violence risk do not appear statistically significant [74].

15.3.5 Anger/Aggression-Focused Therapy

Treatments specifically targeting anger assume the existence of a direct and dynamic relationship between reduction of anger and reduction of aggression [75]. In this perspective, a meta-analytic review confirmed a strong relationship between anger and violence, with higher effect size when violence was evaluated using self-reported measures [76]. Evidence on effectiveness of anger/aggression-focused therapy (AFT) often refers to criminal justice settings, and only a few studies conducted on mental health samples are available [25, 77]. A recent review of published meta-analyses also found that most of the therapies targeting anger and/or aggression are group based or class based rather than based on individual case management, and the therapeutic modality is frequently cognitive behavioural or psychoeducational [78]. A systematic review evaluating the efficacy of structured group interventions in mentally disordered offenders within hospital settings included four pertinent studies [79]. A moderate-to-high effect size was found, but evidence was based on trials open to bias: only one study had a controlled design; sample sizes were small and included heterogeneous participants; heterogeneous and sometimes non-standardised assessments were used across the studies, not including behavioural measures; moreover, two out of four studies failed to provide any statistical data [79]. Regarding studies specifically performed in mental health populations, only two non-randomised trials are available. First, a study conducted in violent male forensic subjects with antisocial personality disorder/conduct disorder with or without SMI evaluated the clinical relevance of aggression control therapy (ACT), a treatment CBT-like programme built on social learning theory [80]. It showed a significant reduction of self-reported aggression outcomes, especially in patients with low psychopathy scores, but the results were based on pre-post-treatment comparisons in the intervention group, rather than on comparisons with controls; this trial could also be considered at high risk of bias for incomplete outcome data. Second, a trial of an adapted CBT-based anger management group was described in a sample of 86 male forensic patients in a high-security hospital, with a history of violent behaviour deriving from anger [81]. Sustained reduction in self-reported feelings of anger and a trend towards improvement in rates of physical aggression were reported among completers, while incidents of verbal aggression were observed to initially increase and then decrease (not below baseline levels) during a 9-month follow-up. However, more research is warranted in order to demonstrate that self-reported reduction in experiences of anger is actually a meaningful indicator of improvement in aggression rates.

15.3.6 Reasoning and Rehabilitation

R&R is a manual-based modified cognitive behavioural programme requiring certified trainers, which has been specifically designed for prisoners (especially medium-to high-risk offenders), developed in Canada for the first time [82]. It is based on the assumption that prisoners have not acquired or neglected cognitive bases and activities necessary to solve life problems in prosocial ways [83]. The aim of the programme is to reduce recidivism rates by addressing issues that lead individuals to risky or criminal behaviour; the treatment focus is therefore on self-control, meta-cognition, interaction and conflict resolution skills, other social skills, enhancement of socially adaptive values, critical reasoning, lateral thinking, coping with anger and other emotions, and recognition and re-framing of maladaptive thoughts. It was observed that R&R may help to reduce recidivism in both institutional and community settings with moderate effect sizes [84], even in the lack of change in the offenders' environment [85]. One of the main problems in using the R&R programme is the low completion rate [25]. Prisoners with psychiatric disorders were often excluded in studies investigating the efficacy of R&R. Among available studies, often affected by high attrition rates (up to 50%), outcomes related to violent attitudes were evaluated using both direct (i.e. re-arrest rates, incidents of verbal and physical aggression, aggressive behaviour rating scales or questionnaires) and indirect measures (i.e. social problem-solving and coping response assessment) [25, 28]. One RCT by Cullen et al. [86] evaluated effectiveness of the standard R&R program in a group of MDOs in a medium-security psychiatric unit on both socio-cognitive skills and criminal attitudes (blame attribution, experience of anger and empathy). Program completers exhibited a significant increase in empathy and ability to manage anger, but differences in incidental verbal aggression rates between treatment groups were no longer significant at the 12-month follow-up. Young et al. [87, 88] investigated treatment outcome and factors predicting completion of a revised version of R&R (R&R2 Mental Health Program—MHP), specifically adapted for offenders with SMI and antisocial youths, consisting of fewer treatment sessions. The authors reported reduced disruptive and violent behaviours among treatment completers when compared to wait-list controls, while treatment completion could be predicted only by mental state/behavioural stability and medication status. The only significant predictor of treatment effectiveness was attitude towards violence. A multisite controlled trial evaluated R&R2MHP compared with standard care among MDOs of medium- and low-safety units, and found reduced aptitude for violence and increased problem-solving skills in the R&R2MHP group [89]. Yip et al. [90] conducted a quasi-experimental controlled study to evaluate the outcome of the R&R2MHP program compared with TAU in patients with schizophrenia, schizoaffective or bipolar disorder in a high-security hospital, and showed consistent findings. In both the Rees-Jones and the Yip studies, the completion rate was greater than in the Cullen study, which may imply that the modified form of R&R can be administered and used at all secure care levels. Jotangia et al. [91] also reported a low dropout rate when administering the R&R2MHP programme to a group of female MDOs in a non-randomised controlled trial, but were not able to demonstrate a significant effect on violence reduction. Using a randomised controlled design, Kingston et al. [92] described the efficacy of another adapted R&R programme (R&R 2: Short Version for Adult) versus standard treatment in a MDO population, with improvements in social skills and various indicators of mental health, but no advantage of R&R2 in reducing recidivism. Finally, R&R adapted for ADHD patients (R&R2 ADHD) was used by Young et al. [93] in patients with severe personality disorders, assuming that the latter had deficits similar to those of ADHD patients. Although it was a limited study for small size, it is possible to consider a positive effect on cognitive functions.

15.3.7 Cognitive Remediation

Cognitive remediation (CR) therapy is a behavioural based training approach designed to help patients with SMI (such as schizophrenia) in improving their cognitive abilities and real-world functioning. Improvement in neurocognition can lead to a reduction in aggressive behaviour, as a secondary outcome [94]. It has been hypothesised that neurocognitive deficits in schizophrenia are the basis of emotion regulation process and a dysfunction in the latter domain could lead to aggressive behaviours, in particular when stressful situations exceed the threshold set by cognitive control systems [94]. Impairments of neurocognition and social cognition experienced by schizophrenia patients accounted for a large portion of the variance of subsequent violent behaviour [95]. In this perspective, CR has the potential to increase cognitive skills and functioning, and consequently the capacity to participate and benefit from other psychosocial interventions focused on violence reduction. Ahmed et al. [94] in a RCT evaluated the effect of computerised cognitive activities versus computer game control activities on psychosocial functioning variables, aggression levels and incidents in a group of patients with schizophrenia and schizoaffective disorder. The group assigned to CR had improvement in large neurocognitive domains, in some functional capacity domains, and a reduction in negative symptoms, agitation and physical and verbal aggression. An improvement in neurocognition has been associated with the reduction of episodes of aggression. CR and other strategies of neurocognitive enhancement could therefore have an action on violent behaviour, by improving the ability to regulate emotions. In a recent systematic review [96], CR and social cognitive training (SCT) effectiveness in reducing aggressive behaviour was proven in different phases of schizophrenia, both on verbal and physical aggressive behaviours, with a persisting effect at a 12-month follow-up after the end of CR. The goal is to reduce impulsiveness and aggression through improving executive functions, verbal memory, social cognition and social functioning. Although further studies are required, CR should be taken into account for an integrated treatment, within the global programmes in managing aggressive behaviour in schizophrenia.

15.3.8 Enhanced Thinking Skills

Enhanced thinking skills (ETS) is one of the most widely used cognitive methods with prisoners, aimed at reducing recidivism rates. It consists of a structured series of exercises designed to modify the thought and behaviour of criminals, through the teaching of interpersonal problem-solving skills. The effectiveness of this method has been repeatedly demonstrated in the reduction of recurrences of violence for prisoners. An observational study compared the effects of ETS and TAU in a group of prisoners with antisocial personality disorder. Outcome measures included aggressiveness, antisocial attitude, anger regulation and social problem-solving abilities, all evaluated using dedicated rating scales. The study showed a beneficial effect of ETS on functioning, though the evidence was not robust due to the absence of a randomised design and the short duration of follow-up [97]. Similar findings were reported in a trial performed among offenders with mixed borderline personality/psychotic disorder, with similar methodological limitations [98].

15.3.9 Psychoeducation

Psychoeducation is an evidence-based, manualised intervention aimed at providing information on nature and treatment of mental disorders, and teaching strategies to cope with them. Group psychoeducation (gPE), always guided by a qualified professional, provides for the possibility to enhance exchange of experiences and mutual support between patients, together with communication and problem-solving skills. Involvement of family members and caregivers is often very important, since a positive effect can be demonstrated on both patients and family members [99]. Furthermore, patients' clinical status (higher or lower dependency) can directly impact family burden [100]. Numerous studies aimed to demonstrate that psychoeducation may increase insight and reduce symptoms of disease, including violent behaviour, also in forensic settings (where psychoeducational programs are not rarely offered). The quality of the evidence seems however low to moderate. Considering schizophrenia patients, the efficacy of gPE was explored in one RCT and in one observational study. These studies reported that psychoeducation improved insight and attitude towards medication, but violence was not directly included as an outcome measure. A recent small and quasi-experimental controlled study evaluated the effectiveness of a combination of family psychoeducation (fPE) and acceptance and commitment therapy in a group of patients with schizophrenia [101]. This combination treatment increased insight and reduced violent behaviour, leading to an improvement in the patients' ability to control their violent attitude. Currently, very little evidence is available on the effects of psychoeducation in antisocial personality disorder and only minor evidence about its efficacy in borderline personality disorder. A RCT tested the efficacy of a brief psychoeducational intervention as a supplement to TAU on antisocial personality disorder within community substance-use disorder treatment centres [102]. The experimental program (Impulsive Lifestyle Counselling—ILC) consisted of six individual sessions, focused on a specific topic: (1) treatment purpose and identification of thoughts and behaviours related to antisocial personality disorder; (2) consequences of impulsive behaviours; (3) link between impulsive behaviours and scales of values and beliefs; (4) concept of "value" and which values can change the lifestyle of the patient; (5) support of social relations; and (6) booster session in which the patient can treat the subjects he/she prefers. Considerable reduction in general aggression and interpersonal aggression was observed in both ILC+TAU and TAU groups, but without statistically significant effects.

15.3.10 Animal-Assisted Therapy

Animal-assisted therapy (AAT) is an intervention involving interaction with animals, since animals appear to have positive effects on mental health. It can also be used among patients with SMI who enact violent and aggressive actions, with stronger evidence regarding equine-assisted therapy (thanks to characteristics of horses, for example imposing and adaptability). Evidence on the matter can be actually derived from a single study, a RCT which was published in 2015 [103]. The study included 90 patients receiving either canine-assisted therapy, equine-assisted therapy, social skills therapy (SST) or TAU. AAT was well tolerated by the patients, with higher efficacy of equine-assisted therapy in reducing aggression incidents and improving aggression scales scores after 3 months with respect to other treatments. However, it should be pointed out that there was great imbalance in baseline aggression levels among treatment arms, with higher baseline severity in the equine-assisted therapy group.

15.3.11 Supported Housing

Supported housing (SH) consists of permanent and supervised housing in residential facilities owned by the community mental health system, with the aim to provide home stability and community integration to individuals in need. Available services can range widely from single-apartment buildings to scattered site services provided by private landlords or supportive services. They are generally included in projects of social or charitable associations. Some studies have shown significant reductions in recurrence rates in prisoners inserted into these structures following release, but no studies have shown yet whether it has a specific benefit for high-risk criminals with personality disorder. A naturalistic study considered the impact of SH in a particular population of men with personality disorder [104]. Lower recurrence rates have been observed in subjects assigned to SH, but the study sample was very small and the design did not imply randomisation (individuals were chosen to receive SH when they lived in a more difficult social context or were unable to live alone). However, this study may indicate that the beneficial effects of SH described on non-psychiatric prisoners can be extended to offenders with personality disorders, but further studies are needed to verify this hypothesis.

15.3.12 Structured Risk Assessment

As previously reported, risk factors for aggressive behaviour can be either static (i.e. previous history of violence) or dynamic (i.e. use of a narcotic substance). Structured approaches to violence risk assessment consist of tools and checklists that aim at preventing forthcoming violent behaviour through the planning of the prompt use of appropriate risk management interventions. Low-risk individuals should receive no or minimal supervision, whereas high-risk individuals usually require intensive and extensive interventions and, ideally, case management. The most common tools are the Historical Clinical Risk Management-20 (HCR-20), the Brøset Violence Checklist (BVC) and the Dynamic Appraisal of Situational Aggression (DASA), which can be used in several different psychiatric settings [105]. These tools have the advantage of minimising the risk of cognitive and situational biases possibly affecting non-structured clinical assessment, but keep at the same time important the role of professionals' clinical experience, not only relying on merely statistical combinations [106]. When evaluating violence risk, it is always important to keep in mind the local violence base rate and the patients' self-report of a violence history, even when applying structured models [107]. Risk prediction is effective only when appropriately accompanied by subsequent risk management strategies [105]. Evidence on the effectiveness of these tools appears to be conflicting: on the one hand, violence assessment tools are a recommended routine step for every psychiatric patient within NICE guidelines [107]; on the other hand, some risk assessment literature tend to focus insufficiently on peculiar patient populations in specific settings [108]. Some authors believe that these tools have only little or no value in discriminating high-risk patients from low-risk patients, given the high frequency and the low specificity of factors associated with violent behaviour [109]. Risk categorisation has some additional limitations, since some patients judged as high risk do not actually commit violence acts. Furthermore, an inaccurate risk assessment can lead to disadvantages, such as unwarranted detention for some patients, failure to treat others and stigma arising from patients being labelled as dangerous [110]. A systematic and meta-analytical review evaluated the predictive accuracy of the most relevant structured instruments for aggressive behaviour in forensic psychiatric hospitals: the predictive accuracy was greater for instruments designed for the prediction of imminent violence, rather than for longer term follow-up periods, especially for screening out low-risk patients [105]. One RCT conducted in a forensic psychiatric sample found that structured risk assessment combined with implementation of a violence management training had a positive impact on inpatient violence incidents [111]. Similar findings were derived from a smaller naturalistic study [112]. One-year observational multicentre study also showed that outpatients with a history of violent behaviour exhibited peculiar characteristics compared to matched controls, and were also prone to carry out additional community violence [3]. Joyal et al. [14] found that among people suffering from SMI and committing violent acts, different subgroups with specific patterns of violence and associated factors could be identified (psychotic, repetitive, institutional, less violent-stabilised); given that, risk assessment tools should target all the different factors associated with violence in the different subgroups.

15.3.13 Addressing Comorbid Substance-Use Disorders

Alcohol/drug misuse is one of the most researched dynamic predictors of aggression or serious violence among MDOs. Substance use can increase the risk of violence in patients with psychiatric disorders [3, 113, 114] through multiple potential pathways, such as direct pharmacological effects, more often at the frontal lobe level [28, 109], exacerbation of psychotic symptoms [115] and non-adherence to treatment [116]. A meta-analysis [115] investigated the relationship between cannabis abuse and violence in psychiatric patients, showing an association. Many different non-pharmacological interventions can be used to address comorbid substance-use disorders in psychiatry, including CBT, motivational interviewing, individual counselling, family therapy and residential programmes [117]. However, only very few studies assessed their efficacy on violence reduction in psychiatric samples; most of the studies addressed the question describing outcomes related to violence only indirectly (i.e. neurocognitive functioning, rehospitalisation) [28]. This was the case of one RCT describing the effects of combined psychiatric and substance-use treatments of individuals with SMI. The already mentioned RCT by Thylstrup et al. [102], conducted on patients with antisocial personality disorder referring to community substance-use disorder treatment centres, described the efficacy of a short-term psychoeducational intervention in addition to TAU on drug use indicators, but no significant differences were found between this treatment and TAU alone in improving self-reported aggression. The authors hypothesised that the intervention could be too brief to impact aggressive behaviour significantly, but similar findings were observed with a more intensive CBT [49]. A systematic review with meta-analysis (including 43 trials) examining the effectiveness of community non-pharmacological treatments for drug using offenders showed that these treatments have some kind of benefit in reducing re-incarceration [118]. Considering that some patients may ask for help for drug/alcohol-use problems, rather than for their behavioural difficulties, further research is warranted to verify the link between improvement in substance use attitudes and effective reduction of violence.

15.3.14 Integrated Approaches and Community Service Programs

Several integrated programmes combining specific treatment approaches and community-based social support services have been developed and promoted, especially in Anglo-American areas, with the aim to improve assessment, treatment and management of patients and offenders suffering from SMI. These programs are worth a particular mention, due to the interest and, sometimes, the criticism they generated over time [119]. They have not been mentioned in previous sections due to the fact that while analysing them it is difficult to get unequivocal data on the potential effectiveness of specific components of the interventions. These programmes are generally delivered by multidisciplinary teams, combining individual and group sessions and comprising both core and tailored interventions. Treatment duration, module and setting are variable. Some of the programmes were initially developed for either specific psychiatric categories of patients or offenders who do not have any mental illness, and were dedicated at a later stage to populations of MDOs [119]. The most interesting and researched approaches include Assertive Community Treatment (ACT) [119–122], Forensic Assertive Community Treatment [123], Dangerous and Severe Personality Disorder (DSPD) programme [124], Chromis violence reduction programme [125], Violence Offender Treatment Programme (VOTP) [126], Involuntary Outpatient Commitment [127] and diversion services [119, 128]. Considering this kind of programmes as a whole, they can potentially enhance the delivery of onward effective care, and appear to have a positive effect themselves on mental state, cognitive skills, global functioning and violence outcomes, even though with different strengths of association depending on many factors. Their effective implementation should be combined with community and tailored services and with monitoring of treatment adherence.

15.4   Summary of Main Results and Evidences

This chapter reviews the available evidence on non-pharmacological interventions (psychological and psychosocial) in reducing aggression and violence (violent attitude, verbal aggression, physical violence) in adults with SMI. We included both the interventions aimed at managing aggression in acute situations, and at preventing and reducing its recurrence over time.

The de-escalation skill application seems to be an important tool for many mental health workers and should help staff to cope actively with acute aggressive behaviours without using physical force. Non-violent conflict management is a way out of passivity, and at the same time avoids provoking violent patients' counter-reactions [29, 43]. It is obvious that de-escalation is not always possible and numerous are the variables to take into consideration in its application such as the environmental context, the staff experience and the severity of aggressive behaviour. Probably different types of aggressive behaviours might require to be managed by different strategies and modalities.

Moreover, a wide number of non-pharmacological interventions have been adopted for SMI offenders with the aim of preventing and reducing violence recurrence in the long term. A limit in this type of studies is that many of the interventions have been borrowed from other populations of offenders, assuming that mentally healthy and MDOs have comparable violence risk factors. The population of MDOs fits actually "halfway" between standard prisoners, who have higher recidivism rates, and standard psychiatric patients, who are generally more insightful and have better compliance to treatment [25]. Currently, a specific evidence on the effectiveness of non-pharmacological interventions in MDOs is weak and not conclusive. In this context, the latest systematic review, performed by Rampling et al. [25], found that the most robust evidence in preventing and managing violence recurrence in SMI was for CBT and modified R&R programme.

As summarised in Table 15.6, other types of non-pharmacological intervention seem to have promising results in preventing aggressive behaviours in SMI, although the results are mostly preliminary and not conclusive. Among them, we believe that DBT, CR, PE and integrated approaches and community service programs may have interesting developments in different SMI populations. Moreover, we think that future research on non-pharmacological approaches in managing and preventing violence among people with SMI should try (1) to overcome several methodological limitations, and (2) to shed light on many issues, which currently remain open and/or controversial. Regarding the first point, the current studies have several limitations and weaknesses, such as the heterogeneity of the population studied (for example, different diagnosis, in- or outpatients, clinical or forensic context), the divergent and not comparable definitions of violence and aggressive behaviour, the different assessment tools, and the contrasting and disparate outcome measures, with both direct and/or indirect indicators.

About the second issue, future research should clarify which are the specific and unspecific effects of the different treatments, the active elements of interventions, the mediators and moderators of their effectiveness, the persistence over time and the role of motivation. It will also be helpful to understand which patients might benefit from which treatment approach and identify possible predictors of individual response. In addition, the rules and methodologies regarding the delivery of different interventions should be better fixed and standardised: indications, timing and duration, frequency of participation in the program, intensity of the training sessions, type of setting, etc. Furthermore, among people with SMI, different subgroups with specific patterns of violence (for example, episodic, repetitive, verbal, physical) and associated factors (for example, categorical diagnosis, the presence of psychotic and/or psychopathic features, the stage of illness, in- or outpatients, clinical or forensic context) should be identified. In this perspective, risk assessment tools should target all the different factors associated with violence in the different subgroups. The new theoretical models developed should consider this complexity, and the information acquired should be used to design treatments that combine effectiveness, efficiency and personalisation, with favourable cost-benefit ratio. Further research should also address the practical applicability of the different techniques in routine clinical practice, in order to assess whether their widespread implementation in mental health services may be recommended.

15.5   Conclusions and Future Directions

The aim of this chapter is to give a critical review about the current research on non-pharmacological interventions in managing, reducing and preventing violence in mental healthcare settings and to start translating the body of evidence into mental health services, clinical and practical. Despite some promising findings, there is the need to design and conduct new and more accurate research in this field, in order to have a more comprehensive picture of why violence occurs and what we can do to minimise it. Violence is a complex phenomenon and requires the analysis of several factors. It is important to remember that aggression management is one of the goals of patient care: it is not something separate and should not be a cause of discrimination. The relationship between SMI and aggression is bivalent: if it is true that mental illness is associated with violent behaviour, it is equally true that psychiatric patients are most frequently victimised. Only an integrated and multifaceted approach involving pharmacotherapy, psychological and psychosocial interventions and attention to environmental circumstances may reduce violence in patients with SMI. Clinical services focusing on early detection, treatment and recovery need continuous funding to be proactive in implementing guidelines and closing the gap between what is possible and what actually occurs in violence management. This task involves developing a strong understanding of the implementation process as well as the roles that actors at different levels must play to effectively bring about practice changes. Future efforts to implement non-pharmacological interventions in managing aggressive behaviours should engage all key stakeholders and adopt a system perspective to reduce inequities in care and make accessible the broadest range of evidence-based services. Moreover, mental health services committed to delivering evidence-based interventions in reducing and preventing violence need to attend to the challenges of enhancing staff skills. In this perspective, a multilevel training, accessible supervision and organisational processes are key to workforce development and programme maintenance. With such a complex phenomenon as violence, success in improving patients' outcomes and staff's working lives will only be achieved through a real collaboration and integration between academic research, clinical practice, judicial system, penitentiary organisation and government policies.

References

1. Choe JY, Teplin LA, Abram KM. Perpetration of violence, violent victimization, and severe mental illness: balancing public health concerns. Psychiatr Serv. 2008;59(2):153–64.
2. Phillips JP. Workplace violence against health care workers in the United States. N Engl J Med. 2016;375(7):e14.

3. Barlati S, Stefana A, Bartoli F, Bianconi G, et al. Violence risk and mental disorders (VIORMED-2): a prospective multicenter study in Italy. PLoS One. 2019;14(4):e0214924.
4. Iozzino L, Ferrari C, Large M, Nielssen O, De Girolamo G. Prevalence and risk factors of violence by psychiatric acute inpatients: a systematic review and meta-analysis. PLoS One. 2015;10:e0128536.
5. Swanson JW, McGinty EE, Fazel S, Mays VM. Mental illness and reduction of gun violence and suicide: bringing epidemiologic research to policy. Ann Epidemiol. 2015;25:366–76.
6. Van Dorn R, Volavka J, Johnson N. Mental disorder and violence: is there a relationship beyond substance use? Soc Psychiatry Psychiatr Epidemiol. 2012;47(3):487–503.
7. Pompili E, Carlone C, Silvestrini C, Nicolò G. Focus on aggressive behaviour in mental illness. Riv Psichiatr. 2017;52(5):175–9.
8. Iennaco JD, Dixon J, Whittemore R, Bowers L. Measurement and monitoring of health care worker aggression exposure. Online J Issues Nurs. 2013;18(1):3.0.
9. Spector PE, Zhou ZE, Che XX. Nurse exposure to physical and nonphysical violence, bullying and sexual harassment: a quantitative review. Int J Nurs Stud. 2014;51(1):72–84.
10. Galiàn-Muños I, Ruiz-Hernàndez JA, et al. User violence and nursing staff burnout: the modulating role of job satisfaction. J Interpers Violence. 2014;31(2):302–15.
11. Gates DM, Gillespie GL, Succop P. Violence against nurses and its impact on stress and productivity. Nurs Econ. 2011;29(2):59–66.
12. Roche M, Diers D, Duffield C, Catling-Paull C. Violence toward nurses, the work environment and patient outcomes. J Nurs Scholarsh. 2010;42(1):13–22.
13. Rubio-Valera M, Luciano JV, Ortiz JM, et al. Health service use and costs associated with aggressiveness or agitation and containment in adult psychiatric care: a systematic review of the evidence. BMC Psychiatry. 2015;15:35.
14. Joyal CC, Côté G, Meloche J, Hodgins S. Severe mental illness and aggressive behaviour: on the importance of considering subgroups. Int J Forens Ment Health. 2011;10:107–17.
15. Wong SCP, Olver ME. Risk reduction treatment of psychopathy and applications to mentally disordered offenders. CNS Spectr. 2015;20:303–10.
16. Fazel S, Zetterqvist J, Larsson H, Långström N, Lichtenstein P. Antipsychotics, mood stabilisers and risk of violent crime. Lancet. 2014;374:1206–14.
17. Large M, Nielsson O. Violence in first-episode psychosis: a systematic review and meta-analysis. Schizophr Res. 2011;125(2-3):209–20.
18. Witt K, Van Dorn R, Fazel S. Risk factors for violence in psychosis: systematic review and meta-regression analysis of 110 studies. PLoS One. 2013;8:e55942.
19. Volavka J. Violence in schizophrenia and bipolar disorder. Psychiatr Danub. 2013;25(1):24–33.
20. Elbogen EB, Mustillo S, Van Dorn R, Swanson JW, Swarts MS. The impact of perceived need for treatment on risk of arrest and violence among people with severe mental illness. Crim Justice Behav. 2007;34:197–210.
21. Müller-Isberner R, Sheilagh H. Evidence-based treatment for mentally disordered offenders. In: Violence, crime and mentally disordered offenders. Chichester: John Wiley & Sons Ltd.; 2000.
22. Economou M, Palli A, Falloon IRH. Violence, misconduct and schizophrenia: outcomes after four years of optimal treatment. Clin Pract Epidemiol Ment Health. 2005;1:3.
23. Nishinaka H, Nakane J, Nagata T, et al. Neuropsychological impairment and its association with violence risk in Japanese forensic psychiatric patients: a case-control study. PLoS One. 2016;11(1):e0148354.
24. Richter MS, O'Reilly K, O'Sullivan D, et al. Prospective observational cohort study of treatment as usual over four years for patients with schizophrenia in a national forensic hospital. BMC Psychiatry. 2018;18:289.
25. Rampling J, Furtado V, Winsper C, Marwaha S, Lucca G, Livanou M, Singh SP. Non-pharmacological interventions for reducing aggression and violence in serious mental illness: a systematic review and narrative synthesis. Eur Psychiatry. 2016;34:17–28.
26. Blackburn R. "What works" with mentally disordered offenders. Psychol Crime Law. 2004;10(3):297–308.

27. Ross J, Quayle E, Newman E, et al. The impact of psychological therapies on violent behaviour in clinical and forensic settings: a systematic review. Aggress Violent Behav. 2013;18:761–73.

28. Quinn J, Kolla NJ. From clozapine to cognitive remediation: a review of biological and psychosocial treatments for violence in schizophrenia. Can J Psychiatry. 2017;62(2):94–101.

29. Hallett N, Dickens GL. De-escalation of aggressive behaviour in healthcare settings: concept analysis. Int J Nurs Stud. 2017;75:10–20.

30. National Institute for Health and Clinical Excellence (NICE). Violence: the short term management of disturbed/violent behaviour in psychiatric in-patient settings and emergency departments national cost-impact report. London: National Institute for Clinical Excellence; 2005.

31. Paterson B, Leadbetter D, Miller G. Workplace violence in health and social care as an international problem: a public health perspective on the total organisational response. Available http://www.nm.stir.ac.uk/documents/ld-integrated-response.pdf; 2004.

32. Bowers L. A model of de-escalation. Ment Health Pract. 2014;17(9):36–7.

33. Davidson J, Wood C. A conflict resolution model. Theory Pract. 2004;43(1):6–13.

34. Leadbetter D, Paterson B. De-escalating aggressive behaviour. In: Kidd B, Stark C, editors. Management of violence and aggression in health care. London: Gaskell; 1995. p. 49–84.

35. Maier GJ, Van Rybroek GJ. Managing counter transference reactions to aggressive patients. In: Eichelman BS, Hartwig AC, editors. Patient's violence and the clinician. Washington DC: American Psychiatric Press Inc.; 1995.

36. De Dreu CKW, Weingart LR. Task versus relationship conflict, team performance, and team member satisfaction: a meta-analysis. J Appl Psychol. 2003;88(4):741–9.

37. Hücker F. Rhetorische Deeskalation. Stuttgart: Boorberg; 1997.

38. Nay WR. Taking charge of anger: how to resolve conflict, sustain relationships, and express yourself without losing control. New York, London: Guilford Publications; 2003.

39. Maier GJ. Managing threatening behaviour: the role of talk down and talk up. J Psychosoc Nurs Ment Health Serv. 1996;34:25–30.

40. Dutschmann A. Aggressionen und konflikte unter emotionaler erregung: deeskalation und Problemlösung (das aggressions-bewaltigungs-programm ABPro). Tübingen DCVT-Verlang; 2000.

41. Miller N, Pedersen WC, Earlywine M, Polock VE. A theoretical model of triggered displaced aggression. Personal Psychol Rev. 2003;7:75–97.

42. Beech B, Leather P. Evaluating a management of aggression unit for student nurses. J Adv Nurs. 2003;44(6):603–12.

43. Richter BD, Warner AT, Meyer JL, Lutz K. A collaborative and adaptive process for developing environmental flow recommendations. River Res Appl. 2006;22(3):297–318.

44. Bowers L, Flood C, Brennan G, LiPang M, Oladapo P. Preliminary outcomes of a trial to reduce conflict and containment on acute psychiatric wards: city nurses. J Psychiatr Ment Health Nurs. 2006;13:165–72.

45. Armelius BA, Andreassen TH. Cognitive-behavioral treatment for antisocial behavior in youth in residential treatment. Cochrane Database Syst Rev. 2007;4:CD005650.

46. National Institute for Health and Clinical Excellence (NICE). Antisocial personality disorder: treatment, management and prevention Volume 77. London, UK: National Collaborating Center for Mental Health; 2009.

47. Gibbon S, Duggan C, Stoffers J, Huband N, Völlm BA, Ferriter M, Lieb K. Psychological interventions for antisocial personality disorder. Cochrane Database Syst Rev. 2010;6:CD007668.

48. Rodrigo C, Rajapakse S, Jayananda G. The 'antisocial' person: an insight in to biology, classification and current evidence on treatment. Ann Gen Psychiatry. 2010;9:31.

49. Davidson K, Tyrer P, Tata P, et al. Cognitive behaviour therapy for violent men with antisocial personality disorder in the community: an exploratory randomized controlled trial. Psychol Med. 2009;39:569–77.

50. Làtalovà K, Praško J. Aggression in borderline personality disorder. Psychiatry Q. 2010;81:239–51.

51. Timmermann IGH, Emmelkamp PMG. The effects of cognitive behavioral treatment for forensic inpatients. Int J Offender Ther Comp Criminol. 2005;49(5):590–606.
52. Hughes G, Hogue T, Hollin C, Champion H. First-stage evaluation of a treatment programme for personality disordered offenders. J Forensic Psychiatry. 1997;8:515–27.
53. Gerhart JI, Ronan GF, et al. The moderating effects of Cluster B personality traits on violence reduction training: a mixed-model analysis. J Interpers Violence. 2013;28(1):45–61.
54. Ronan G, Gerhart J, Bannister D, Udell C. Relevance of a stage of change analysis for violence reduction training. J Forensic Psychiatry Psychol. 2010;21(5):761–72.
55. Wykes T, Steel C, Everitt B, et al. Cognitive behavior therapy for schizophrenia: effect sizes, clinical models and methodological rigor. Schizophr Bull. 2008;34(3):523–37.
56. Garrett M, Lerman M. CBT for psychosis for long-term inpatients with a forensic history. Psychiatr Serv. 2007;58(5):712–3.
57. Frommberger U, Hamann K, Kammerer J, et al. A feasibility study on violence prevention in outpatients with schizophrenia. Int J Law Psychiatry. 2018;58:54–62.
58. Haddock G, Barrowclough C, Shaw JJ, et al. Cognitive-behavioural therapy v. social activation therapy for people with schizophrenia and a history of violence: randomized controlled trial. Br J Psychiatry. 2009;194(2):152–7.
59. Hodel B, West A. A cognitive training for mentally ill offenders with treatment resistant schizophrenia. J Forensic Psychiatry. 2003;14(3):554–68.
60. Hornsveld RH, Nijman HL. Evaluation of a cognitive-behavioural program for chronically psychotic forensic inpatients. Int J Law Psychiatry. 2005;28(3):246–54.
61. Yates KF, Kunz M, Khan A, et al. Psychiatric patients with histories of aggression and crime five years after discharge from a cognitive-behavioral program. J Forensic Psychiatry Psychol. 2010;21(2):167–88.
62. Bateman A, O'Connell J, Lorenzini N, Gardner T, Fonagy P. A randomized controlled trial of mentalization-based treatment versus structured clinical management for patients with comorbid borderline personality disorder and antisocial personality disorder. BMC Psychiatry. 2016;16:304.
63. Taubner S, White LO, Zimmermann J, Fonagy P, Nolte T. Attachment-related mentalization moderates the relationship between psychopathic traits and proactive aggression in adolescence. J Abnorm Child Psychol. 2013;41(6):929–38.
64. Kuokkanen R, Lappalainen R, et al. Metacognitive group training for forensic and dangerous non forensic patients with schizophrenia: a randomized controlled feasibility trial. Crim Behav Ment Health. 2014;24(5):345–57.
65. Low G, Jones D, Duggan C, Power M, Macleod A. The treatment of deliberate self-harm in borderline personality disorder using dialectical behaviour therapy: a pilot study in a high security hospital. Behav Cogn Psychother. 2001;29:85–92.
66. McCann RA, Ball EM, Ivanoff AM. Dialectical behaviour therapy with an inpatient forensic population: the CMHIP forensic model. Cogn Behav Pract. 2000;7:447–56.
67. Trupin EW, Stewart DG, Beach B, Boesky L. Effectiveness of a dialectical behavior therapy program for incarcerated female juvenile offenders. Child Adoles Ment Health. 2002;7(3):121–7.
68. Scheel KR. The empirical basis of dialectical behaviour therapy: summary, critique and implications. Clin Psychol Sci Pract. 2000;7:1.
69. Linehan MM, Armstrong HE, Suarez A, Allmon D, Heard HL. Cognitive-behavioural treatment of chronically parasuicidal borderline patients. Arch Gen Psychiatry. 1991;48:1060–4.
70. Linehan MM, Heard HL, Armstrong HE. Naturalistic follow-up of a behavioural treatment for chronically parasuicidal borderline patients. Arch Gen Psychiatry. 1993;50:971–4.
71. Evershed S, Tennant A, et al. Practice-based outcomes of dialectical behaviour therapy (DBT) targeting anger and violence, with male forensic patients: a pragmatic and non-contemporaneous comparison. Crim Behav Ment Health. 2003;13:198–213.
72. Keulen-de Vos M, Bernstein DP, Clark LA, et al. Validation of the schema mode concept in personality disordered offenders. Legal Criminol Psychol. 2017;22(2):420–41.

73. Tarrier N, Dolan M, Doyle M et al. Exploratory randomized clinical trial of schema modal therapy in the personality disorder service at Ashworth Hospital. UK: Ministry of Justice (Research Series 5/10); 2010.
74. Bernstein D, Nijman H, Karos K, Keulen-de Vos M, et al. Schema therapy for forensic patients with personality disorders: design and preliminary findings of a multicenter randomized clinical trial in the Netherlands. Int J Forensic Ment Health. 2012;11:312–24.
75. Rice ME, Harris GT, Varney GW, Quinsey VL, Cyr M. Planning treatment programmes in secure psychiatric facilities. Law Ment Health. 1990;6:159–87.
76. Chereji SV, Pintea S, David D. The relationship of anger and cognitive distortions with violence in violent offenders' population: a meta-analytic review. Eur J Psychol Appl Legal Context. 2012;4(1):1–98.
77. Henwood KS, Chou S, Browne KD. A systematic review and meta-analysis on the effectiveness of CBT informed anger management. Aggress Violent Behav. 2015;25:280–92.
78. Lee AH, Di Giuseppe R. Anger and aggression treatments: a review of meta-analyses. Curr Opin Psychol. 2018;19:65–74.
79. Duncan EAS, Nicol MM, Ager A, Dalgleish L. A systematic review of structured group interventions with mentally disordered offenders. Crim Behav Ment Health. 2006;16:217–41.
80. Hornsveld RH, Nijman HL. Aggression control therapy for violent forensic psychiatric patients: method and clinical practice. Int J Offender Ther Comp Criminol. 2008;52(2):222–33.
81. Wilson C, Gandolfi S, Dudley A, et al. Evaluation of anger management groups in a high-security hospital. Crim Behav Ment Health. 2013;23:356–71.
82. Ross R, Fabiano E. Time to think: a cognitive model of delinquency prevention and offender rehabilitation. Johnson City, TN: Institute of Social Sciences and Arts, Inc.; 1985.
83. Berman AH. The reasoning and rehabilitation program: assessing short- and long-term outcomes among male Swedish prisoners. J Offender Rehabil. 2004;40(1/2):85–103.
84. Tong LS, Farrington DP. Effectiveness of "Reasoning and Rehabilitation" in reducing reoffending. Psicothema. 2008;20:20–8.
85. Joy Tong L, Farrington D. How effective is the "reasoning and rehabilitation" programme in reducing reoffending? a meta-analysis of evaluations in four countries. Psychol Crime Law. 2006;2(1):3–24.
86. Cullen A, Clarke A, Kuipers E, et al. A multisite randomized trial of a cognitive skills programme for male mentally disordered offenders: violence and antisocial behaviour outcomes. J Consult Clin Psychol. 2012;80(6):1114–20.
87. Young S, Chick K, Gudjonsson G. A preliminary evaluation of reasoning and rehabilitation 2 in mentally disordered offenders (R&R 2M) across two secure forensic settings in the United Kingdom. J Forensic Psychiatry Psychol. 2010;21(4):490–500.
88. Young S, Das M, Gudjonsson G. Reasoning and Rehabilitation cognitive skills programme for mentally disordered offenders: predictors of outcome. World J Psychiatry. 2016;6(4):410–8.
89. Rees-Jones A, Gudjonsson G, Young S. A multi-site controlled trial of a cognitive skills program for mentally disordered offenders. BMC Psychiatry. 2012;12:44.
90. Yip V, Gudjonsson G, et al. A non-randomised controlled trial of the R&R2MHP cognitive skills program in high risk male offenders with severe mental illness. BMC Psychiatry. 2013;13:267.
91. Jotangia A, Rees-Jones A, et al. A multi-site controlled trial of the R&R2MHP cognitive skills program for mentally disordered female offenders. Int J Offender Ther Comp Criminol. 2015;59(5):539–59.
92. Kingston DA, Olver ME, McDonald J, Cameron C. A randomised controlled trial of a cognitive skills programme for offenders with mental illness. Crim Behav Ment Health. 2018;28:369–82.
93. Young S, Hopkin G, Perkins D, et al. A controlled trial of a cognitive skills program for personality-disordered offenders. J Atten Disord. 2013;17(7):598–607.
94. Ahmed AO, Hunter KM, Goodrum NM, et al. A randomized study of cognitive remediation for forensic and mental health patients with schizophrenia. J Psychiatr Res. 2015;68:8–18.

95. O'Reilly K, Donohoe G, Coyle C, et al. Prospective cohort study of the relationship between neuro-cognition, social cognition and violence in forensic patients with schizophrenia and schizoaffective disorder. BMC Psychiatry. 2015;10(15):155.

96. Darmedru C, Demily C, Franck N. Cognitive remediation and social cognitive training for violence in schizophrenia: a systematic review. Psychiatry Res. 2017;251:266–74.

97. Doyle M, Khanna T, Lennox C, Shaw J, Hayes A, et al. The effectiveness of an enhanced thinking skills programme in offenders with antisocial personality traits. J Forensic Psychiatry Psychol. 2013;24(1):1–15.

98. Tapp J, Fellowes E, Wallis N, Blud L, Moore E. An evaluation of the Enhanced Thinking Skills (ETS) programme with mentally disordered offenders in a high security hospital. Legal Criminol Psychol. 2009;14:201–12.

99. Chan SW, Yip B, Tso S, Cheng B, Tam W. Evaluation of a psychoeducation program for Chinese clients with schizophrenia and their family caregivers. Patient Educ Couns. 2009;75(1):67–76.

100. Paranthaman V, Satnam K, Lim J, Amar-Singh HS, Sararaks S, et al. Effective implementation of a structured psychoeducation programme among caregivers of patients with schizophrenia in the community. Asian J Psychiatr. 2010;3(4):206–12.

101. Komala EPE, Keliat BA, et al. Acceptance and commitment therapy and family psycho education for clients with schizophrenia. Enferm Clin. 2018;28(Supl1 Part A):88–93.

102. Thylstrup B, et al. Psycho-education for substance use and antisocial personality disorder: a randomized trial. BMC Psychiatry. 2015;15:285.

103. Nurenberg JR, Schleifer SJ, Shaffer TM, et al. Animal-assisted therapy with chronic psychiatric inpatients: equine-assisted psychotherapy and aggressive behaviour. Psychiatr Serv. 2015;66(1):80–6.

104. Bruce M, Crowley S, et al. Community DSPD pilot services in South London: rates of reconviction and impact of supported housing on reducing recidivism. Crim Behav Ment Health. 2014;24:129–40.

105. Ramesh T, Igoumenou A, Vazques Montes M, Fazel S. Use of risk assessment instruments to predict violence in forensic psychiatric hospitals: a systematic review and meta-analysis. Eur Psychiatry. 2018;52:47–53.

106. Brook M. Structured approaches to violence risk assessment: a critical review. Psychiatric Annals. 2017;47(9):454–9.

107. Commane C, Toal F, Mullen P, Ogloff J. Take home notes: risk assessment and management of violence in general adult psychiatry. CPD Online; 2019.

108. Douglas T, Pugh J, Singh I. Risk assessment tools in criminal justice and forensic psychiatry: the need for better data. Eur Psychiatry. 2017;42:134–7.

109. Nielssen O. Preventing violence in schizophrenia. Evid Based Psychiatr Care. 2015;1:15–8.

110. Large M, Ryan C, Callaghan S, Paton M, Singh S. Can violence risk assessment really assist in clinical decision-making? Aust N Z J Psychiatry. 2014;48:286–8.

111. Abderhalden C, Needham I, Dassen T. Structured risk assessment and violence in acute psychiatric wards: randomized controlled trial. Brit J Psychiatry. 2008;193(1):44–50.

112. Kaunomäki J, Jokela M, et al. Interventions following a high risk assessment score: a naturalistic study on a Finnish psychiatric admission ward. Health Serv Res. 2017;17:26.

113. Fazel S, Långström N, Hjern A, et al. Schizophrenia, substance abuse, and violent crime. JAMA. 2009;301(19):2016–23.

114. Sokya M. Substance misuse, psychiatric disorder and violent and disturbed behaviour. Br J Psychiatry. 2000;172:345–50.

115. Dellazizzo L, Potvin S, Beaudoin M, Luigi M, et al. Cannabis use and violence in patients with severe mental illnesses: a meta-analytic investigation. Psychiatry Res. 2019;274:42–8.

116. Volavka J, Citrome L. Heterogeneity of violence in schizophrenia and implications for long-term treatment. Int J Clin Pract. 2008;62(8):1237–45.

117. Lubman DI, King JA, Castle DJ. Treating comorbid substance use disorders in schizophrenia. Int Rev Psychiatry. 2010;22(2):191–201.

118. Perry AE, Woodhouse R, Neilson M, et al. Are non-pharmacological intervention effective in reducing drug use and criminality? A systematic and meta-analytical review with an economic appraisal of these interventions. Int J Environ Res Public Health. 2016;13:966.
119. Vanderloo MJ, Butters RP. Treating offenders with mental illness: a review of the literature. Utah Criminal Justice Center, University of Utah; 2012.
120. Stevens H, Agerbo E, Dean K, et al. Reduction of crime in first-onset psychosis: a secondary analysis of the OPUS randomized trial. J Clin Psychiatry. 2013;74(5):e439–44.
121. Walsh E, Gilvarry C, Samele C, et al. Reducing violence in severe mental illness: randomized controlled trial of intensive case management compared with standard care. BMJ. 2001;323:1–5.
122. Wilson D, Tien G, Eaves D. Increasing the community tenure of mentally disordered offenders: an assertive case management program. Int J Law Psychiatry. 1995;18:61–9.
123. Morrissey J, Meyer P, Cuddeback G. Extending assertive community treatment to criminal justice settings: origins, current evidence, and future directions. Community Ment Health J. 2007;43(5):527–44.
124. Tyrer P, Duggan C, Cooper S, Crawford M, et al. The successes and failures of the DSPD experiment: the assessment and management of severe personality disorder. Med Sci Law. 2010;50:9.
125. Tew J, Dixon L, Harkins L, Bennett A. Investigating changes in anger and aggression in offenders with high levels of psychopathic traits attending the Chromis violence reduction programme. Crim Behav Ment Health. 2012;22:191–201.
126. Braham L, Jones D, Hollin C. The Violent Offender Treatment Program (VOTP): development of a treatment program for violent patients in a high security psychiatric hospital. Int J Forensic Ment Health. 2008;7:157–72.
127. Swartz MS, Bhattacharya S, et al. Involuntary outpatient commitment and the elusive pursuit of violence prevention: a view from the United States. Can J Psychiatry. 2017;62(2):102–8.
128. Scott DA, McGilloway S, et al. Effectiveness of criminal justice liaison and diversion services for offenders with mental disorders: a review. Psychiatr Serv. 2013;64(9):843–9.